BEHAVIOURAL SCIENCES AND THEIR RELEVANCE TO COMMUNITY HEALTH

Dr. Ahmed Taha

ALLIED
HEALTH
PRESS

Behavioural Sciences and their Relevance to Community Health

Author: **Dr. Ahmed Taha**

Allied Health Press
4164 Lakeshore Road
Burlington ON L7L 1A4
Canada
www.alliedhealthpress.com
Email: orders@arclereducation.com

ISBN: 978-1-77956-253-1

Allied Health Press publishes wide variety of books and eBooks. For more information about Allied Health Press and its products, visit our website at www.alliedhealthpress.com

ABOUT THE AUTHOR

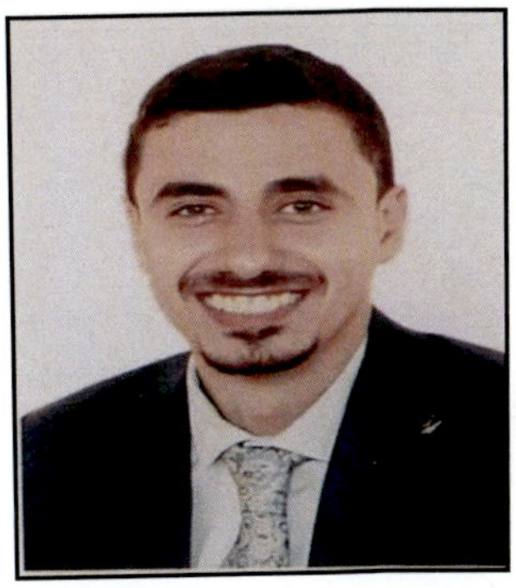

Dr. Ahmed Taha Abdel Sattar, MD, M.Sc. (c), MBChB, is a distinguished graduate of Fayoum University with a GPA of 4 (Summa Cum Laude). Currently a Teaching Assistant in Ophthalmology at Fayoum University Hospital, he has over 14 peer-reviewed publications with 100+ citations and five years of experience in international medical publications. Committed to advancing medical knowledge and patient care, he mentors future healthcare professionals while providing compassionate care to patients.

Word Roots, Prefixes, and Suffixes by Chapter

Chapter 1 Behavioral Sciences

a- not, without: abiotic

bio- life, living: biodiversity

-ology study of: biology

de- away from, down: deductive reasoning

Chapter 2 Community Health

Algia Pain

BX biopsy

Eu- Good; Well

Necr/o- Death

-asthenia weakness

Chapter 3 Role of Social and Behavioral Science in Public Health

epi-, on, upon

-ation, process

anthropo-, human

path(o)-, disease

psych-, of or pertaining to the mind

bio-, life

Chapter 4 Health Communication

dis not, opposite of

mis wrongly

un not

inter between

pre before

non not

super above

Chapter 5 Cardiovascular and Lymph Vascular Systems

Somn- Somnambulism

Dys- Dysfunction

Insomn- Insomnia

Hypno- Hypnotherapy

Noct- Nocturnal

Chapter 6 Tobacco Control and Prevention

Im- Mortal

-ity Immortality

-al Illogical

-able Non-biodegradable

Chapter 7 Mental Health and Community Well-being

Ment-: "mind" or "intellect."

-al: "relating to."

-ment: often indicating "action or process."

-al: often indicating "related to."

Chapter 8 Prevention of Sexually Transmitted Diseases and HIV

Sexu Sexual

Path/o Pathogen

Genit/o Genital

Infect Infection

Retrovir Retroviral

Chapter 9 Women's and Adolescent Health

-ago attack, diseased state or condition

alg/e, alg/o pain

andr/o male

-ase enzyme

asthen-, -asthenia weakness, lack of strength

cadaver/o dead body

carot/o stupor, sleep

Chapter 10 Obesity and Nutrition

phago Eat, Feed

Troph Food, nutrition, nourish

adi-, lip(o)- Fat

corp-, soma- Body

-in Protein

Table of Contents

LIST OF FIGURES

LIST OF TABLES

PREFACE

Each year, two-thirds of global deaths are attributed to noncommunicable diseases, which stem from genetic, physiological, environmental, and behavioral factors. Behavior significantly impacts health; for instance, many noncommunicable disease risk factors, like smoking and sedentary lifestyles, are behaviorally driven. The overuse of antibiotics in human health care is a primary yet preventable cause of antimicrobial resistance. While hand hygiene is a highly effective measure to prevent infection spread, many individuals fail to maintain adequate hand hygiene, even when water, and soap are readily available. It is important not to simply attribute these issues to a lack of knowledge or awareness; they are fundamentally behavioral issues, and nearly all health challenges involve individual behavior.

When we refer to behavioral elements, we mean health problems or outcomes that can be influenced by specific health-related actions taken by individuals or communities. These behaviors are crucial not only for protecting against health emergencies but also for accessing services, and promoting better health.

To effectively address global, and local health challenges, and achieve the Sustainable Development Goals, the United Nations must understand how, and why people, and communities behave in their particular contexts. As the leading global public health authority, the World Health Organization (WHO) cannot achieve its ambitious goal of improving global health, and the health of over 7 billion people without a comprehensive understanding of health-related behaviors. Thus, we have established a Behavioral Science Unit at WHO, and dedicate this theme issue of the Bulletin of the World Health Organization to this field.

Human behaviors, and decision-making are complex, influenced by cognitive, social, and environmental factors. Behavioral science is the evidence-based study of human behavior, and its drivers, helping anticipate how people will respond to health programs, and policies. Over the past decade, the integration of behavioral science has bolstered the success of numerous public policies, and programs across various sectors, including health, consumer protection, education, energy, environment, and taxation.

However, behavioral science has yet to become a fundamental component of daily practice in most public health work, remaining an underutilized resource. Barriers to adopting behavioral theories, and approaches include practical challenges such as limited capacity, funding, and time. Additionally, policymakers, and technical managers still lack confidence in the effectiveness, sustainability, and replicability of these interventions.

These barriers have hindered the integration of behavioral science into public health policy. Overcoming these challenges requires more research, investment, and stronger collaboration across sectors. Despite an encouraging increase in behavioral research, its application to global health remains limited and often reflects the research agendas of high-income countries.

As members of the broader public health community, we must improve our ability to listen to and observe people and their needs. This necessitates the rigorous collection of behavioral data to understand, for instance, why our minds resort to heuristics—mental shortcuts—when faced with overwhelming or unclear information, or when making difficult decisions.

Utilizing behavioral insights is ultimately an exercise in humility. It requires experts, and policymakers to challenge each other's knowledge, biases, and preferences, and to incorporate behavioral evidence into health-related decisions that each of us makes daily.

This book explores the role of behavioral sciences in understanding, and addressing community health issues. It examines the various behavioral theories, and approaches, highlighting their relevance to promoting health, and preventing disease at the community level. The book covers a wide range of topics, including health behavior change, social determinants of health communication, and community-based interventions. It aims to provide a comprehensive overview of how behavioral sciences can inform public health practice and policy, ultimately improving the health and well-being of communities.

This book serves as a valuable resource for public health practitioners seeking to apply behavioral science principles in their work. It provides practical insights and strategies for designing and implementing community health programs. Community health workers will find the book to be a useful guide for understanding the behavioral aspects of health and disease, helping them to better support and educate community members.

Researchers in the field of public health and behavioral sciences will benefit from the book's comprehensive review of current knowledge and research findings, guiding future research directions. Students and educators in public health and related fields will find the book to be a valuable learning tool, providing a solid foundation in the role of behavioral sciences in community health.

Chapter 1

BEHAVIORAL SCIENCES

Contents

Introduction

The behavioral sciences study how creatures in the natural world interact behaviorally with one another and with their cognitive processes. It entails the methodical study and analysis of both animal and human behavior through mathematical modeling, controlled scientific experiments, and naturalistic observation. It makes an effort to reach valid, impartial conclusions by careful formulation and observation. Psychobiology, criminology, anthropology, sociology, psychology, economics, and cognitive science are a few examples of behavioral sciences. Broadly speaking, the main goal of behavioral science is to make generalizations about how society and human behavior interact and influence one another.

Orientation and Directional Terms

Term	Definition	Illustration
Alzheimer's disease	Alzheimer's Disease (AD) is the most common form of dementia worldwide (60–70% of all dementia cases) and is a progressive neurodegenerative disorder.	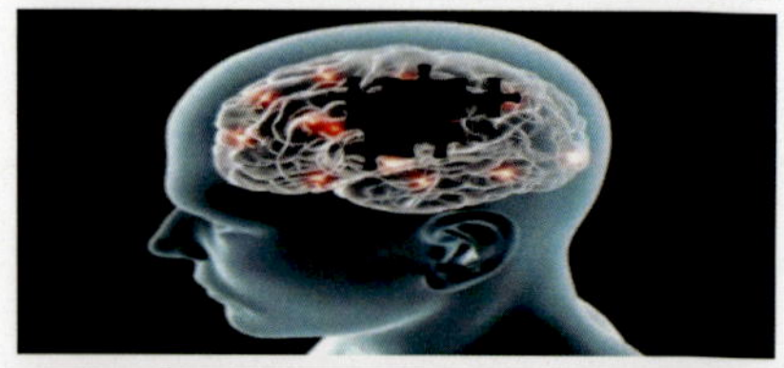
Central Nervous System	The central nervous system (CNS) is comprised of the brain and spinal cord. The three broad functions of the CNS are to take in sensory information, process information, and send out motor signals.	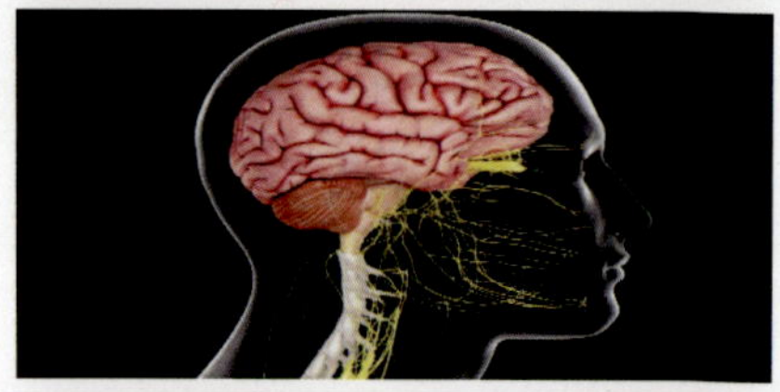
Mental disorder	A mental disorder is a mental or behavioral pattern that causes significant distress or impairment in a person's functioning. Mental disorders can affect a person's thinking, perceptions, mood, or behavior.	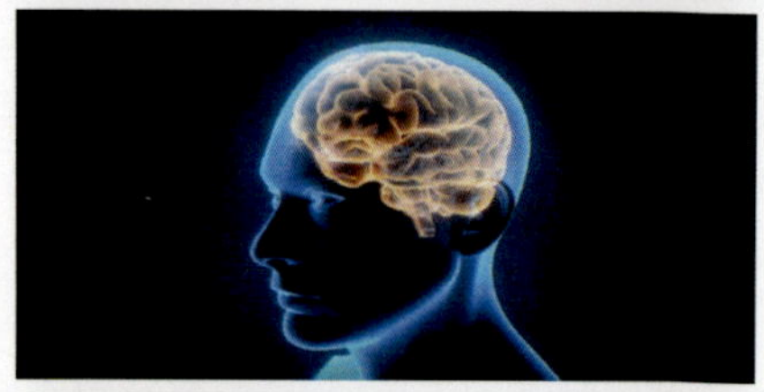
Neurotransmitters	Neurotransmitters are chemical messengers within your body. They transmit cellular signals from neurons (i.e., nerve cells) to various target cells in muscles, glands, or other nerves.	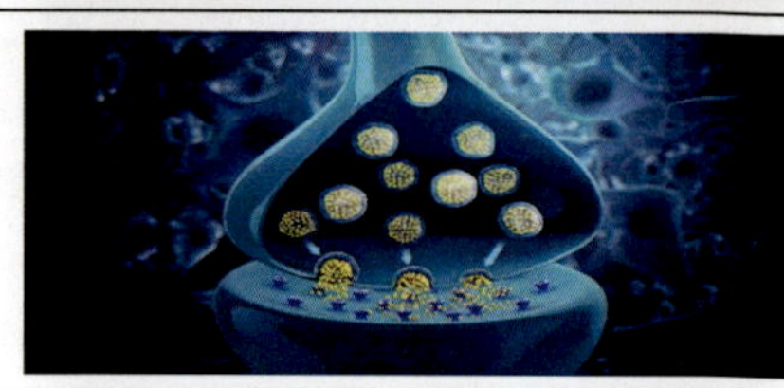
Peripheral nervous system	The peripheral nervous system (PNS) is a network of nerves that runs throughout the body, head, and neck, and is responsible for carrying messages to and from the central nervous system (CNS).	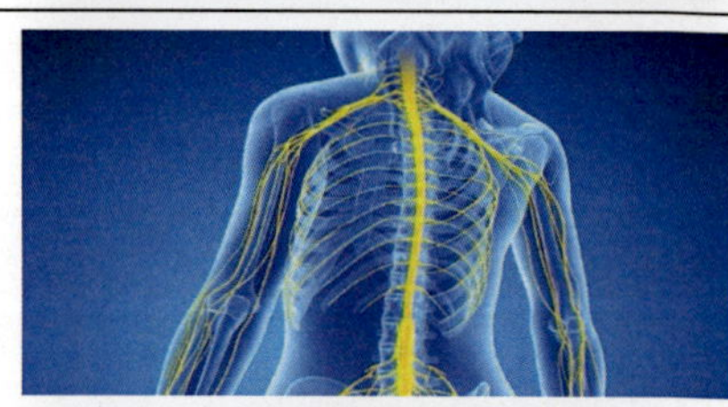
Psychiatric Disorders	A psychiatric disorder is a mental illness diagnosed by a mental health professional that greatly disturbs your thinking, moods, and/or behavior and seriously increases your risk of disability, pain, death, or loss of freedom.	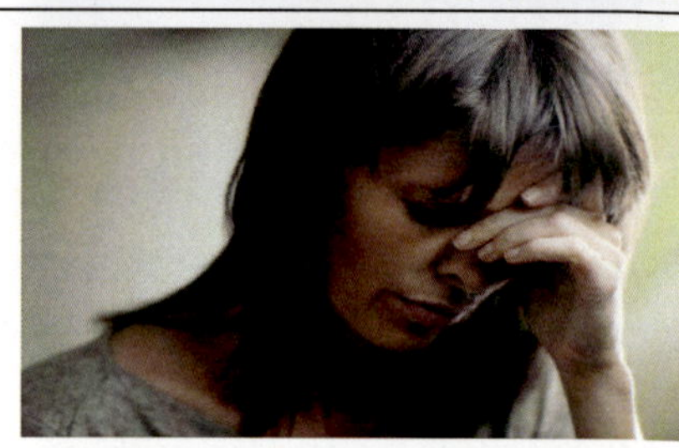

1.1. Definition and Scope of Behavioral Sciences

Behavioral sciences employ an interdisciplinary approach to study human behavior and comprehend human needs within the larger context of societal issues. The behavioral sciences encompass a variety of fields such as Sociology, Anthropology (excluding Archaeology), Technical Linguistics, Psychology, Anthropology (excluding Physiological Psychology), and the behavioral facets of Economics, Geography, Law, Psychiatry, and Political Science.

Luthans has shown the relationship between behavioral science and other disciplines as follows:

- Arts and Sciences;
- Humanities;
- Physical Sciences;
- Biological Sciences;
- Social Sciences.Economics;
- History;
- Political Science;
- Behavioral Science;
- Anthropology;
- Sociology;
- Psychology.

Behavioral science takes a whole systems approach to understanding behavior, viewing humans as products of socio-psychological, and cultural factors rather than viewing individuals in isolation. Therefore, this science examines human behavior in light of the social and cultural context, interpersonal orientation, psychological framework, and group influence. This aids in the solution of issues brought about by the complexity of the human condition.

1.1.1. Difference Between Behavioral Sciences and Social Sciences

The terms social sciences and behavioral sciences are frequently used interchangeably. These two broad fields are related and both investigate systematic processes in behavior, but they are different in how much different aspects of behavior are scientifically analyzed.

The behavioral sciences use an abstraction of empirical data to study how organisms in a social system make decisions and communicate with one another. This encompasses a variety of disciplines, including social neuroscience and psychology.

On the other hand, social sciences offer an insightful framework for examining how the social organization affects individual and group structural adjustment, allowing researchers to better understand how a social system function. Sociology, economics, history, counselling, public health, anthropology, and political science are among the disciplines that they usually cover.

1.1.2. Categories of Behavioral Sciences

The two main subcategories of behavioral sciences are social communication sciences and neural decision sciences. The fields of study that are primarily concerned with the decision-making and personal functioning that enable organisms to survive in social environments are collectively referred to as decision sciences. These include social neuroscience, anthropology, psychology, cognitive science, organization theory, and psychobiology.

However, the disciplines that investigate how organisms communicate and how those strategies interact with one another in a given environment are included in the communication sciences. These encompass disciplines such as social networks, sociology, anthropology, organizational behavior, and organization studies.

Studying animal and human behavior is the focus of the scientific field known as behavioral science. Behavioral science examines how people behave as well as how societies, groups, and cultures behave as well as the processes that may lead to particular behaviors. This field and the social sciences overlap greatly, which can occasionally cause confusion. The social sciences are more likely to concentrate on structural systems and cultures, whereas behavioral science is more likely to examine the interactions within and between organisms that determine behavioral trends.

Several tools are available to behavioral scientists for data collection. Among the most effective methods are controlled, ethical experiments intended to push the limits of acceptable behavior and investigate the motivations underlying behavior, as well as individual and group observation. Because people are interested in how the environment influences behavior, research in this field can take a multidisciplinary approach, incorporating elements of many social sciences as well as more rigorous sciences like chemistry, neurology, and even geology.

Behavioral scientists use their findings in a multitude of contexts. To match animals appropriately and create habitats that will allow the animals to live as naturally as possible within the facility, zoological parks and breeding programs frequently rely heavily on behavioral science. Marketers closely monitor this area to discover what drives consumer behavior and how purchasing patterns emerge. There is a great deal of interdisciplinary collaboration between social scientists and behavioral scientists, and social scientists are also interested in behavioral science.

Numerous findings from behavioral studies on humans, animals, and even plants have been made; some of these findings have very serious ramifications. For instance, professionals in the public health domain have acquired the ability to incorporate behavioral science into their work in order to encourage individuals to seek medical attention and adopt healthy habits. Behavioral science may be used by psychologists and other mental health specialists in their patient care. For example, if a person seeks cognitive behavioral therapy to treat a phobia, the treatment plan will be created with behavioral science findings in mind.

A rewarding career in behavioral science may be found by those with an interest in the behavior of humans and animals. Since the work primarily entails patient observation and in-depth study of subjects, it calls for patience and a keen eye for detail. Communication and scientific skills are also highly valued. For instance, studies of subjects like social networking, behavioral economics, and memetics are studied in this field, along with subjects like neurology and biology.

1.2. Relevance of Behavioral Sciences in Health

Medical science cannot handle the complexity on its own. The socio-behavioral sciences need to be a major component of health care professionals' education in order to be sufficient and effective.

1.2.1. Socio-Behavioral Science Inputs

Healthcare professionals' education should include input from the following behavioral sciences.

1) Geography
- Society and its ecology.
- Human settlement patterns.
- Human movements/migrations and the spread of disease physical geography and health sanitation.
- Environmental pollution.
- Town and regional planning and health.
- Spatial patterns of health systems, morbidity, and mortality.

2) Social Anthropology
- Marriage, family, descent and kinship culture, symbols and symbolism.
- Language and socio-linguistics.
- Belief systems including religion.
- Diets, food habits, taboos and health/ ill health behavior.
- Human development cycle and associated health problems Indigenous political and economic systems value systems.
- Social institutions and norms.

3) Sociology
- Society and the social system.
- Social differentiation and stratification -age, sex, class, caste.
- Social mobility.
- Poverty, inequality, exploitation and alienation demography.
- Criminology.
- Urban and rural societies.
- Racial and ethnic relations.
- Groups and group behavior.
- Status, roles and access to scarce resources social control.

4) Psychology
- The psychic and mental processes.
- Ego, personality and social behavior.
- Feelings.
- Emotions.
- Crisis and coping with personal/ emotional and social disorders.
- Motivations.
- Attitudes.
- Stress (frustration, threat, conflict, aggression, depression, anxiety).

5) Political Science
- Government structure and processes.
- Public Administration.
- Bureaucracy.
- Use of power in society.
- Pluralism and democracy.
- Interest pressure groups.
- Political parties.
- Policy formulation and execution.
- Political socialization and behavior.
- Politics and law in society.
- International politics and economy and the super powers.

6) Economics
- Production, distribution and consumption of goods and services.
- Markets and the relation of supply to demand.

- Budgets and national income and expenditure.
- Taxation and social amenities.
- Labor, employment, underemployment and unemployment.
- Cost-benefit analysis.
- Economic determination of human behavior.
- Economic changes and health conditions.

These topics give students a sufficient understanding of both the art and science of medicine, which include the social organization of medical care in specific cultural contexts and health delivery systems.

Each of the aforementioned topics is only pertinent and useful when spoken of informally and explanatorily about the phenomenon of health or ill health in a specific society, aside from offering a sufficient cultural and social context for understanding and resolving health problems and lacking the depths that will transform the health care professionals into specialists.

Therefore, each topic should be approached as "in" rather than "of" medicine, in line with the analytical distinction that Strauss made between sociology "of" medicine—that is, the study of medicine to shed light on sociological issues—and sociology "in" medicine, which is primarily concerned with the sociological causes and explanations of issues like illnesses, diseases, and patients' preferences for specific pharmacies and medical facilities. Collectively, the topics should provide a body of knowledge about the organization of the health care delivery system and the connection between social structure and health or illness in specific societies, serving as frameworks for comprehending and analyzing behavior related to health and illness.(Bartres et al., 2002; Baxter et al., 1999)

1.3. The Biological Bases of Behavior

Similar to physical health, emotional well-being is the outcome of an intricate interplay between environmental, social, and biological factors. At any time in a person's life, aberrations or distortions in one or more of these influences can lead to health disorders of any kind. Distinguishing biological from social and environmental factors in the etiology of psychiatric illness presents theoretical challenges.

Because of this, the phrase "organic mental disorder," which was once used to characterize behavioral symptoms whose causes lay outside of the emotional spectrum, is no longer frequently used. Furthermore, over the past few decades, advancements in neurophysiology and neuroimaging have demonstrated that neuroanatomical and neurochemical factors have a significant influence on psychiatric function. The contributions of these and other biological elements to the expression of typical behavior and its abnormalities are the main topics of this section.

1.3.1. Genetics of Behavior

It is commonly known that genetic factors play a part in the emergence of physical ailments like cancer, diabetes, and heart disease. The manifestation of behavior and its disorders are also significantly influenced by genetic factors. It is more difficult to separate genetic from social and environmental etiologies in behavioral disorders than in physical disorders because behavioral disorders are expressed in and therefore confused by the social setting. Adoption, twin, and family risk studies are among the research instruments that can be used to distinguish and identify these factors.

1.3.1.1. Research Studies

The etiology of disorders can be distinguished between genetic and non-genetic risk factors through the use of family risk studies. The prevalence of a behavioral disorder or trait in the proband—the relatives of an affected individual—is compared to the general population to determine how common it is. A disorder would be expected to have a higher concordance rate (i.e., genetic component) if it has a genetic component. The disorder is more common in close relatives of those who have it than in more distant relatives or the general public, if concordant, the disorder affects both relatives.

Genetic factors associated with disorders are also identified through twin studies. These studies are predicated on the idea that, compared to dizygotic twins, who are only genetically similar to one another, the probability of both twins having a disorder will be higher in monozygotic twins due to their shared genetic composition. Furthermore, whether the twins are raised in separate adoptive homes or in the same home, this assumption should remain valid. This hypothesis is strongly supported by anecdotal evidence and documented findings from twin studies for a wide range of behavioral and psychiatric traits and disorders.

1. **Psychiatric Disorders:** Empirical research indicates that major psychiatric disorders like bipolar disorder and schizophrenia have a genetic component. While approximately 1% of the general population suffers from each of these disorders, individuals who have a close genetic relationship to someone who has bipolar disorder or schizophrenia are more likely to develop these disorders than those who have more distant relationships (Table 1.1). Additionally, recent research indicates that the volume of brain regions recognized to be associated with schizophrenia symptoms (e.g., grey matter in language regions and frontal lobes)) are more similar in monozygotic twin pairs than in dizygotic twin pairs (Thompson et al., 2001).

Table 1.1. *Risk of Developing Schizophrenia and Bipolar Disorder in Relatives of Patients*

RELATIONSHIP TO PATIENT	APPROXIMATE RISK FOR SCHIZOPHRENIA (%)	APPROXIMATE RISK FOR BIPOLAR DISORDER (%)
No relationship (general population)	1	1
First-degree relative (sibling, dizygotic twin, child or parent) of a patient with the disorder	10	20
Child of two parents with the disorder	40	60
Monozygotic twin of a patient with the disorder	50	75

Source: *Barbara Fadem. Behavioral Science in Medicine. Lippincott Williams & Wilkins. ISBN 978–1-60913–664–2.*

Some studies have linked chromosomal markers on chromosomes 1, 7, 8, and 22 to schizophrenia, although it has been challenging to correlate these markers with specific psychiatric illnesses. Recently, a genetic variation in the dysbindin gene on chromosome 6 has also been linked to schizophrenia markers (Shi et al., 2009; Straub et al., 2002), chromosome 8, and a neuregulin 1 gene genetic variant (Stefansson et al., 2002), as well as genes linked to disrupted glutamate transmission on chromosomes 13 and 21 (Chumakov et al., 2002). It's interesting to note that velocardiofacial syndrome, a condition linked to a higher risk of schizophrenia, shares markers with chromosome 22's long arm (Table 1.2). Furthermore, recent research indicates that chromosome 3, specifically 3p21.1, contains a locus associated with an increased risk for major depressive disorder and bipolar disorder.

Table 1.2. *Behavioral Manifestations of Chromosomal Neuropsychological Disorders*

CHROMOSOME	DISORDER	BEHAVIORAL MANIFESTATIONS
1	Alzheimer's disease	Depression, anxiety, early onset dementia (before age 60)
4	Huntington's disease	Erratic behavior, psychiatric symptoms (e.g., depression), dementia
5	Sotos syndrome	Intellectual impairment, phobias, hyperphagia
7	Williams syndrome	Hypersociality, intellectual disability, behavioral problems, hypotonia
8	Cohen syndrome	Autistic behavior, intellectual disability
9	Dystonia musculorum deformans/ torsion dystonia (DYT1 gene)	Major depressive disorder, learning problems
	Tuberous sclerosis	Seizures, cognitive impairment, autistic behavior
11	Acute intermittent porphyria	Manic behavior, psychosis
12	Phenylketonuria	Attention deficit/hyperactivity disorder
13	Wilson's disease	Depression, personality changes, thought disorders
14	Alzheimer's disease	Depression, anxiety, early onset dementia
15	Chromosome 15 inversion-duplication syndrome	Seizures, autistic behavior, hypotonia
	Prader-Willi/Angelman syndrome	Intellectual disability, hypotonia, rage, stubborness, self-injury
16	Tuberous sclerosis	Seizures, cognitive impairment, autistic behavior
17	Neurofibromatosis-1	Cognitive impairment, autistic behavior
	Charcot-Marie–Tooth disease	Peripheral neuropathy, neuropathic pain
	Smith-Magenis syndrome	Intellectual disability, impaired expressive language, stereotyped behavior, clinging and dependency, seizures
18	Tourette's disorder	Discontrol of language and movements May be mistaken for a behavior disorder
19	Alzheimer's disease (site of the Apo E_4 gene)	Depression, anxiety, late onset dementia (over 60 years of age)
21	Progressive myoclonic epilepsy Alzheimer's disease (associated with Down's syndrome)	Cognitive regression, aphasia, intellectual disability Early onset dementia
22	Metachromatic leukodystrophy	Personality changes, psychosis, dementia
	Neurofibromatosis-2	Hearing impairment
	DiGeorge/velocardiofacial syndrome	Schizophrenia, bipolar disorder, psychomotor retardation, language delay, ADHD, seizures
X	Fragile X syndrome	Autistic behavior
	Kallman syndrome	No sense of smell, lack of sex drive, depression, anxiety, fatigue, insomnia
	Lesch-Nyhan syndrome	Self-mutilation and other bizarre behavior, intellectual disability
	Rett syndrome	Autistic behavior, hand-wringing, breathing abnormalities

Source: Barbara Fadem. Behavioral Science in Medicine. Lippincott Williams & Wilkins. ISBN 978–1-60913–664–2.

The genesis of personality traits is also influenced by genetic factors. For instance, monozygotic twins have a higher concordance rate for personality traits like distractibility, activity level, fearfulness, and responsiveness to stimulation than dizygotic twins. These elements also contribute to the genesis of personality disorders, which are diagnosed when a person's personality traits significantly hinder their ability to function in social or professional contexts.

Based on commonalities in their presentations, personality disorders are grouped into three clusters. Each of the clusters' patient relatives tends to have distinct mental health issues when compared to the general population. Patients with cluster B personality disorders (histrionic, narcissistic, antisocial, and borderline) are more likely to have relatives with major depressive and substance-abuse disorders, whereas patients with cluster A personality disorders (schizoid, schizotypal, and paranoid) are more likely to have relatives with psychotic disorders like schizophrenia. Anxiety disorders in relatives have been linked to personality disorders in Cluster C (avoidant, obsessive-compulsive, and dependent) (Bouchard, 2007).

2. **Neuropsychiatric Conditions:** Numerous neuropsychiatric conditions have a strong genetic component to their etiology. For instance, family risk studies reveal that while only 10% of nonrelatives have Alzheimer's disease, 25% to 50% of close relatives of those who have the condition eventually get it. Additionally, the concordance rate for Alzheimer's disease is higher in monozygotic twins than in dizygotic twins.

Alzheimer's disease has been associated with multiple chromosomes. Alzheimer's disease and chromosome 21 (amyloid precursor protein gene) are most commonly associated because people with Down's syndrome (trisomy 21) who survive past the age of 40 eventually exhibit behavioral and neuroanatomical signs of Alzheimer's disease. Alzheimer's disease has also been connected to chromosomes 1 (presenilin 1 gene) and 14 (presenilin 2 gene), especially in the early onset form that manifests before the age of 60. Additionally, apolipoprotein E_2 (Apo E_2) alleles on chromosome 19 appear to be less common, whereas the presence of the E_4 allele (Apo E_4) appears to be associated with a higher risk of Alzheimer's disease, especially in women (Bartres-Faz et al., 2002). Table 1.2 contains specific chromosomal associations for additional neuropsychiatric symptoms and disorders.

Two other neuropsychiatric disorders that have a strong genetic component are Tourette's syndrome and Huntington's disease. Huntington's disease is a fatal autosomal-dominant disorder linked to an abnormal gene on the short arm of chromosome 4. The disorder has a 50% chance of developing in the offspring of one affected parent. Genetic anticipation is another feature of Huntington's disease (as well as Fragile X syndrome), which causes the illness to manifest earlier and with more severe symptoms in subsequent generations. Tourette's disorder affects a large portion of its patients' family members, and monozygotic twins are more likely than dizygotic twins to have concordance in the condition.

3. **Substance-Abuse Disorders:** Many people think that a person's poor social choices or lack of self-control are what lead to substance abuse disorders. While abusers undoubtedly face social challenges, a growing body of research indicates that substance abuse disorders, including alcoholism, may also have a genetic component. Evidence of genetic associations in

alcoholism includes the following findings:

- The concordance rate for alcoholism is about twice as high for monozygotic twins as it is for dizygotic twins.
- Adopted children in adulthood tend to show the drinking patterns characteristic of their biological rather than their adoptive parents.
- Alcoholism is about four times more prevalent in the biological children of alcoholics than of non-alcoholics.

Moreover, there is a correlation between the sex and age of onset of the genetic component of alcoholism; sons of alcoholics are more susceptible than their daughters, especially if the sons start abusing alcohol before the age of 20.

Genetic factors are also linked to cocaine abuse. Early in this century, (McHugh et al., 2002), it was demonstrated that a polymorphism in the prodynorphin gene's promoter region was linked to defense against cocaine abuse.

1.3.2. Behavioral Neuroanatomy

The central nervous system (CNS) and the peripheral nervous system (PNS) make up the human nervous system. The brain (cerebral hemispheres, basal ganglia, and thalamus), brainstem (pons, medulla, and midbrain), and spinal cord make up the central nervous system (CNS). Somatosensory (afferent), motor (efferent), and autonomic neurons make up the PNS. The CNS and PNS are anatomically distinct, but they collaborate in their functions.

1.3.2.1. The Cerebral Cortex

The cerebral cortex is part of the brain most directly linked to behavior, though subcortical regions are also involved. The functional division of the cortex into sensory, motor, and association areas can be made; these areas work together to influence behavior in the end.

Anatomically speaking, the cortex can also be separated into limbic lobes, which house the medial portions of the frontal, temporal, and parietal lobes, as well as frontal, temporal, parietal, and occipital lobes. The primary neuropsychiatric roles of these and other cortical regions are demonstrated by behavioral changes observed in patients with brain lesions brought on by illness, trauma, or surgical procedures.

The frontal lobes have lateralized emotional-behavioral functions. While lesions to the right prefrontal area are more likely to cause signs of elevated mood, lesions to the left prefrontal area, both cortical and subcortical, can cause depression. Similarly, positive mood is linked to activation of the left prefrontal cortex and stress is linked to activation of the right prefrontal cortex, according to fMRI studies (Davidson & Irwin, 1999).

1.3.2.2. Limbic Lobe

The limbic lobe is also known as the limbic system because the neurons that make up its circuits are crucial to emotion. Its main roles include controlling the activity of the autonomic nervous system (ANS) and mediating between the hypothalamus and cerebral cortex. The Papez circuit, also known as the limbic system, was initially defined by Papez in 1937 and subsequently extended to encompass additional regions. This circuit comprises the hippocampus, fornix, amygdala, septum, cingulate gyms, part of the thalamus, and other associated structures (Figure 1.1). Additionally, the limbic system affects the hypothalamus, which in turn affects hormone secretion and endocrine regulation of emotions. Anomalous behavior is caused by damage to the limbic lobe, specifically the amygdala and hypothalamus. According to recent neuroimaging research, patients with schizophrenia have smaller volumes of limbic structures like the hippocampus and amygdala than they do of the prefrontal cortex.

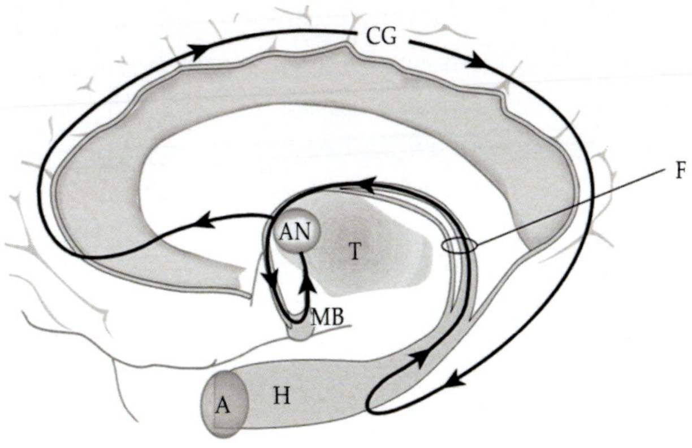

Figure 1.1. *Papez circuit. A, amygdala; AN, anterior nucleus of the thalamus; CG, cingulate gyrus; H, hippocampus; MB, mamillary body; F, fornix; T, thalamus. The arrow represents the anatomy of the loop believed to be involved in the processing of emotions. (Reprinted with permission from Filley, C. M. (2011). Neurobehavioral anatomy (3rd ed.). Niwot, CO: University Press of Colorado.).*

Source: *Barbara Fadem. Behavioral Science in Medicine. Lippincott Williams & Wilkins. ISBN 978-1-60913-664-2.*

1.3.2.3. The Basal Ganglia

Information from the entire cerebral cortex is received by the basal ganglia nuclei, which then projects it to the frontal lobes via the thalamus. There are four structural components of the basal ganglia:

- Striatum (containing the caudate nucleus and the putamen);
- Pallidum (also called the globus pallidus);
- Substantia nigra; and
- Subthalamic nucleus.

The purpose of the basal ganglia is to convert the intention to move into actual movement. Neuropsychiatric disorders that cause damage to its nuclei can cause motor symptoms. For instance, damage to the substantia nigra or excessive striatal activity can cause Parkinsonian symptoms like akinesia, bradykinesia, or the inability to initiate or continue movement. The involuntary, erratic movements (chorea) of Huntington's disease are linked to under activity of the striatum and shrinkage of the caudate nucleus with loss of Y-aminobutyric acid (GABA)-ergic neurons. Tourette's syndrome is also linked to damage to the caudate, while conditions characterized by abrupt, uncontrollable limb movements are caused by lesions of the pallidum and subthalamic nucleus.

Human immunodeficiency virus (HIV) infection of the brain can eventually result in cognitive and psychiatric symptoms like depression, apathy, withdrawal, and memory loss, in addition to motor difficulties.

Table 1.3. *Grading Deep Tendon Reflexes*

GRADE	DESCRIPTION
0	No response; always abnormal
1+	A slight but definitely present response; may or may not be normal
2+	A brisk response; normal
3+	A very brisk response; may or may not be normal
4+	A tap elicits a repeating refles (clonus); always abnormal

Source: Barbara Fadem. Behavioral Science in Medicine. Lippincott Williams & Wilkins. ISBN 978-1-60913-664-2.

Ataxia, elevated motor tone, and elevated deep tendon reflexes are among the motor issues that HIV patients experience (Table 1.3). Diffuse brain disease, specifically white matter demyelination and cerebellar atrophy is the cause of these problems together (Klunder et al., 2008).

1.3.2.4. Hemispheric Specialization

The right side of the body is managed by the left side of the brain. The left hemisphere of the brain is referred to as the dominant hemisphere since the right hand is preferred by about 90% of people. The anterior commissure, habenular commissure, hippocampal commissure, and corpus callosum are among the structures that facilitate communication between the cerebral hemispheres. Empirical research employing individuals who have undergone surgical division of the corpus callosum to address severe epilepsy or who have experienced injury to only one side of the brain, reveals that the hemispheres are functionally lateralized.

As language function is linked to the left hemisphere, impairment of speaking, writing, and reading skills occurs in nearly all right-handed individuals and in the majority of left-handed individuals as well. The right hemisphere, also known as the non-dorninant hemisphere, is mainly linked to perception. It is also linked to spatial relations, body image, music and face recognition, puzzle solving, map reading, and artistic and musical ability. Although right hemisphere damage typically has no direct effect on intelligence or personality, it can have motor sequelae and indirect effects on behavior.

The way the brain functions varies depending on a person's sex. For instance, women seem to have better interhemispheric communication than men and typically have larger corpus callosum and anterior commissure. Women usually use both hemispheres during verbal tasks, while men only activate one hemisphere (Figure 1.2) (Shaywitz et al., 1995). Men's more developed right hemispheres could help to explain some of the consistently observed male advantage in spatial task performance (Halpern, 2000).

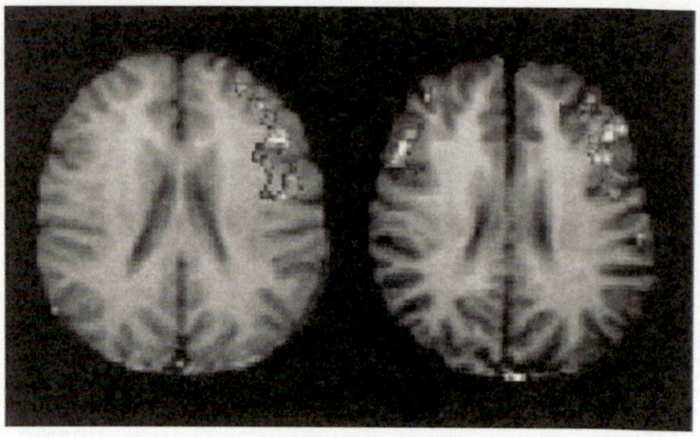

Figure 1.2. *Composite functional magnetic resonance images (fMRI) of male and female brains. These composite fMRI images in males (left image) and females (right image) show the distribution of activation of a cognitive task this case, phonological processing involving identifying whether nonsense words (e.g., lee! and jeet) rhymed or not. Males show unilateral activation in the left inferior frontal gyrus, whereas females show activity in both the left and right inferior frontal gyri.*

Source: Barbara Fadem. Behavioral Science in Medicine. Lippincott Williams & Wilkins. ISBN 978–1-60913–664–2.

1.3.2.5. Memory and Language

Knowing facts and their meanings is known as declarative or explicit memory (e.g., knowledge about individuals or locations) and is deliberately retrieved. Semantic and episodic memory are two categories of explicit memory. The information stored in implicit or non-declarative memory pertains to the execution of an action (e.g., bicycle riding) and is unconsciously recalled. Working memory and procedural memory are examples of implicit memory types. Time-based classifications can also be applied to memory. For instance, memory held for a few seconds is known as immediate or short-term recall. Memory stored for minutes to a lifetime is known as long-term recall. Recent memory is that portion of long-term recall that is retained for hours or days (e.g., your lunch), recent history is retained for the previous month (e.g., knowledge of the present), while remote memory refers to the distant past (e.g., your first-grade teacher's name).

There are two types of amnesia or memory loss: retrograde and anterograde. The loss of previously acquired knowledge is known as retrograde amnesia, and it is most commonly linked to the temporal lobes and other declarative episodic memory-related brain regions. Anterograde amnesia makes it difficult for the affected person to pick up new knowledge. Recent events and facts are not retained, even though prior knowledge and routines are typically retained. Anterograde amnesia is usually caused by injury to the hippocampal region and its surrounding structures. Damage to regions of the basal forebrain, particularly the nucleus basalis of Meynert, which produces acetylcholine (ACh), or to the medial thalamic nuclei, which are impacted in Korsakoff's syndrome along with the mammillary bodies, may also be the cause.

One could argue that language is a human-only ability. The early years of childhood are crucial for the development of language skills, which are necessary for social communication throughout life. Language deficits known as aphasias are caused by damage to particular areas of the brain.

1.3.2.6. Consciousness, Coma, and Brain Death

The brain regions most directly involved in arousal and consciousness are the reticular formation, a network of neurons in the brainstem, and the thalamus. Relatively small, localized lesions of either of these structures, especially the reticular formation, can cause profound loss of consciousness or coma, non-sleep loss of consciousness that lasts for a long time, as opposed to cortical lesions (especially left-sided lesions), which must be extensive to cause loss of consciousness (Kandel et al., 2000). Coma can also be brought on by lesions that damage the brainstem and thalamus's connections. The Glasgow Coma Scale allows consciousness levels to be rated on a range of 3 to 15.

There is no conscious cognitive function in a patient in a profound coma. A patient in a persistent vegetative state, on the other hand, might seem to be awake and have their eyes open, but they are unaware of other people and their surroundings. The decision of whether to keep a patient in a persistent vegetative state on life support is a crucial ethical one in medicine because of this simulation of consciousness.

1.3.2.7. Peripheral Nervous System

Outside of the central nervous system (CNS), the PNS is home to sensory, motor, and autonomic fibers. These include the cranial, spinal, and peripheral ganglia nerves. Motor information is sent from the CNS to the PNS and sensory information is sent from the PNS to the CNS.

1.3.2.8. The Autonomic Nervous System

The PNS region most directly linked to behavior is the ANS. The sympathetic branch of the ANS is heavily involved in responding to stress, while the parasympathetic branch primarily maintains homeostasis and conserves resources. Together, these divisions provide innervation to the internal organs and synchronize emotional responses with visceral responses, including blood pressure, heart rate, and secretion of peptic acid. The development and progression of physical illnesses like hypertension, peptic ulcer disease, and rheumatoid arthritis are linked to the exacerbation of these visceral responses as a result of psychological stress.

1.3.2.9. The Hypothalamus

Between the thalamus and the pituitary gland, the hypothalamus plays a crucial role in the biological regulation of emotion, especially anger and aggression. The hypothalamus plays a crucial role in maintaining homeostasis, particularly in controlling body temperature and eating and drinking habits. Damage to the hypothalamic satiety center, the ventromedial nucleus, causes increased appetite and obesity, while damage to the lateral nucleus causes decreased appetite and weight loss. Another function of the hypothalamus is to synchronize the pituitary gland and ANS activity.

The pituitary gland, which controls gonadal hormone secretion, mediates the function of hypothalamus in controlling adult sexual activity. Research on animals demonstrates that gonadal hormone exposure during perinatal life causes permanent sex differences in the volume of specific hypothalamic nuclei in males and females. Certain research indicates that comparable anatomical sex differences in these nuclei are linked to human sexual orientation (LeVay, 1991, 2010).

1.3.3. Neurotransmission

Chemical messengers called neurotransmitters play a key role in nervous system cell function at all levels. It is thought that interactions and imbalances among these messengers in the brain lead to emotions and psychopathology. Amino acids, peptides, and biogenic amines (monoamines) are the three main classes of neurotransmitters. Presynaptic terminals synthesize amino acids and biogenic amines, while neuronal cell bodies synthesize peptides. Other substances, such as endocrine hormones, can also serve as neurotransmitters.

Neuron membrane proteins called postsynaptic and presynaptic receptors are able to identify particular neurotransmitters. The neurotransmitter is released upon stimulation of the presynaptic neuron, crosses the synaptic cleft (i.e., the space between the presynaptic neuron's axon terminal and the postsynaptic neuron's dendrite), and binds to receptors on the postsynaptic neuron. When a neurotransmitter increases the likelihood that a neuron will fire, it is said to be excitatory; when it decreases this likelihood, it is said to be inhibitory.

1.3.3.1. Regulation of Neurotransmitters

Mood and behavior are strongly correlated with the concentration of neurotransmitters in the synaptic cleft. There are active and passive mechanisms that influence this concentration. Neurotransmitters leave the synaptic cleft passively by diffusing into nearby tissue after being released by the presynaptic neuron. Active removal is achieved by either degradation by enzymes like acetylcholinesterase (AChE) or reuptake by the presynaptic neuron. There is evidence that regulates neural responsiveness not only through neurotransmitter availability but also through variations in the number of receptors or their affinity (sensitivity) for particular neurotransmitters (neuronal plasticity) and the efficiency with which a neurotransmitter signal is converted into a message.

Postsynaptic receptors can modify the metabolism of neurons through the utilization of second messengers like cyclic adenosine monophosphate and guanosine monophosphate, lipids like diacylglycerol, and Ca^{2+} when they are stimulated by neurotransmitters. In addition to neurotransmitters, eicosanoid metabolites and gases such as nitric oxide may also function as second messengers.

Common psychiatric diseases and conditions

are linked to changes in the availability of particular neurotransmitters (Table 1.4). For some of these disorders, pharmacologic agents that normalize neurotransmitter availability are linked to symptom relief.

Table 1.4. *Neuropsychiatric Conditions Associated Neurotransmitter Activity, and Implicated Brain Areas*

NEUROPSYCHIATRIC SYMPTOM	NEUROTRANSMITTER (MAJOR METABOLITE) ACTIVITY INCREASED (↑) OR DECREASED (↓)	PRIMARY BRAIN AREAS IMPLICATED IN SYMPTOM PRODUCTION	OTHER BRAIN AREAS IMPLICATED
Depression	Norepinephrine (MHPG) (↓), serotonin (5-HIAA) (↓), dopamine (HVA) (↓)	Left prefrontal cortex	Limbic system
Mania	Dopamine (HVA) (↑),GABA (↓)	Right prefrontal cortex	Limbic system
Psychosis	Dopamine (HVA) (↑), serotonin (5-HIAA) (↑), glutamate (↑ or ↓)	Bilateral prefrontal cortex	Limbic system
Anxiety	GABA (↓), serotonin (5-HIAA) (↓), norepinephrine (MHPG) (↑)	Locus ceruleus, prefrontal cortex (particularly in OCD)	Right parahippocampal gyrus
Dementia	ACh (↓), glutamate (↑)	Hippocampus	Nucleus basalis of Meynert (ACh production)

HVA, homovanillic acid; 5-HIAA, 5-hydroxyindoleacetic acid; GABA, γ-aminobutyric acid; MHPG, 3-methoxy-4-hydroxyphenyl-glycol.

Source: Barbara Fadem. Behavioral Science in Medicine. Lippincott Williams & Wilkins. ISBN 978-1-60913-664-2.

1.3.3.2. Biogenic Amines

Catecholamines, indolamines, ethylamines, and quaternary amines are examples of biogenic amines, also known as monoamines. According to the monoamine theory of mood disorders, abnormalities in mood are caused by changes in monoamine receptors and altered monoamine activity.

1.3.3.3. Dopamine

One catecholamine called dopamine plays a role in the etiology of Parkinson's disease, depression, the conditioned fear response, and the "rewarding" nature of drugs of abuse. The pathophysiology of schizophrenia and other psychotic disorders has also been linked to dopamine.

There are at least five different subtypes of dopamine receptors known to exist: D_1, D_2, D_3, D_4, and D_5. While the D_1 and D_4 subtypes of the D_2 receptor are implicated in the action of more recent, atypical antipsychotics like clozapine, the D_2 receptor subtype appears to be the primary site of action for traditional antipsychotic agents. The nigrostriatal tract, tuberoinfundibular tract, and mesolimbic-mesocortical tract are the three main dopaminergic tracts in the brain (Figure 1.3).

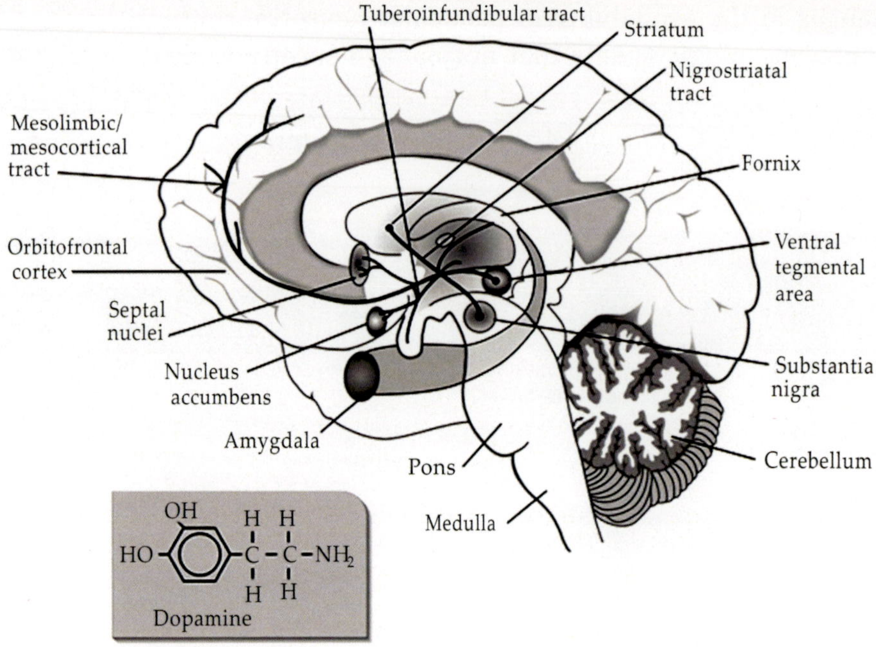

Figure 1.3. *Distribution of dopaminergic axons in the CNS. Most dopamine containing fibers arise from the substantia nigra (which projects to the striatum) and the ventral tegmental area.*

Source: Barbara Fadem. Behavioral Science in Medicine. Lippincott Williams & Wilkins. ISBN 978-1-60913-664-2.

Parkinson's disease is characterized by the degeneration of the nigrostriatal tract, which is involved in the regulation of muscle tone and movement. Parkinsonian symptoms can therefore arise from treatment with traditional antipsychotic medications that block postsynaptic dopamine receptors receiving input from the nigrostriatal tract.

Dopamine inhibits the anterior pituitary's secretion of prolactin by acting on the tuberoinfundibular tract. Antipsychotic medications that block dopamine receptors inhibit this inhibition, which raises prolactin levels and causes side effects like breast enlargement, galactorrhea, and dysfunction in the sexual organs.

The mesolimbic-mesocortical tract, which projects into the limbic system and prefrontal cortex, is linked to psychotic symptoms and may play a part in emotional expression. Positivity in the symptoms (e.g., anxiety) is linked to hyperactivity of the mesolimbic tract (e.g., hallucinations) and mesocortical tract hypoactivity accompanied by adverse symptoms (e.g., indifference) of schizophrenia (Stahl, 2008).

The ventral tegmental area to the nucleus accumbens is a significant dopaminergic pathway in the brain (Figure 1.3). This pathway is activated after abusing certain drugs, indicating that it plays a role in the rewarding and addictive properties of these substances.

1.3.3.4. Norepinephrine

A catecholamine, norepinephrine affects mood, anxiety, arousal, memory, and learning. Noradrenergic neurons produce dopamine similarly to dopaminergic neurons. Dopamine is synthesized and then converted to norepinephrine by the enzyme dopamine beta-hydroxylase, which is found in noradrenergic neurons. The locus ceruleus (Figure 1.4) is the most significant of the nuclei in the upper brainstem that house the majority of noradrenergic neurons, which number about 10,000 per hemisphere of the brain.

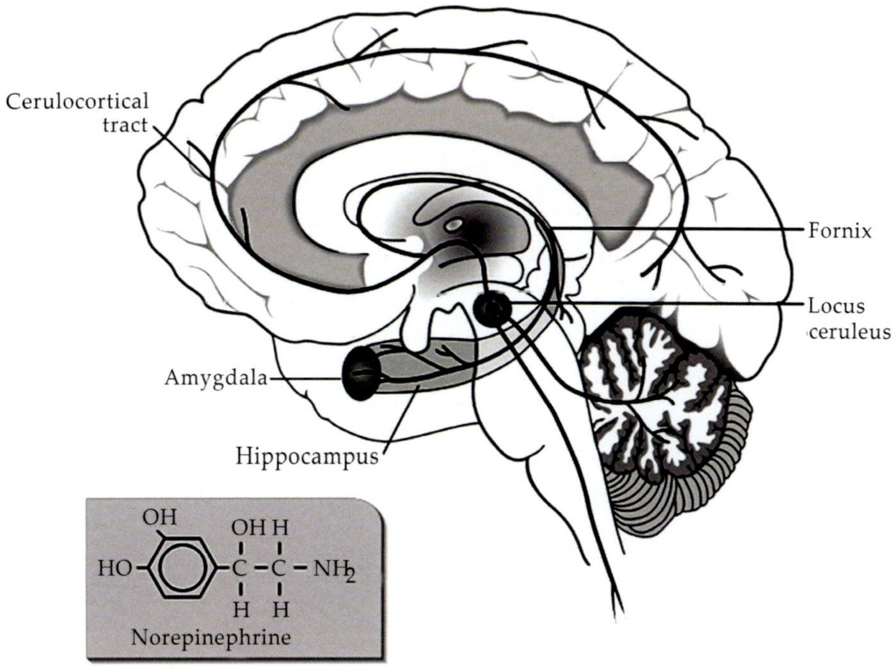

Figure 1.4. *Distribution of noradrenergic axons in the CNS. Most noradrenaline-containing fibers arise from the locus ceruleus and are distributed throughout the CNS.*

Source: Barbara Fadem. Behavioral Science in Medicine. Lippincott Williams & Wilkins. ISBN 978-1-60913-664-2.

1.3.3.5. Serotonin

An indolamine called serotonin affects mood, appetite, sleep, sensitivity to pain, sexuality, and impulse control. The enzyme tryptophan hydroxylase and an amino acid decarboxylase both convert the amino acid tryptophan into serotonin, also referred to as 5-hydroxytryptamine, during the synthesis of serotonin. Anatomically, the dorsal raphe nucleus in the upper pons and lower midbrain houses the majority of serotonergic cell bodies in the brain (Figure 1.5).

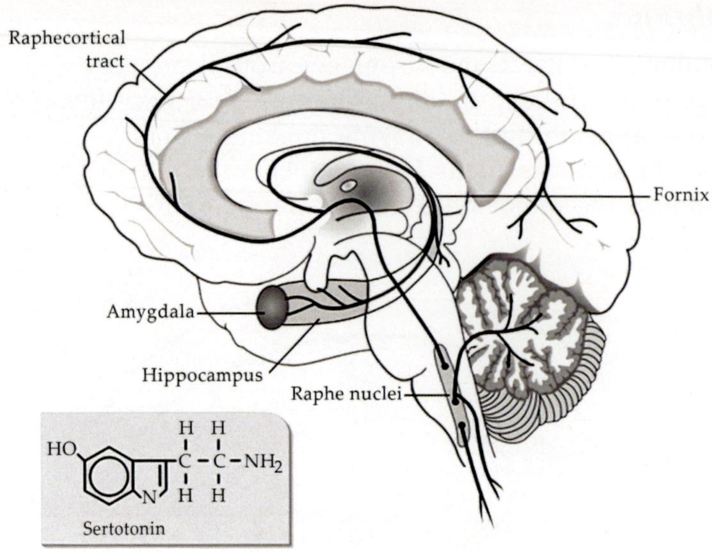

Figure 1.5. *Distribution of serotonergic axons in the CNS. Most serotonin-containing fibers arise from the raphe nuclei and are distributed throughout the CNS.*

Source: Barbara Fadem. Behavioral Science in Medicine. Lippincott Williams & Wilkins. ISBN 978–1-60913–664–2.

Elevated levels of serotonin in the brain are linked to both beneficial and negative outcomes, including enhanced mood and sleep, reduced sexual function (especially delayed climax), and psychotic symptoms at elevated levels. As a result, more recent antipsychotic drugs aim to restore normalcy to both the dopaminergic and serotonergic systems. Reduced serotonin availability is linked to chronic pain syndromes, violent behavior, poor impulse control, depression, anxiety disorders like OCD, and alcoholism. The majority of antidepressants currently on the market increase serotonin and other biogenic amine availability in the synaptic cleft through various mechanisms.

1.3.3.6. Acetylcholine (ACh) and Histamine

Neurotransmitters implicated in behavior and the unsettling side effects of psychoactive medication are histamine, an ethylamine, and ACh, a quaternary amine.

Neuron-skeleton-muscle junctions use ACh. With the aid of the enzyme choline acetyltransferase, cholinergic neurons produce ACh from acetyl coenzyme A and choline. ACh is broken down by the enzyme AChE into choline and acetate. Cholinergic mechanisms are essential to cognitive functioning and are likely involved in mood disorders, though they are not the cause of them. Cognitive disorders like Alzheimer's disease are caused by loss of cholinergic neurons or decreased availability of ACh due to decreased production of the synthesizing enzyme choline acetyltransferase. Reduced availability of ACh is also linked to symptoms of movement disorders, sleep disorders, and Down syndrome. While there is currently no medication that can restore lost function in Alzheimer's patients, some patients may experience a delay in the disease's progression by using medications like galantamine (Razadyne), rivastigmine (Exelon), and donepezil (Aricept) that block AChE's activity.

Nicotinic ACh receptors are less important in behavior and the adverse effects of psychoactive substances than muscarinic ACh receptors. The traditional anticholinergic side effects of antipsychotics and tricyclic antidepressants, such as dry mouth, blurred vision, urinary hesitancy, and constipation, are caused by the blockade of muscarinic receptors by these medications.

Psychoactive substances also change histamine's availability. Common side effects of medications like antipsychotics and tricyclic antidepressants, like drowsiness and increased appetite that results in weight gain, are partially caused by histamine-receptor blockade.

1.3.3.7. Other Neurotransmitters Involved in Behavior

The majority of brain synapses are involved in the action of amino acid neurotransmitters, including glutamate, glycine, and GABA. These and other neuropeptides, like endogenous opioids, influence behavior.

1. **Amino Acids:** GABA, the primary inhibitory neurotransmitter in the central nervous system, is intimately linked to anxiety symptoms. GABA is produced when glutamate is decarboxylated by the enzyme glutamate decarboxylase. GABA transaminase then removes the GABA from the synapse through reuptake. How well-working anti-anxiety medications like benzodiazepines (e.g., diazepam [Valium]) and tranquilizers (e.g., secobarbital [Seconal]) are based on their capacity to raise GABA's affinity for its binding site, enabling chloride to enter the cell. Consequently, the neuron experiences hyperpolarization and inhibition, leading to a reduction in neuronal firing and, ultimately, anxiety.

The main excitatory neurotransmitter in the central nervous system is glutamate. Glutamate can be produced by cells that require it, even though it is a non-essential amino acid. Citric acid cycle and glycolytic intermediates are produced via its synthetic pathways. Mechanisms of cell death, memory formation, epilepsy, and neurodegenerative diseases have all been linked to glutamate. Particular changes in the major glutamate receptor, N-methyl-D-aspartate (NMDA), have been connected to symptoms of schizophrenia. Psychotic symptoms are induced in healthy volunteers by drugs that block NMDA receptors (Tamminga and Frost, 2001). Additionally, genes linked to the development of schizophrenia are linked to NMDA-receptor pathway disruption (Chumakov et al., 2002). The processes of learning and memory are also mediated by NMDA receptors. Calcium ions enter the neuron as a result of sustained elevation of glutamate activating NMDA receptors. Because of excitotoxicity, long-term excessive calcium exposure causes nerve cell degeneration and death. Alzheimer's patients can now receive approval for the use of memantine (Namenda), an NMDA receptor antagonist that eventually prevents this calcium influx.

An inhibitory neurotransmitter mainly found in the spinal cord is glycine. It functions both independently and as a glutamate regulator.

2. **Neuropeptides:** Among the neuropeptides influencing behavior are endogenous opioids, i.e., endorphins and enkephalins. These brain-produced neurotransmitters influence mood and addiction in addition to reducing pain and anxiety.

The placebo effect (i.e., subjective reactivity to inactive pharmaceutical agents) could be mediated by the dopaminergic and endogenous opioid systems (Finnis et al., 2010,). For instance, it has been shown that placebo-induced release of endogenous dopamine in the striatum of

Parkinson's disease patients can be inhibited by prior treatment with an opioid-receptor blocker such as naloxone (Sher, 1997).

1.4. The Psychological Bases of Behavior

The foundation of the psychodynamic theory is the notion, first put forth by Sigmund Freud and then expanded upon by others, that forces originate from processes that people are unaware of affect behavior. Though these unconscious forces prevent thoughts and feelings from entering consciousness, they are also dynamic and influence people's decisions, feelings, and actions all their lives. This idea of the dynamic unconscious serves as the foundation for many psychotherapeutic interventions, including psychoanalysis and related therapies.

The terminology used in psychodynamic theory is defined and explained in this section. The ideas of personal defense mechanisms and transference reactions between the physician and patient are the main topics of discussion. The connection between these theoretical ideas and standard medical practice may not be immediately apparent. Nonetheless, being aware of these concepts can assist medical professionals in interpreting and handling seemingly contradictory, aggressive, or even self-destructive behavior in their patients.

1.4.1. Freud's Theories of the Mind

To explain his theories about behavior, Freud created the topographic theory of the mind early in his career. The structural theory was developed by him later in his career.

1.4.1.1. Topographic Theory

The unconscious, preconscious, and conscious levels make up the three levels of the mind according to topographic theory. Repressed ideas and emotions that are unavailable to the conscious mind are stored in the unconscious mind.

The primary process of thinking that the unconscious employs is linked to primal urges, wish fulfilment, instant gratification, and pleasure-seeking. It lacks a sense of time and logic. Adults suffering from psychotic disorders as well as young children exhibit primary process thinking.

Memories that are easily accessible but not instantly available are stored in the preconscious mind. Preconscious material includes things like the names of the cranial nerves, which are accessible for exams but not immediately memorable to a medical student.

Thoughts that an individual is presently aware of reside in the conscious mind. It works closely with the preconscious mind, but it is not able to access the unconscious mind like the preconscious mind does. The conscious mind is capable of delaying gratification and employs secondary process thinking, which is rational, mature, and time-oriented.

Whether it is possible to determine whether the unconscious mind exists at all is one question that the topographic theory poses. Freud proposed that dreams, which stand for the satisfaction of irrational unconscious urges and wish fulfilment, are one piece of evidence supporting the existence of the unconscious.

Additional instances of unconsciousness include parapraxes, also known as Freudian slips, which are verbal or auditory errors that disclose an individual's actual but unconscious emotions, and hypnosis, a psychotherapy method that circumvents the conscious mind to unveil information from the unconscious (Table 1.5).

Table 1.5. *Freud's Proof of the Unconscious*

PROOF	EXAMPLE
Dreams	A man who has personally unacceptable sexual feelings for his therapist, Dr. Freud, dreams that he is walking naked down a street named "Sigmund Road"
Parapraxes	A woman who unconsciously fears the responsibilities of a new and lucrative position states, "My new job is a landmine … I mean a goldmine"
Hypnosis	Under hypnosis, a woman who has no conscious memory of the event reveals that she was sexually abused as a child by her father

Source: Barbara Fadem. Behavioral Science in Medicine. Lippincott Williams & Wilkins. ISBN 978-1-60913-664-2.

1.4.2. Structural Theory

The id, ego, and superego are the three components of the mind according to Freud's structural theory. In essence, each of the three components is unaware. Innate sexual and aggressive drives are part of the id, which is present from birth. It is not affected by the outside world and is governed by primary process thinking. The ego regulates the id's expression and uses defense mechanisms to shape it to fit the needs of the outside world. The ego makes it possible to maintain fulfilling interpersonal connections and, by reality testing (i.e., continuously assessing what is legitimate and then applying that to actual situations), allows an individual to preserve a sense of reality regarding their own body and the outside world. The superego, which also regulates id impulses, emerges at the age of six and stands for moral principles and conscience.

When the id's desires threaten to overpower the ego and superego's authority, conflict results. When this happens, the ego uses the active defense mechanism of repression to drive the id impulses and undesirable emotions further into the unconscious. Sadly, information that is forced into the unconscious seldom goes down well. This material affects the person's emotional state, leading to dissociative and somatic symptoms as well as psychiatric symptoms like anxiety and depression, even though the person may not be aware of its content. Psychoanalysis is the therapeutic method that Freud created to retrieve and consciously deal with this suppressed material. He noticed that patients' upsetting psychological symptoms disappeared after receiving psychoanalysis treatment. Freud was adamant that unconscious conflicts were not the root cause of psychotic disorders like schizophrenia. His hypothesis—which was validated by further research—was that psychotic disorders were organic in nature and could not be treated with psychoanalytic methods.

1.4.3. Defense Mechanisms

People defend themselves against emotional pain in a similar way to how they would defend against physical pain—albeit unconsciously. Their methods, which Freud referred to as defense mechanisms, function by preventing conflict from entering the conscious mind. By reducing anxiety, this protection aids in the person's ability to maintain equilibrium, safety, and self-worth.

Defense mechanisms are frequently used by people in need of medical and mental health care to cope with the pain and anxiety brought on by their conditions. Therefore, these mechanisms may be beneficial to the patient. Defense mechanisms, however, can eventually be detrimental if they keep a patient from getting treatment or from following doctor's orders.

1.4.3.1. Mature and Less Mature Defense Mechanisms

An individual's coping style and personality are strongly correlated with the type of defense mechanism they employ. Regression is a defense mechanism used, for instance, by someone who, when under stress from illness, tends to become demanding and childlike.

There are different levels of maturity in defense mechanisms. A person with less developed defense mechanisms is shielded from anxiety and unpleasant emotions, but at a great social cost. The same purpose is fulfilled by mature defense mechanisms, but at little societal cost. For instance, a man verbally abuses his own office assistant as a way to deal with his unrecognized anger toward his employer through the less developed defense mechanism of displacement. On the other hand, the same man could manage his anger by playing a hard game of racquetball, which is a mature defense mechanism of sublimation.

There may even be social advantages to developed defense mechanisms. A man who is low on self-esteem uses the defense mechanism of altruism to make himself feel better about himself when he gives of his time to visit hospitalized patients. Besides sublimation and altruism, other developed defense strategies include humor and suppression.

The goal of humor is to communicate deeply uncomfortable emotions without adding to the discomfort. For instance, a patient may joke about Viagra (sildenafil citrate) if he is uncomfortable discussing his erectile dysfunction. A person willfully pushes anxiety-inducing or socially unacceptable emotions out of conscious awareness through suppression, a defense mechanism that involves some aspects of consciousness. Suppression is a defense mechanism used, for instance, by a prostate cancer patient who willfully switches topics in his mind when he starts to consider the possibility of a relapse while still seeking the proper medical attention for his condition.

1.4.3.2. Common Defense Mechanisms in Medical Patients

The most fundamental form of defense is repression; other forms of defense are only employed when repression is ineffective. Both repression and denial are common defense mechanisms employed by medical patients, and they are closely related. When a patient experiences repression, they unintentionally reject a part of their inner reality. When someone is in denial, they unintentionally reject a part of the outside world. For instance, a cocaine addict who uses repression does not feel guilty about their addiction because they do not acknowledge themselves or remember that their drug use has lasted for years rather than months. By employing denial, he maintains that he can quit taking the drug whenever he wants, despite evidence to the contrary.

Regression and undoing are two more defense strategies that sick patients frequently exhibit. When a patient practice undoing, she thinks she can magically change the past and make up for bad behavior by adopting good behavior now, like making amends or owning up to her mistakes. For instance, a woman whose intravenous drug addiction has left her terminally ill with AIDS decides to stop taking the drug and joins a support group where she discloses that she stole money to buy the drug. This same woman may exhibit regression, returning to childlike behavior patterns such as pouting, whining, and demanding that family members give her more attention, while she is in the hospital due to complications from her illness.

1.4.3.3. Rationalization, Intellectualization, and Isolation of Affect

People, both educated and ignorant, employ coping strategies to ward off unpleasant feelings. But intelligent people typically have defense mechanisms that make use of the higher order mental processes. These processes include affect isolation, intellectualization, and rationalization. When someone rationalizes, they unintentionally change how they see something to make its unfavorable outcome seem plausible. A blind person employing this defense mechanism would be someone who thinks they have supernormal hearing again. Intellectualization is the process of avoiding unpleasant feelings by using reason. This defense mechanism is employed by the pilot of a doomed flight who explains to the passengers the technical details of the engine failure. When considering or summarizing an emotional event, a person who uses isolation of affect does not consciously feel any emotion. When discussing the death of a loved one, the person who remains emotionless has cut himself off from the tragic occasion.

1.4.3.4. Somatization and Dissociation

Somatoform and dissociative disorders are characterized by dramatic defense mechanisms called somatization and dissociation. Somatization is the unconscious process by which an individual experiences and expresses physical symptoms in order to cope with negative emotions. A class of illnesses known as somatoform disorders exhibit physical symptoms devoid of a strong enough biological foundation. When someone dissociates, they mentally divide a portion of their awareness from reality and may even lose track of what has actually happened. For instance, a teenager suffering from dissociative amnesia, a form of dissociative disorder, lacks conscious memory of a car accident in which he was driving and his girlfriend was killed, even though he is unharmed.

1.4.3.5. Defense Mechanisms and Psychopathology

Aspects of psychopathology can be explained by certain defense mechanisms. For example, the defense mechanism of identification (in this case, identification with the aggressor) may have caused the person to unintentionally model himself after a powerful figure in his past, which could account for the tendency of some abused children to grow up to be abusers. Even though the case study illustrates a negative result, if the person utilizes a loving, supportive figure from the past as a role model for his behavior, identification can have a positive outcome.

Attributing one's own personally unacceptable feelings to others is a defense mechanism known as projection, and its use has been linked to psychopathology, paranoia, and even to common prejudice. Projecting is a way for the man with unconscious homosexual impulses to keep himself from acknowledging his own personally unacceptable homosexual feelings when he starts to mistakenly believe that his male boss is making sexual advances toward him.

Some people tend to categorize people or situations as either wonderful or terrible. By using this defense mechanism, the person using it to avoid confronting the uncertainty that comes with the realization that everyone possesses both good and bad traits. Patients suffering from borderline personality disorder frequently resort to splitting as a defensive strategy.

Acting out is the act of avoiding feelings that one finds personally unacceptable by acting in a way that attracts attention and is frequently socially inappropriate. It is more prevalent in teenagers and can lead to social and intellectual dysfunction. A 14-year-old boy who has never been in trouble before may be expressing his melancholy and anxiety over his parents' divorce by talking back to the teacher and failing classes.

Hypocrisy is the term used to describe someone who intentionally acts amiably toward someone they dislike. It is an example of the defense mechanism of reaction formation if it is done unintentionally because you find it personally unacceptable to dislike that person. A woman who uses reaction formation is one who unconsciously resents the duties of childrearing and spends excessive amounts of money on expensive gifts and clothes for her kids.

1.4.4. Transference Reactions

Adult relationships and attitudes are inadvertently shaped by early relationships that individuals had with significant others, including parents. This transference, or modeling, is especially strong in relationships with individuals whose roles were originally filled by their parents. In their interactions with teachers, doctors, and psychotherapists, among other caregivers, people frequently exhibit strong transference reactions. In some forms of psychotherapy, an analysis of these reactions gives the therapist information about the patient's previous significant relationships.

Transference may change behavior and judgment in patient-physician relationships because it heightens emotionality. This change may come about in a good or bad way. Positive transference can lead to the patient having irrational faith in the physician. If strong, the patient can become overly idealistic or even start feeling attracted to the doctor sexually. Negative transference, on the other hand, occurs when a patient's expectations and wishes are not met, leading to the patient becoming bitter or hostile toward the physician. This subliminal animosity may lead to disregard for medical advice.

Transference reactions toward patients also occur in doctors. These responses are a result of countertransference, which is the result of the doctor's significant prior relationships. When a patient brings up a close friend or relative, the doctor may experience countertransference reactions. They frequently happen when a physician is attending to a friend, relative, or coworker. Countertransference can impair medical judgment in both situations and result in a patient responding inappropriately. (Berntson et al., 2009; Bouchard et al., 2007).

1.5. Evolving Models of Health Care

Health care refers to the process of enhancing an individual's physical and mental well-being through the identification, diagnosis, treatment, mitigation, or cure of disease, illness, injury, and other conditions. Health professionals and other related health fields provide healthcare.

1.5.1. Health, Disease, Sickness, and Illness

According to the World Health Organization (WHO), a patient's capacity to manage daily tasks and achieve full physical, social, and emotional functioning is a key indicator of their state of physical, mental, and social well-being. When health is at its best, one can lead a life that is characterized by psychological well-being, zestful activity, spiritual serenity, and competence. Disease is the body's way of expressing dysfunction. Disease is identified and categorized according to the kind of organ damage (e.g., liver cirrhosis, myocardial infarction), by a functional deficit (e.g., diabetes), or by malfunctions in the homeostatic system (e.g., autoimmune disorder, infectious disease). The term "sickness" describes the actions of a person who feels as though they have a disease or functional impairment. It is possible for someone to feel ill without having a diagnosed illness. On the other hand, a person may be ill but not act or feel sick. One becomes the sick person in relation to the rest of the community when they are thought of as sick or when they feel sick. This releases an individual from the duty to carry out daily responsibilities blamelessly (i.e., to request a sick day). Nonetheless, the ill person has duties to: (1) seek and accept assistance; and (2) follow professional or culturally advised regimens that promote recovery.

A patient's experience as a whole, including their feelings, behaviors, perceptions of their condition, and reactions from others, is embodied by their illness. Reactions differ based on the individual's position in the family or community, which is influenced by cultural norms and expectations. How the patient behaves and how the community as a whole reacts depends on beliefs about how or why the illness occurred (explanatory models) and how the illness progresses.

1.5.2. Risk and Prevention

Risky behaviors such as these present direct health risks (e.g., careless driving, smoking), as well as a number of environmentally harmful circumstances (e.g., contaminants in the environment, tainted water). Lower risk behaviors or unsuccessful attempts at prevention (e.g., a diet heavy in fat, inactivity). As certain risk factors (e.g., race, and genetic composition) cannot be changed, and a person's lifestyle has a big influence on many risk factors (e.g., diet) and can therefore be changed. Additional risk factors that may or may not be modifiable include occupation, social class, religious beliefs, and cultural customs. These factors can have complex effects on one's health. The notion of health care encompasses not only the management of illness but also the prevention of disease, trauma, and disease as well as the promotion of health. In addition to using medical procedures, healthcare providers aim to alter patients' attitudes, behaviors, social and cultural norms, and surroundings in order to accomplish these objectives. Such work necessitates an understanding of these factors' interactions, their effects on patients' health, and the strategies for effectively modifying them.

Primary prevention refers to actions taken to safeguard, advance, and preserve health. These include the worries of experts in public health, whose job is to monitor the environment, encourage workplace safety, and improve sanitation. In medical settings, primary prevention entails counselling patients on personal habits like eating a healthy diet, exercising frequently, keeping a normal weight, abstaining from drugs and alcohol, and refraining from other risky behaviors like smoking. Many different kinds of health professionals may be in charge of secondary prevention, which entails actions like medical surveillance, health screening, immunization, and harm reduction to strengthen resistance to or lessen the effects of risk factors.

1.5.3. Evolving Approaches to Health Care

According to archeological findings, people have been providing medical care for at least the last 30,000 years. Early human theories about illness included observable natural explanations like weather patterns and individual actions, as well as unobservable, enigmatic, or supernatural explanations like sorcery. Using oils, tonics, and herbs whose curative or healing qualities would have been discovered empirically over time, or simply accepting fate, were likely the naturalistic treatments. Due to the long history of religious and medical integration, illnesses caused by supernatural forces were treated with rituals that were interpreted and carried out by priests or Shamans who understood the relationships between the mystical and natural realms.

During the Babylonian era, some 6,000 years ago, theories regarding health care and the human body were first documented. The Code of Hammurabi outlined the various surgical procedures that had to be carried out, along with a pricing schedule and consequences for malpractice. Five millennia ago, Egyptian medical records detailed the symptoms of heart, eye, and stomach problems; they also addressed wounds, fractures, and dislocations, and they recognized that brain lesions could lead to the paralysis of the corresponding side of the body.

Many modern medical procedures are derived from the major systems of traditional Chinese, Ayurvedic, and Greek medicine that emerged between 1,500 and 500 BC. Despite regional and cultural divides, knowledge was freely exchanged throughout the ancient world via trade and conquest, leading to the development of universal ideas that served as the cornerstone of each of these systems:

1. The universe is an integrated whole that is subjected to laws governing all phenomena including human behavior and health.
2. The individual is an integrated system of physical, mental, cultural, and spiritual qualities.
3. Health is a state of balance (homeostasis) between the individual and the outside world, and among the elements, humors, and forces within the individual.
4. All living things are endowed with a life force composed of vital energies that must be kept in balance (e.g., male/female, yin/yang) to maintain optimal health.
5. Disease results from disruption or imbalance within the life force, an imbalance between the life force and external events (stress), or an imbalance among humors and bodily functions.
6. Symptoms represent the body's efforts to restore balance and health.
7. Healers supplement or strengthen the body's efforts to restore balance by applying treatments based on universal principles.

The study of ethnomedicine is based on these conceptions of health and illness, which are derived from indigenous cultural beliefs. It also shows an understanding of some of the ideas present in both conventional and alternative medical systems. The interplay and interdependence of etiological factors, the idea of "balance" or homeostasis, the impact of stress, and an understanding of the healer's role are examples of common or universal principles.

Hippocrates (460 BC), who is credited with founding the first medical school devoted to the scientific study of medicine, is the author of many modern health care concepts. Up until the work of Galen, a Roman practitioner in the second century AD who compiled the medical knowledge of his time and started anatomical and physiological investigations, Hippocratic medicine was the ultimate standard for medical knowledge and professional ethics. Galen was limited by his religious beliefs to performing dissections only on animals. As a result, while he made substantial contributions to our understanding of how the respiratory, circulatory, digestive, and neurological systems function, many of his anatomical findings turned out to be incorrect.

Galen established the idea that people with a background in pathology, or physicians, should be the primary healers in society by claiming that lesions in particular body organs caused dysfunctions. This assertion laid the scientific groundwork for allopathic medicine. Galenic remedies were founded on the law of opposites; that is, illnesses were treated with drugs or other measures that had the opposite effect of the symptom. These methods were only tangentially related to his scientific research.

Galenic medicine dominated medical dogma for 1,400 years despite its shortcomings. Due to the translation and preservation of Roman, Greek, and Arabic texts, Galen's work was rediscovered in Europe. Despite its widespread influence on most major medical systems, its dissemination paradoxically impeded scientific advancement. Even though it's likely that the law of opposites helped some cases (e.g., applying cooling remedies in fever cases), it frequently served as justification for harmful and inappropriate "treatments" like bloodletting, purging, indiscriminate enemas, and other intrusive and toxic practices.

Significant advancements in the field of medicine were made possible by the Renaissance and later Age of Enlightenment, which were characterized by a return to reason, critical discourse, and experimental inquiry. Important discoveries about the physical, mechanical, and chemical functions of the human body were made during the seventeenth century thanks to advances in the natural sciences, but for a while, the evolution of medical procedures was not greatly influenced by these scientific findings. Galenism faced more challenges, which confirmed the doctor's role in promoting and supporting the body's natural healing processes. As a result, homeopathic, osteopathic, naturopathic, and chiropractic medicine were developed.

1.5.3.1. Biomedical Model – Discipline Specific

Systematic observation, objective measurement, and experimental testing of theories formed the scientific basis of medicine by the end of the 19th century. These exercises were designed and instructed in the context of particular fields, including pathology, microbiology, physiology, and pharmacology. The corresponding clinical procedures became increasingly complex and condition-specific over time. For instance, developments in microbiology demonstrated that germs caused illness and could be managed with vaccination, antiseptics, and sterilization.

Despite these developments, medicine and medical education remained archaic due to Galenism's lingering effects and a lack of investigation into the effectiveness of different procedures. But as medical science advanced at the start of the 20th century, a thorough investigation of the caliber of medical education in North America was eventually conducted. The Carnegie Foundation published the Flexner Report in 1910, which provided a critical assessment of the scientific curricula offered in all US and Canadian medical schools. Higher standards for medical education based on scientific methodology and the biological sciences were recommended in the report. These suggestions turned into the biomedical model's defining standards, giving medicine a discipline-specific identity. Flexner minimized, if not completely disregarded, the contributions that the social and behavioral sciences have made to medicine. As a result, post-Flexnerian medicine lost some of its focus on the larger behavioral and social context of illness and health care and instead became primarily biomedical.

Although the field of biomedicine grew quickly at the start of the 20th century, important academic fields continued to raise awareness of the drawbacks of a purely biological approach, particularly public health and the behavioral sciences of anthropology, psychology, and sociology. The effects of extreme stress on soldiers' health during the two world wars have highlighted the role that psychosocial factors play in illness and treatment outcomes. Though valuable, their distinctive methodologies too frequently limited rigorous social science studies of the contextual determinants of health and healthcare processes. In order to investigate the relationship between psychosocial factors and biological processes in the genesis or causation of both illness and disease, researchers lacked the necessary instruments. The intellectual tide began to turn again in the middle of the 1970s, with the goal of incorporating a broad range of approaches and perspectives into the multidisciplinary study of health and illness.

1.5.3.2. Biopsychosocial Model – Multidisciplinary

George Engel wrote "The Need for a New Medical Model: A Challenge for Biomedicine," which was published in Science in 1977. In 1980, he conducted additional research on the model and published an article in the American Journal of Psychiatry titled "The Clinical Application of the Biopsychosocial Model." Engel claimed that the biopsychosocial model distinguished itself from the biomedical model by acknowledging two things: (1) a hierarchical structure of biological and social systems that contribute to the disease and illness experience; and (2) multiple determinants of disease and the ensuing illness process. The systems hierarchy and levels of organization were as follows:

- Biosphere;
- Society–nation;
- Culture–subculture;
- Community;
- Family;
- Two-person;
- Person (experience & behavior);
- Nervous system;
- Organs/organ systems;
- Tissues;
- Cells;
- Organelles;
- Molecules;
- Atoms;
- Subatomic particles.

Every system was considered a part of a higher order, abstract system. As a result, when one system changes, so do other systems, especially those that are closest to it. Within the framework of the biopsychosocial model, the behavioral and social sciences held equal significance to the biological sciences in comprehending the determinants of illness. Consequently, scholars shifted their attention towards pinpointing particular psychosocial factors that are linked to particular diseases or illnesses.

1.5.4. Clinical Application of the Biopsychosocial Model

A kidney donor will continue to have normal renal functioning because people can survive with just one kidney and still function normally physiologically. In the biological model, a donor regains full health following surgery. The biopsychosocial model, in contrast, focuses on the psychosocial aspects of the conditions of both the donor and the recipient. For example, this model acknowledges that if a donor knows the recipient benefited from the donation, the community commends the donor for the gift, and the donor believes the recipient will fully recover, then the donor's recovery and sense of self-worth may be facilitated, even enhanced. The model acknowledges, however, that the donor may experience emotional harm or other impairment upon learning that they are only receiving one kidney; furthermore, the donor may feel less appreciated if their gratitude is not sufficiently conveyed. Such views could hinder a person's ability to fully recover functionally.

The principles of the biopsychosocial model of care are as follows: education is necessary to reassure a donor of their biological integrity; knowledge of the benefits to the recipient will reinforce a donor's sense of self-worth; and the support of family and community is essential to recovery and return to a state of full health. These principles apply even in the absence of a need for biomedical intervention beyond appropriate postoperative care for a donor.

1.5.4.1. Integrated Sciences Model – Interdisciplinary

The determinants of health are not just a set of discrete psychosocial and biological variables, each of which is linearly correlated with a particular health outcome, nor are they limited to hierarchically related discipline-specific systems. Instead, several etiological factors that constantly interact through intricate mechanisms and interconnected processes determine one's state of health (see Figure 1.6). The biological processes involved in the etiology of the condition, the psychosocial factors influencing these processes, as well as the mechanisms by which biological and psychosocial factors interact to determine health outcomes, must all be identified in order to determine the determinants of disease and illness. A number of interdisciplinary fields (see Table 1.6), where behavioral and biological scientists collaborate by combining theoretical and methodological efforts, have grown as a result of efforts to identify these mechanisms of bio-behavioral interaction.

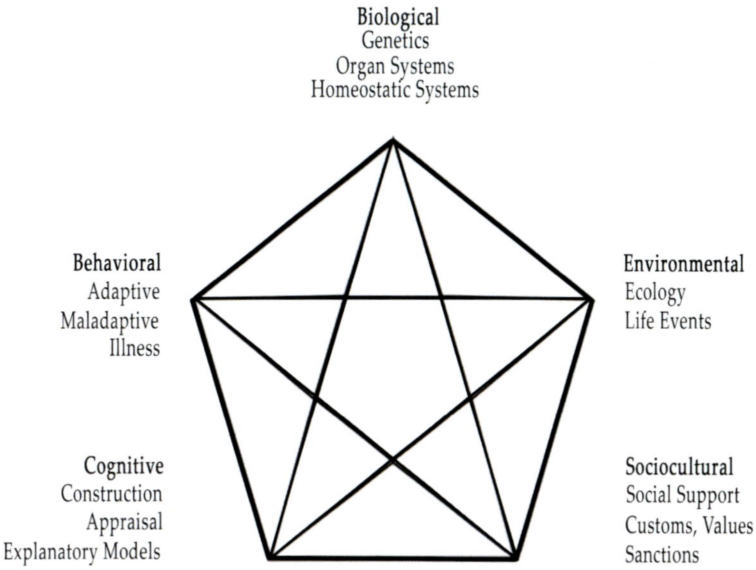

Figure 1.6. *The integrated sciences model.*

Source: Olle Jane Z. Sahler John E. Carr Julia B. Frank, and João V. Nunes. The Behavioral Sciences and Health Care. Hogrefe. ISBN 9781616764869.

Table 1.6. *Interdisciplinary Research Fields in Health Care*

Genomic sciences	Seek to identify the genetic processes associated with normal and abnormal development and functioning, and the mechanisms by which these processes influence, and are influenced by, human behaviors, social and biological functioning, and environmental interaction.
Cognitive neurosciences	Seek to determine the brain structures and neuroendocrine mechanisms that contribute to, and are influenced by, specific cognitive processes (perception, learning, memory, problem solving).
Social neurosciences	Seek to determine the specific biological systems and mechanisms that implement social processes and behaviors, and the mechanisms by which those social processes modify and influence organ-based, neural, neuroendocrine, and immunological functions.
Psychoneuroimmunology	Seeks to define the mechanisms by which stressful events and emotional responses influence neurological and immune system functioning.

Source: Olle Jane Z. Sahler John E. Carr Julia B. Frank, and João V. Nunes. The Behavioral Sciences and Health Care. Hogrefe. ISBN 9781616764869.

These research partnerships show how the biopsychosocial model has developed from a multidisciplinary perspective that saw the biological and behavioral sciences as separate from each other, despite their equal importance. Instead, the biopsychosocial model has evolved to emphasize three key areas: (1) the interdependence of biological and behavioral processes; (2) the mechanisms underlying their interaction; and (3) the integration of biological and behavioral scientific concepts, theories, and principles into a more integrated sciences model.

The evolution of the human brain is largely responsible for the survival of the human species. The brain and its corresponding neuroendocrine subsystem have evolved over many eons in response to genetic abnormalities and epigenetic events, giving Homo sapiens the ability to survive in harsh environments. These skills enabled the organism to deal with threats from various domains by adapting, avoiding, anticipating, and planning in response to experience and reflexivity. Humans eventually developed the capacity to relate to, work with, take care of, and communicate with other humans. These kinds of functions give our species incredible resources for surviving and controlling its surroundings.

All biological and psychosocial phenomena are seen as functionally interactive and interdependent in an integrated sciences model (ISM). The universal scientific principles and processes of homeostasis, stress, adaptation, learning, development, and genetic modification are all included in the principles of interaction. It is possible to see the individual as a complex adaptive organism with homeostatic abilities that allow for adaptation to environmental, cognitive, sociocultural, and behavioral challenges in addition to biological ones (see Figure 1.6). Each domain's homeostatic challenges add to the condition of the individual and cause adaptive responses in the other domains. Similar to the initial biopsychosocial model, modifications in one domain have an impact on all others since the organism is continuously working to preserve optimal balance, or homeostasis, both within and between domains.

1.5.4.2. Integrated Sciences Mode

1. The human organism possesses an integrated network of homeostatic systems enabling it to adapt to any challenge to homeostasis from biological, behavioral, cognitive, sociocultural, and environmental domains. This homeostatic network is regulated by the brain and associated neuroendocrine systems.
2. Any challenge to homeostasis constitutes "stress" and initiates a multivariate stress response.
3. Variables within each domain interact with those in other domains via diverse bio-behavioral mechanisms. Hence, stress in one domain initiates responses in all domains.
4. Challenges to the organism are ongoing, and this interactive system is constantly evolving as it is continuously adapting.
5. Diseases and disorders are byproducts of the failure of the homeostatic stress response system. Therefore, accurately addressing the differential role of stress conditions and other risk factors in each domain is essential to determining the best intervention strategy.
6. Treatment of the disease may alleviate or, in turn, initiate new stress responses within any of the domains of variables.

1.5.5. Stress – The Engine of Adaptation

Stress is defined as any disturbance to homeostasis. This phrase, which has physics roots, describes the multidisciplinary idea of a system under stress (i.e., the overall consequences of any difficulty in any field). In other domains, adaptive responses are triggered by stress or biological, developmental, environmental, behavioral, cognitive, or sociocultural challenges to homeostasis. The organism tries to resolve, cope with, and learn from the stressful condition. Thus, stress is the engine that drives adaptation, the raison d'être for the evolution of the brain's remarkable capabilities and, therefore, is not necessarily destructive. Rather, the level of stress influences the type, intensity, and result (adaptive or maladaptive) of the stress response. Every college student is aware of the inverted U-shaped curve that illustrates the correlation between productivity and stress. Insufficient challenge or stress can erode motivation and lead to subpar performance. Excessive stress or challenge can demotivate people to work hard and hinder productivity. Stress that is at its ideal level inspires and motivates without overwhelming. Individual health is defined by the adaptive success of the stress response in this intricate network of homeostatic systems; disease or disorder is a result of its maladaptive breakdown or dysfunction. Paradoxically, an excessive stress response can also be a cause of illness and dysfunction, as in the case of autoimmune disorders, in which the host body is attacked by the immune system, which is meant to defend against external pathogens.

1.5.6 Integrated Assessment

A thorough investigation of the distinct and combined effects of biological, behavioral, cognitive, sociocultural, and environmental risk factors should be part of the assessment process. The healthcare provider can use this information to learn more about the biobehavioral mechanisms and processes that may be suitable targets for treatment because they contribute to a specific disorder. The intricacy and interconnectedness of the variables causing smoking addiction are demonstrated by an integrated sciences model, which explains why therapies that concentrate solely on one area (e.g., altering a smoker's mentality) or a single factor (e.g., banning tobacco advertising) are probably doomed to failure. Treating as many of the contributing factors as possible maximizes the likelihood of changing complexly determined health behaviors. Mr. Howard and Dr. Knight, as described in the example, decided on a multimodal approach and agreed to implement the following strategies:

- **Biological:** Nicotine patches to counter nicotine dependence;
- **Behavioral:** Alternative work break and stress relief activities such as taking a walk, social gatherings in nonsmoking venues, stress management training, and meditation;
- **Cognitive:** Explaining to others (e.g., young people) how smoking is harmful; exposure to high-profile, high-status nonsmokers;
- **Sociocultural:** Encouraging the family to praise, reward, and reinforce nonsmoking; encouraging membership in a "smoke-enders" group; pursuing cultural and sports activities that preclude smoking behavior;
- **Environmental:** Make smoking materials and opportunities less accessible (e.g., restrict access to tobacco and limit smoking to inconvenient and uncomfortable places).

A treatment plan that is multimodal as opposed to one that is focused on a single domain is likely to produce better results. Multimodal perspectives provide more flexibility in treatment strategizing because some interventions may et al., not always be useful or worthwhile. Additionally, a particular factor may not be a good target for treatment even though it may be important in the etiology of the condition (e.g., new medications increase the chances of survival for HIV/ AIDS patients; however, behavioral treatment of the social and psychological aspects of the illness remains a primary goal of disease management). (Carr et al., 1999; Chumakov et al., 2002).

A Closer Look

Clinical Application of an Integrated Sciences Model

Frank Howard has been diagnosed with chronic obstructive pulmonary disease (COPD) and advised by his physician, Dr. Elizabeth Knight, to give up smoking. Working collaboratively, Dr. Knight and Mr. Howard carefully review Mr. Howard's lifestyle to identify variables or situations that influence his smoking. Reviewing each of the domains shown in Figure 1.6, they come up with the following information:

- **Biological:** While he recognizes the implication of a diagnosis of COPD, Mr. Howard's nicotine dependence is making it difficult for him to quit smoking.
- **Behavioral:** The stress relief he experiences is a strong incentive for smoking.
- **Cognitive:** He previously believed he could quit anytime he chose. The knowledge that smoking contributes to his COPD is powerful, but not enough by itself to deter his behavior, although he is now willing to consider a change in smoking behavior.
- **Sociocultural:** Previous role models and cultural sanctions had strong reinforcing value, but Mr. Howard is now getting increasing social and familial support for not smoking.
- **Environmental:** Tobacco had been readily accessible and smoking opportunities available and reinforcing. However, as the cost of tobacco has increased and places and opportunities for smoking have decreased, Mr. Howard is becoming more open to change.

Summary

- The behavioral sciences explore the cognitive processes within organisms and the behavioral interactions between organisms in the natural world. It involves the systematic analysis and investigation of human and animal behavior through naturalistic observation, controlled scientific experimentation, and mathematical modeling. It attempts to accomplish legitimate, objective conclusions through rigorous formulations and observation.
- Behavioral Sciences is the knowledge of human behavior with an interdisciplinary approach to understanding human needs in the context of wider societal problems. Behavioral Sciences include Sociology, Anthropology (minus Archaeology), Technical Linguistics, and most of Physical Anthropology, Psychology (minus Physiological Psychology), and behavioral aspects of Sociology, Economics, Geography, Law, Psychiatry, and Political Science.
- Like physical health, emotional health is a result of complex interactions among biological, social, and environmental influences. Disorders of health of either type result from aberrations or distortions in one or more of these influences at any time in a person's life. Theoretical difficulties exist when trying to separate biological social and environmental factors in the etiology of psychiatric illness.
- The role of genetic influences on the development of physical conditions such as heart disease, diabetes, and cancer is well documented. Genetic influences are also important in the display of behavior and its disorders. Because behavioral disorders are expressed in and thus are confounded by the social setting, it is more difficult in behavioral than in physical disorders to isolate genetic from social and environmental etiologies.
- Neurotransmitters are chemical messengers that are closely involved in cellular function at all levels of the nervous system. Emotions and psychopathology are believed to result from interactions and imbalances among these messengers in the brain. The three major classes of neurotransmitters are the biogenic amines (monoamines), amino acids, and peptides.
- Psychodynamic theory is based on the idea, cast by Sigmund Freud and modified later by others, that behavior is influenced by forces derived from processes of which individuals are not aware. Although these unconscious forces keep thoughts and emotions out of consciousness, they are at the same time dynamic and affect peoples' choices, emotions, and behavior throughout life. Psychotherapeutic treatments, such as psychoanalysis and related therapies, are based on this concept of the dynamic unconscious.
- Health care is the improvement of health via the prevention, diagnosis, treatment, amelioration or cure of disease, illness, injury, and other physical and mental impairments in people. Health care is delivered by health professionals and allied health fields.
- The World Health Organization (WHO) defines health as a state of physical, social, and mental well-being, measured by the patient's ability to cope with everyday activities, and fully function physically, socially, and emotionally. At its optimal level, good health provides for a life marked by spiritual serenity, zestful activity, a sense of competence, and psychological well-being.
- Disease is the manifestation of impaired bodily functions. Disease is recognized and classified by the type of organ damage (e.g., cirrhosis of the liver, myocardial infarction),

by functional impairment (e.g., diabetes), or by homeostatic system failures (e.g., infectious disease, autoimmune disorder).

- Sickness refers to those behaviors manifested by an individual who believes that they are suffering from a disease or functional impairment.
- Illness represents the totality of a patient's experience: how a patient feels, how a patient behaves and perceives their condition, and how others respond. Responses vary according to the person's place within the family or community, as shaped by cultural beliefs and expectations.

References

1. Bartres-Faz, D., Junque, C., Moral, P., López-Alomar, A., Sanchez-Aldeguer, J., & Clemente, I. C. (2002). Apolipoprotein E gender effects on cognitive performance in age-associated memory impairment. *Journal of Neuropsychiatry and Clinical Neurosciences, 14*(1), 80–83. https://doi.org/10.1176/jnp.14.1.80.
2. Baxter, L. R. (1999). Functional imaging of brain systems mediating obsessive-compulsive disorder. In D. S. Charney, E. J. Nestler, & B. S. Bunney (Eds.), *Neurobiology of Mental Illness* (pp. 534–547). Oxford University Press.
3. Berntson, G. G., & Cacioppo, J. T. (2009). *Handbook of Neurosciences for the Behavioral Sciences*. Wiley. https://doi.org/10.1002/9780470478509.
4. Bouchard, T. J., Jr. (2007). Genes and human psychological traits. In P. Carruthers, S. Laurence, & S. Stich (Eds.), *The Innate Mind: Foundations for the Future* (Vol. 3, pp. 81–99). Oxford University Press.
5. Carr, J. E. (1999). Proposal for an integrated sciences curriculum in medical education. *Teaching and Learning in Medicine, 10*(1), 3–7. https://doi.org/10.1207/S15328015TLM1001_1.
6. Chumakov, I., Blumenfeld, M., Guerassimenko, O., Cavarec, L., Palicio, M., Abderrahim, H., & Schizophrenia Working Group. (2002). Genetic and physiological data implicating the new human gene G72 and the gene for L-amino acid oxidase in schizophrenia. *Proceedings of the National Academy of Sciences, 99*(21), 13675–13680. https://doi.org/10.1073/pnas.212514299.
7. Cuff, P. A., & Vanselow, N. A. (2004). *Improving Medical Education: Enhancing the Behavioral and Social Science Content of Medical School Curricula*. National Academies Press.
8. Davidson, R. J., & Irwin, W. (1999). The functional neuroanatomy of emotion and affective style. *Trends in Cognitive Sciences, 3*(1), 11–21. https://doi.org/10.1016/S1364-6613(98)01265-0.
9. de la Fuente-Fernandez, R., Ruth, T. J., Sossi, V., Schulzer, M., Caine, D. B., & Stoessl, A. J. (2001). Expectation and dopamine release: Mechanism of the placebo effect in Parkinson's disease. *Science, 293*(5532), 1164–1166. https://doi.org/10.1126/science.1060950.
10. Engel, G. L. (1977). The need for a new medical model: A challenge for biomedicine. *Science, 196*(4286), 129–136. https://doi.org/10.1126/science.847460.
11. Finnis, D. G., Kaptchuk, T., Miller, F., & Benedetti, F. (2010). Biological, clinical and ethical advances of placebo effects. *The Lancet, 375*(9715), 686–695. https://doi.org/10.1016/S0140-6736(09)61706-8.
12. Freud, A. (1966). *The Ego and the Mechanisms of Defense* (Rev. ed.). International Universities Press.

13. Gazzaniga, M. S. (2010). *The Cognitive Neurosciences* (4th ed.). MIT Press.
14. Goldstein, R. Z., & Volkow, N. D. (2002). Drug addiction and its underlying neurobiological basis: Neuroimaging evidence for the involvement of the frontal cortex. *American Journal of Psychiatry, 159*(10), 1642–1652. https://doi.org/10.1176/appi.ajp.159.10.1642.
15. Halpern, D. F. (2000). *Sex Differences in Cognitive Abilities* (3rd ed.). Lawrence Erlbaum Associates.
16. Harlow, J. M. (1868). Recovery after severe injury to the head. *Publications of the Massachusetts Medical Society, 2*, 327–346.
17. Kandel, E. R., Schwartz, J. H., & Jessell, T. M. (2000). *Principles of Neural Science* (4th ed.). Appleton and Lange.
18. Klunder, A. D., Chiang, M. C., Dutton, R. A., Lee, S. E., Toga, A. W., Lopez, O. L., & Alzheimer's Disease Neuroimaging Initiative. (2008). Mapping cerebellar degeneration in HIV/AIDS. *Neuroreport, 19*(16), 1655–1659. https://doi.org/10.1097/WNR.0b013e328316e59c.
19. LeVay, S. (1991). A difference in hypothalamic structure between heterosexual and homosexual men. *Science, 253*(5023), 1034–1037. https://doi.org/10.1126/science.1899707.
20. LeVay, S. (2010). *Gay, Straight and the Reason Why: The Science of Sexual Orientation*. Oxford University Press.
21. McHugh, P. F., Kellogg, S., Bell, K., Schluger, R. P., Leal, S. M., & Kreek, M. J. (2002). Potentially functional polymorphism in the promoter region of the prodynorphin gene may be associated with protection against cocaine dependence or abuse. *American Journal of Medical Genetics, 114*(4), 431–434. https://doi.org/10.1002/ajmg.10479.
22. Nestler, E. J., Hyman, S. E., & Malenka, R. C. (2001). *Molecular Neuropharmacology*. McGraw-Hill.
23. Shaywitz, B. A., Shaywitz, S. E., Pugh, K., Constable, R. T., Skudlarski, P., Fulbright, R. K., & Gore, J. C. (1995). Sex differences in the functional organization of the brain for language. *Nature, 373*(6515), 607–609. https://doi.org/10.1038/373607a0.
24. Sher, L. (1997). The placebo effect on mood and behavior: The role of the endogenous opioid system. *Medical Hypotheses, 48*(4), 347–349. https://doi.org/10.1016/S0306-9877(97)90005-1.
25. Shi, J., Levinson, D. F., Duan, J., Sanders, A. R., Zheng, Y., Pe'er, I., & Wang, S. (2009). Common variants on chromosome 6p22.1 are associated with schizophrenia. *Nature, 460*(7256), 753–757. https://doi.org/10.1038/nature08111.
26. Stahl, S. M. (2008). *Stahl's Essential Psychopharmacology* (4th ed.). Cambridge University Press.
27. Stefansson, H., Sarginson, J., Kong, A., Yates, P., Steinthorsdottir, V., Gudfinnsson, E., & Gudbjartsson, D. F. (2002). Association of neuregulin 1 with schizophrenia confirmed in a Scottish population. *American Journal of Human Genetics, 72*(1), 83–87. https://doi.org/10.1086/340199.
28. Straub, R. E., Jiang, Y., MacLean, C. J., Ma, Y., Webb, B. T., Myakishev, M. V., & Morrow, B. (2002). Genetic variation in the 6p22.3 gene DTNBP1, the human ortholog of the mouse dysbindin gene, is associated with schizophrenia. *American Journal of Human Genetics, 71*(2), 337–348. https://doi.org/10.1086/341510.

29. Tamminga, C. A., & Frost, D. O. (2001). Changing concepts in the neurochemistry of schizophrenia. *American Journal of Psychiatry, 158*(9), 1365–1366. https://doi.org/10.1176/appi.ajp.158.9.1365.

30. Teasdale, G., & Jennett, B. (1974). The Glasgow coma scale. *The Lancet, 2*(7872), 81–83. https://doi.org/10.1016/S0140-6736(74)91639-0.

31. Thompson, P. M., Cannon, T. D., Narr, K. L., van Erp, T. G. M., Poutanen, V. P., Huttunen, M., & Toga, A. W. (2001). Genetic influences on brain structure. *Nature Neuroscience, 4*(12), 1253–1258. https://doi.org/10.1038/nn759.

Chapter

2

COMMUNITY HEALTH

Contents

Introduction

Community health nursing, a vital component of public health, focuses on promoting and protecting the health of populations. Nurses in this field work in diverse settings, including schools, clinics, and community centers, addressing a wide range of health issues from disease prevention to health education. They play a crucial role in identifying community health needs through assessments and collaborating with other health professionals to develop and implement strategies to meet these needs. Emphasizing preventive care, community health nurses educate individuals and groups on healthy lifestyles, manage chronic diseases, and ensure access to healthcare services. By advocating for vulnerable populations and working to eliminate health disparities, community health nurses contribute significantly to improving overall community well-being and fostering a healthier, more informed society.

The function of any community includes its members' sense of belonging and shared identity, values, norms, communication, and supporting behaviors. Some communities who may share almost everything, while other communities (large, scattered and composed of individuals) who may share only there common interests and involvement in certain goals.

A community is often defined by its geographic boundaries and is thus called a geographic community. For example, a city, town, or neighborhood is a geographic community. A community demarcated by geographic boundaries becomes a clear target for analysis of health needs to form basis for planning health programs and a geographic community is also easily mobilized for action. Community can also be identified by a common interest or goal. A collection of people, although they are widely scattered geographically, can have an interest or goal that binds the members-together called common interest community. (e.g., Disabled individual scattered throughout a large city may emerge as a community through a common interest in their need for improved wheelchaired access or other handicapped facilities).

Orientation and Directional Terms

Term	Definition	Illustration
Community Health Nursing	Community health nursing is the synthesis of nursing and public health practice applied to promote and protect the health of the population.	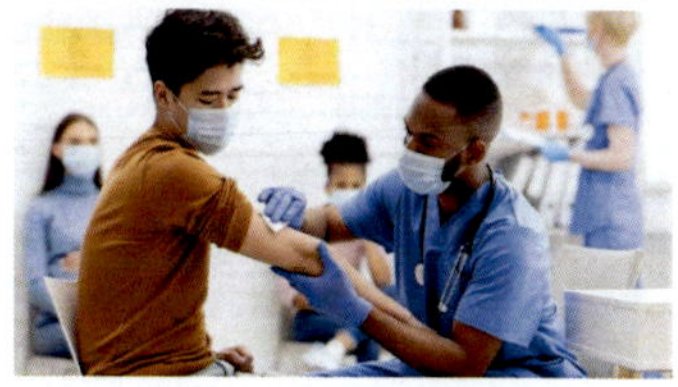
Heath System	The health system consists of all organizations, people, and actions whose primary intent is to promote, restore, or maintain health. This includes efforts to influence determinants of health as well as more direct health-improving activities.	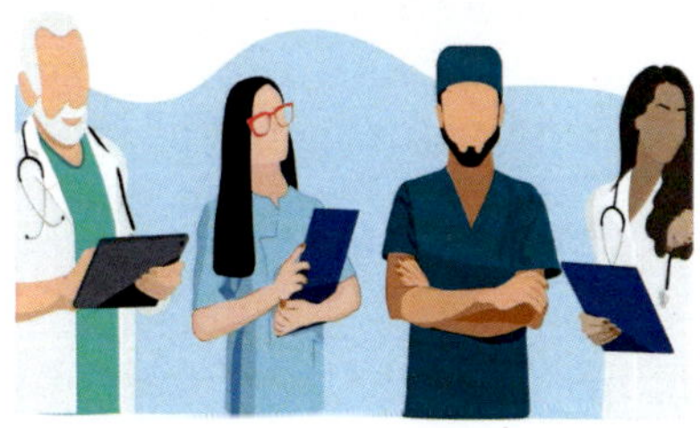
Myocardial Infarction (MI)	Myocardial infarction (MI), colloquially known as "heart attack," is caused by decreased or complete cessation of blood flow to a portion of the myocardium. Myocardial infarction may be"silent," and go undetected, or it could be a catastrophic event leading to hemodynamic deterioration and sudden death.	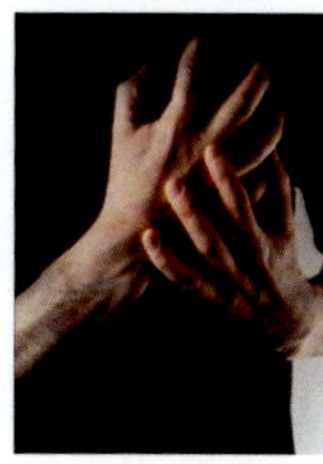 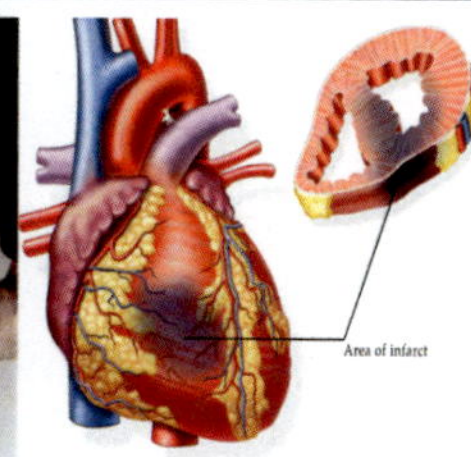
Public Health	Public health, the art and science of preventing disease, prolonging life, and promoting physical and mental health, sanitation, personal hygiene, control of infectious diseases, and organization of health services.	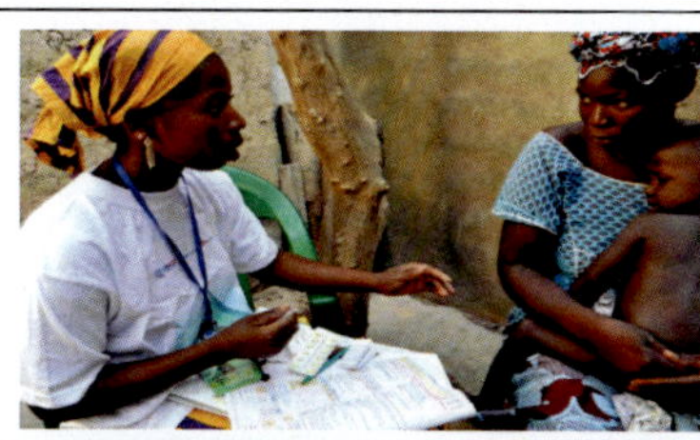
Substance Abuse	Substance abuse, also known as drug abuse, is the use of a drug in amounts or by methods that are harmful to the individual or others. It is a form of substance-related disorder. Differing definitions of drug abuse are used in public health, medical, and criminal justice contexts.	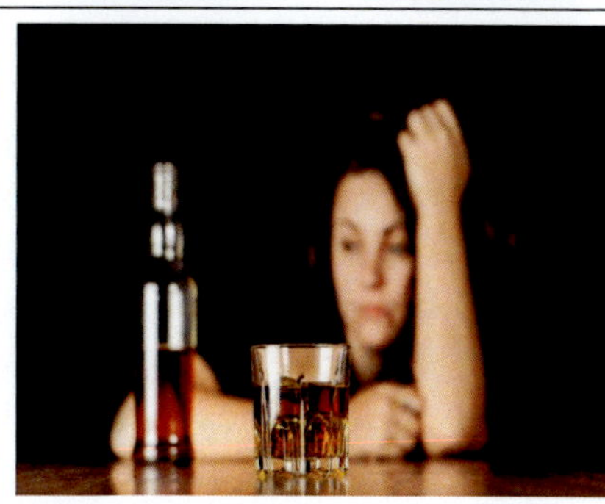

2.1. Definitions of Health and Community

Health is a multifaceted concept that encompasses the physical, mental, and social well-being of an individual, not merely the absence of disease or infirmity. According to the World Health Organization (WHO), health is "a state of complete physical, mental, and social well-being and not merely the absence of disease or infirmity." This holistic view recognizes that various factors, including environmental, social, and psychological elements, contribute to a person's overall health. Health is dynamic and can be influenced by lifestyle choices, access to healthcare, and the presence of supportive networks and environments.

A healthy body suggests that the body functions mechanically. The ability to think clearly and coherently is referred to as mental health, and it is related to how you feel, think, and approach problems. A person in good mental health is able to coexist with others, recognize their needs, and build relationships that are fulfilling for both parties. Social health refers to the ability to:

- Make and maintain relationships with others.
- Interact well with people and the environment.

The ability to adjust to changing circumstances, to growing older and maturing, to heal from injuries, to endure pain, and to peacefully face death is referred to as health (Illich, 1975). A system's (such as a cell, organism, family, or society) capacity to adapt to a wide range of environmental challenges (Brody and Sobel, 1981). According to Lamberton (1978), the antithesis of both health and illness is nothing at all. Moreover, death is seen as a normal aspect of development and growth rather than the ultimate sickness. According to her, a person's relationship with the environment has a significant impact on both health and sickness. One further way to think of health is as a foundation for daily existence. It's a good idea to highlight one's physical capabilities as well as social and personal resources.

A community is a collection of people who regularly interact and work together, sharing similar interests, and values, or living close to one another. Communities can be characterized by several factors, such as location (like a town or neighborhood), identity (like race or religion), or interests (like social or professional groups). Members' sense of camaraderie and belonging is frequently what defines them. Beyond geographical limits, the idea of community encompasses online communities where people come together to pursue common interests and objectives. Through pooled resources, support networks, and cultural norms, a community can significantly influence the health behaviors and outcomes of its members.

2.1.1. The Three Features of a Community

A community has three features, location, population, and social system.

1. **Location:** every physical community carries out its daily existence in a specific geographical location. The health of the community is affected by this location, including the placement of the service, the geographical features.
2. **Population:** consists of specialized aggregates, but all of the diverse people who live within the boundary of the community.
3. **Social System:** the various parts of communities' social system that interact and include the heath system, family system, economic system and educational system.

2.1.2. Health and Wellness

Each views health differently in their way. Some people may have one or more diagnosed illnesses, but they may still describe their health as good. This is so because everyone's perception of health is influenced by their values and expectations. This unique variability must be taken into account when conceptualizing health. A person in good health is dynamic; they are always adjusting to changes in their internal and external environments. For instance, even if they have a respiratory infection, a person may think they are well.

Wellness is a lifestyle aimed at achieving physical, emotional, intellectual, spiritual, and environmental well-being. The use of wellness measures can increase stamina, energy, and self–esteem, then enhance the quality of life.

Individual variability is also accommodated by the concept of wellness. A person's physical, emotional, psychological, social, and spiritual well-being can all be considered to be in balance. This is known as wellness. This condition is dynamic. Everybody would define wellness according to their standards. The actions that support well-being and ward off disease are known as wellness behaviors. These include things like managing stress, being aware of what to eat, and maintaining physical fitness.

2.1.3. Models of Health

There are multiple interpretations of health, with some models focusing solely on the presence or absence of specific illnesses, while others emphasize holistic health beliefs, wellness, and a more comprehensive approach.

2.1.3.1. Clinical Model

According to this model, disease is the opposite of health because it is defined as the lack of indications and symptoms of an illness or injury. According to this model, Dunn described health as a condition of relative homeostasis and a relatively passive state of freedom from illness. Therefore, illness is something that an individual experiences. Many medical professionals base their diagnosis of a patient's health on the presence or absence of disease-related signs and symptoms.

2.1.3.2. Host –Agent – Environment Model

This model helps to identify the cause of an illness. In this model:

i. **Host:** Refers to the person (or group) who may be at risk for or susceptible to an illness.

ii. **Agent:** is any factor (internal or external) that can lead to illness by its presence.

iii. **Environment:** refers to those factors (physical, social, economic, emotional, spiritual) that may create the likelihood or the predisposition for the person to develop disease.

In this model health and illness depends on the interaction of these three factors (Figure 2.1).

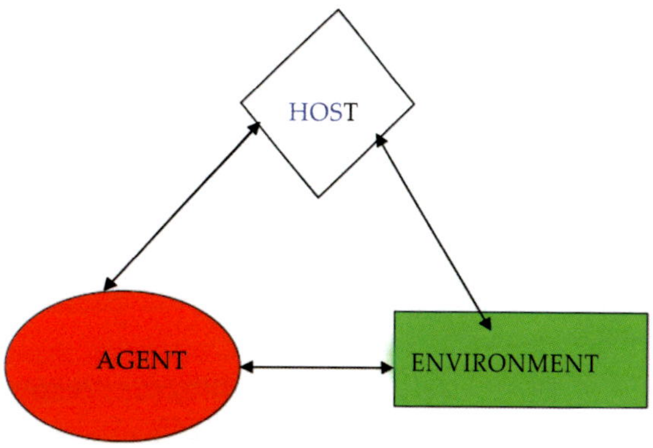

Figure 2.1. *Host – agent – environment model.*

Source: https://www.cartercenter.org/resources/pdfs/health/ephti/library/lecture_notes/nursing_students/comm_hlth_nsg_final.pdf.

2.1.3.3. Health Belief Model (HBM)

There is a relationship between a person's beliefs and actions. Factors that influence a person's beliefs:

- ·Personal expectations about health and illness.
- Earlier experience with illness or health.
- Age and development state.

A person's ideas, convictions, and attitudes regarding health and illness are referred to as their health beliefs. They could be founded on reality or erroneous expectations, common sense or myths, accurate information, or misinformation. Health beliefs typically have a positive or negative impact on health behavior.

- Addresses the relationship between person's beliefs and behavior.
- Provides a way of understanding and predicting how clients will behave about their health and how they will comply with health care therapies. Figure 2.2 shows the health-belief model.

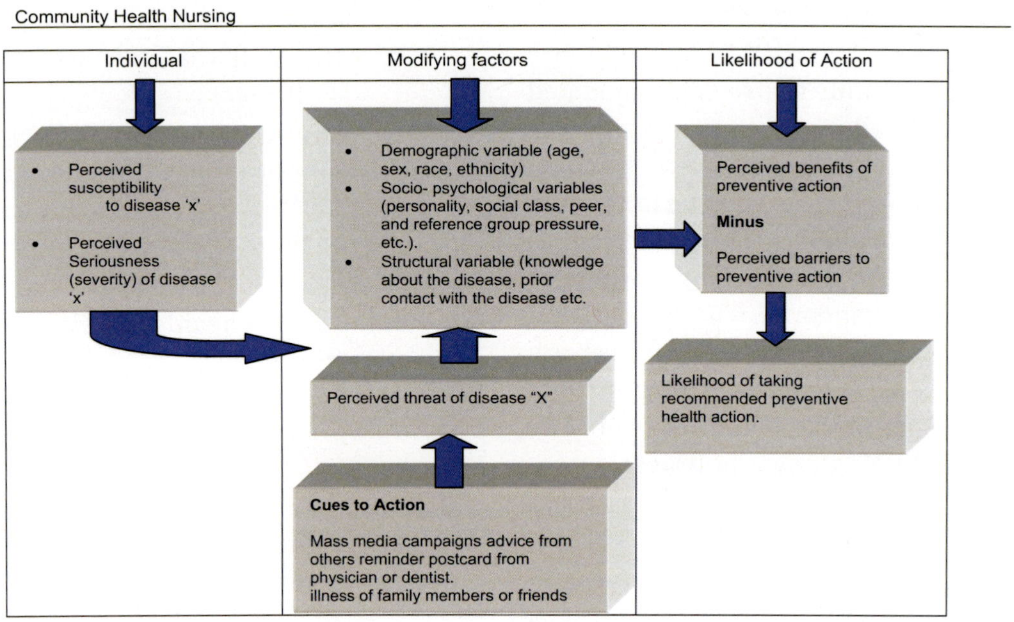

Figure 2.2. *Health- belief model.*

Source: https://www.cartercenter.org/resources/pdfs/health/ephti/library/lecture_notes/nursing_students/comm_hlth_nsg_final.pdf.

2.1.3.3.1. Components in HBM

1. **The First Component (Individual Perception):** The perception of an individual's vulnerability to illness: for example, a family history of coronary heart disease (CHD),

especially if a parent or both siblings passed away from myocardial infarction (MI) in the fourth decade of life.

2. **Second Component (Modifying Factors):** The degree of seriousness of the illness as perceived by an individual. Psychological and demographic factors, the perceived danger of the illness, and cues to take action all impact and alter this perception.
3. **Third Component (Likelihood of Action):** The probability of an individual taking preventive action is determined by how they perceive the advantages and obstacles associated with doing so. The preventive measure could involve changing one's lifestyle, adhering more closely to prescribed medications, or seeking out medical guidance or care.

2.1.3.3.2. Implication of HBM to Nursing

Helps nurses to understand factors influencing client's

- Perception;
- Beliefs and Behaviors;
- Plan care that will most effectively assist the client in maintaining or restoring health and preventing illness.

2.1.3.4. High–Level Wellness Model

Dunn (1961) stated that a person's health is acknowledged as a continuous process that leads to optimal functioning. The individual, family, and community are all involved in this process. According to Dunn, experiencing a high level of wellness is when a person is glowing with health, full of vitality, and has the energy to burn. In these moments, the world seems like a magnificent place.

2.1.3.5. Holistic Health Model

Although holism is viewed as a "new" paradigm for health, it is not at all novel. Throughout history, the humanities, western political tradition, and major religions have all placed a strong emphasis on holism. A different perspective on health known as holism recognizes and values how a person's mind, body, and spirit interact with their surroundings. The term holism, which comes from the Greek holos (whole), was coined in Holism and Evolution by South African philosopher Jan Christian Smuts in 1926. Smuts saw holism as the antidote to modern science's atomistic methodology. An atomistic approach disassembles things, dissecting the individual piece by piece to comprehend the bigger picture by dissecting the individual atom or molecule. The foundation of holism is the idea that no human being—or even component of a person—can be completely comprehended by studying them in isolation from their surroundings. People are thought of as constantly shifting energy systems. The organism and the system in which it lives are viewed as greater than and distinct from the sum of their parts, as the Figure 2.3 below demonstrates.

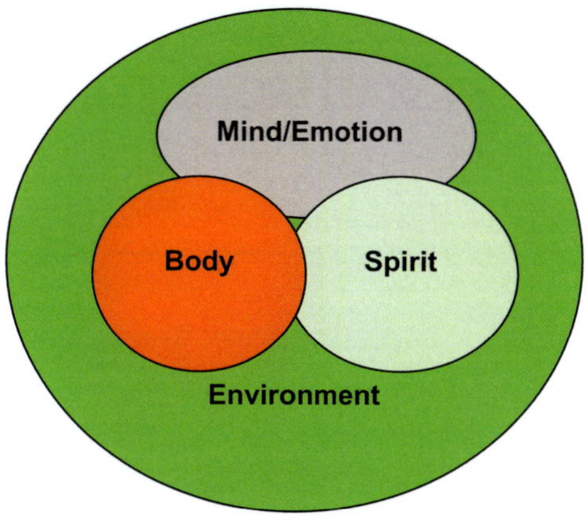

Figure 2.3. *Schematic representation of holism.*

Source: https://www.cartercenter.org/resources/pdfs/health/ephti/library/lecture_notes/nursing_students/comm_hlth_nsg_final.pdf.

2.1.4. Health and Illness

Community-based nursing care prioritizes health promotion and illness prevention over illness cure. As a result, this holistic approach is very different from acute care. The quantity and kind of medical services provided, as well as the size of the hospital, are not considered to be factors in improving health. The goal of care in an acute care setting is typically to address urgent medical issues. In the community, care is provided with an emphasis on maximizing each person's capacity for self-care, irrespective of their health status. The client is in charge of making decisions about their care and providing it. The client's capacity to function takes precedence when health is the central theme of care. Programs that are community-based and educational can be created to address lifestyle issues. Strategies for protecting public health are related to legislative or environmental actions that protect sizable populations. Protecting one's health requires a communal approach. Counselling, screening, vaccinations, and chemoprophylactic treatments for individuals in clinical settings are examples of preventive services.

The prevention focus is a key concept of community-based nursing. Prevention is conceptualized on three levels:

- Primary prevention level;
- Secondary prevention level; and
- Tertiary prevention level.

2.1.5. Health – Illness Continuum

A visual representation of the differences between the views of traditional medicine and high-level wellness is provided by the wellness-illness continuum (Travis & Ryan, 1988). There are no illness indications or symptoms at the neutral point. A person's health deteriorates when they move to the left. A person with wellness-oriented goals aspires to move rightward, toward high-level wellness, rather than just staying at the neutral point, which is more absence of disease.

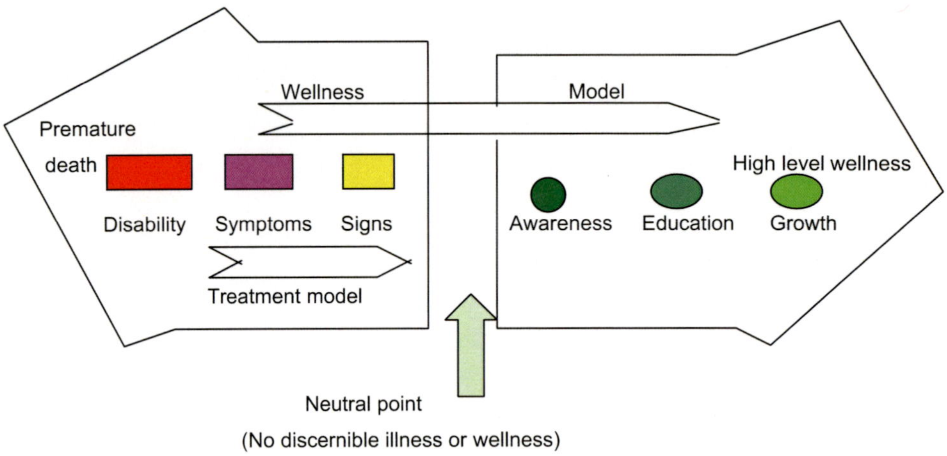

Figure 2.4. *Illness – wellness continuum model.*

Source: https://www.cartercenter.org/resources/pdfs/health/ephti/library/lecture_notes/nursing_students/comm_hlth_nsg_final.pdf.

This individual assesses how their life is currently being conducted, gains knowledge of the available options, and moves closer to self-actualization by pursuing these options in the pursuit of extreme well-being. Figure 2.4 shows the illness – wellness continuum model.

2.1.6. Community Health Practice

It is a component of the greater public health initiative, which aims to protect and enhance the health of particular groups of people and communities. Community health practice incorporates six basic elements:

1. Promotion of Health
    - It includes all efforts that seek to move people closer to optimal well-being or a higher level of wellness.
    - It is the combination of educational and environmental supports for action and condition of living conducive to health.
2. **Treatment of Disorders**: It focuses on the illness end of the continuum and is the remedial aspect of community health practice. This is practiced by:
    - Direct service to people with health problems; e.g., home visits for elderly people, chronic illness, etc.
    - Indirect service; e.g., assisting people with health problems to obtain treatment and referral.
    - Development of a program to correct unhealthy conditions; e.g., alcoholism, drug abuse, etc.
3. **Rehabilitation**: It involves efforts which seek to reduce disabilities, as much as possible, and restore functions; e.g., stroke rehabilitation.
4. Evaluation
    - It is the process by which the practice is analyzed, judged, and improved according to established goals and standards.
    - It helps to solve problems and provides direction for future health care planning.
5. **Research**: It is a systematic investigation that helps to discover facts affecting community health and community health practices, solve problems, and explore improved methods of health services.

2.1.7. Community Health Nursing

It is described as the integration of public health and nursing practice to preserve and improve population health. It is a subspecialty of nursing that concentrates on the healthcare requirements of groups, communities, and especially vulnerable populations. It is an ongoing, all-encompassing practice that is aimed at every community member group. It incorporates public health and community practice with all the fundamental components of professional, clinical nursing. To enhance community health, it integrates the body of knowledge from professional nursing theories and public health science (Weir et al., 2010).

2.1.7.1. Characteristics of Community Health Nursing

Six important characteristics of community health nursing are particularly salient to the practice of this specialty.

1. It is a specialty field of nursing.
2. Its practice combines public health with nursing.
3. It is population-focused.
4. It emphasizes wellness and other than disease or illness.

5. It involves inter-disciplinary collaboration.
6. It promotes the client's responsibility and self-care.

2.1.7.2. Community Settings Nursing Care

Community health nursing encompasses a broad range of contexts and involves the promotion, prevention, maintenance, restoration, coordination, management, and assessment of care for individuals, families, and groups, including communities (Lancaster, S.). Regardless of an illness or injury, the goal of care in community settings is to maximize each person's potential for self-care. The client is in charge of providing care and overseeing healthcare divisions. Nursing care was also affected by the changes in health care services. The community and particularly the home are altered. The goal of care is to improve the client's quality of life and encourage activities that maximize their level of comfort, rather than to solve problems through treatment.

2.1.7.3. Acute Care Setting

Those receiving intensive hospital care are referred to by this term. The goal of care in an acute care setting is typically to address urgent medical issues. When a patient needs extremely technical care, an acute care setting within a hospital can also be utilized as an ambulatory clinic or for day surgery patients. Numerous of these patients have illnesses that could be fatal, necessitating constant care and close observation. Acute nursing care differs from community-based nursing care as a result.

2.1.8. Public Health Nursing

It is the art and science of organizing community efforts to promote health, prevent disease, and extend life. Public health nursing is the provision of nursing services with an emphasis on population health promotion. It is aimed to:

- improve sanitation;
- control of community epidemics;
- prevent the transmission of infection;
- provide education about the basic principles of personal hygiene;
- organize medical and nursing services for early diagnosis, prevention and treatment of diseases.

2.2. Historical Development of Community Health Nursing

Understanding the origins and influencing factors that shaped community health's evolution over time is helpful before one can fully comprehend the nature of the field or define its practice. The field of community health nursing has developed over centuries through adaptability and expansion. Its approach was modified to meet the demands of a shifting society, but its original objective of bettering community health has never changed. The development of community health nursing has been impacted by shifts in public health, nursing, and society over several years. It is now evident from tracking the field's development that public health nursing has always played a leadership role. Nurses in this specialty have provided leadership in:

- planning and developing programs;
- shaping policy;
- administration; and
- the application of research to community health.

Four general stages mark the development of public health or community health nursing.

- The early home care stage.
- The district nursing stage.
- The public health nursing stage.

- The community health nursing stage.

2.2.1. Early Home Care Stage

For many centuries, female friends and family members cared for the ill at home. Reducing suffering and fostering healing were the main goals of this care (Kalish & Kalish, 1986). Religious and humanitarian organizations laid the foundation for home care nursing in the past. The Elizabethan Poor Law, enacted in England in 1600, gave the underprivileged and disabled access to nursing and medical care. In Paris, Saint. In 1617, Vincent DePaul founded the Sisters of Charity, a lay organization whose mission is to assist the underprivileged and destitute. Their work established the groundwork for contemporary community health nursing by emphasizing the training of nurses, overseeing their care, and identifying the root causes and solutions of clients' issues (Bullough & Bullough, 1978).

The set back of these services were:

- Social approval following the reformation caused a decline in the number of religious orders with subsequent curtailing of nursing care for the sick and poor.
- High maternal mortality rates prompted efforts to better prepare midwives and medical students.
- The Industrial Revolution created additional problems; among them were epidemics, high infant mortality, occupational diseases, injuries, and increasing mental illness both in Europe and America.

Florence Nightingale (1820–1910) started her work in response to the appalling conditions, which were present at the time. A significant portion of the groundwork for contemporary community health nursing practice was established by Florence Nightingale's outstanding achievements. Community health nursing now follows Nightingale's lead due to her vision and successful attempts at health reform, as well as her concern for populations at risk.

2.2.2. District Nursing

The official organization of visiting nursing, also known as district nursing, was the next step in the development of community health nursing. Even in those early days, district nurses considered cleanliness and a healthy lifestyle important for their patients, even though their primary focus was on the sick. They were referred to by Nightingale as "health nurses." One of the things that set district nursing apart early on, and later on, the specialty of public health nursing, was its focus on prevention and health nursing. The care of individuals was the primary focus of district nurses' work. Under the direct supervision of a doctor, district nurses took temperatures and pulse rates and administered basic medical care to the sick and impoverished. They also taught family members how to take care of the sick and how to maintain good personal hygiene, diet, and lifestyle choices.

Problems of district nursing:

- Increased number of immigrants;
- Increased crowded city slums;
- Inadequate sanitation practices;
- Unsafe and unhealthy working conditions.

Nevertheless, nursing educational programs at that time did not truly prepare district nurses to cope with their patients, multiple health, and social problems.

2.2.3. Public Health Nursing Training

District nursing began to focus on the health and welfare of the general public at the turn of the century, rather than just the impoverished.

This renewed focus was a result of increased public health awareness. Specialized initiatives like infant welfare helped to advance nursing education, provided the public with healthcare and health education, and allowed nurses to work more independently (Bullough & Bullough 1978). The contributions of Lillian D. Wald (1867–1940) to public health nursing were significant. Her primary goal was to assist the underprivileged. The public health nursing stage was defined by service to the public with the family targeted as the primary unit of care. Wald's emphasis on illness prevention and health promotion through health education and nursing intervention as well as her use of epidemiological methodology established these actions as hallmarks of public health nursing practice.

2.2.4. Community Health Nursing

As public health nurses carried on with their work in public health by the late 1960s and early 1970s, the term "community health nursing" emerged, marking the beginning of a new era. In the community, numerous other nurses were not necessarily in the public health field. To give a name that covered all nurses in the community, their practice settings included community-based clinics, doctor's offices, workplaces, schools, etc.

The distinction between community health nursing and public health nursing was unclear. In 1984, the Division of Nursing organized a consensus conference on the fundamentals of Public Health Nursing practice and education in Washington, DC. Despite the terms being used interchangeably, many in the field understood them to mean different things (1985). This group concluded that the term "community health nursing" encompasses all nurses who practice in the community, regardless of their level of education. One way to conceptualize public health nursing as a subset of community health nursing is as a generalist practice for nurses with baccalaureate-level training in basic public health and as a specialized practice for those with master's-level or higher training. Some of these unresolved issues are still being debated today, having begun in the 1980s and continuing to this day.

The integration of nursing and public health sciences with an emphasis on population health promotion and protection remains the definition of public health nursing. Public health nursing and community health nursing are terms that are interchangeable and describe a specialized population-focused nursing practice that incorporates both nursing services and public health sciences.

A possible distinction between the two terms might be to view community health nursing as a beginning level of specialization and public health nursing as an advanced level. Whichever term is used to describe this specialty, the fundamental issues and defining criteria remain as:

- Are the populations and communities the target of practice?
- Are the nurses prepared in public health and engaging in public health practice?

2.2.4.1. The Specialty of Community Health Nursing

The two characteristics of any specialized nursing practice are:

- Specialized knowledge and skills; and
- Focus on a particular set of people receiving the service.

Community health nursing likewise possesses these two qualities. Community health nursing is a specialty that adds public health knowledge and skills to address the needs and issues of communities, with a focus on vulnerable populations and communities. To create a practice that is community-based and population-focused, community health nursing, as a specialty, blends nursing and public health sciences (Williams, 1992). To improve the health of communities and vulnerable populations, professional nursing theories and the body of knowledge from the public health sciences are synthesized (American Public Health Association, 1992). The philosophical orientation and practice of community health nursing are distinct due to their foundation in both public health and nursing sciences.

2.2.4.2. Factors Influenced the Growth of Community Health Nursing

Even though many factors influenced the growth of community health nursing, six are particularly significant:

1. Advanced Technology

- As technological innovation increased, health care services and nutrition improved, and lifestyle changed, community health nursing has become grown and developed to meet the needs of the communities.
- Advanced technology industrialization.
- Large-scale employment and urbanization.
- High urban population density.
- Many health-related problems.
- Community health nursing growth and development.

2. Progress in Causal Thinking

- Germ theory disease causation (single cause ⍰ single effect).
- Tripartite view of disease causation (i.e., agent, host, environment).
- Multiple disease causation approach (multiple cause ⍰ multiple effect).

The way community health nurses control health problems by looking at all potential causes and then focusing on strategic causal points has changed significantly as a result of the advancements made in the study of causality, especially in epidemiology.

3. **Changes in Education**: People usually have a better understanding of health when their awareness of their surroundings grows. People believe they have the right to know and to inquire about the rationale behind the care they receive as a result. Planning for clients has given way to collaboration with clients for community health nurses.
4. **Consumer Movement**: Consumers demanding quality service seek more comprehensive and co-coordinated care. This movement has stimulated some basic changes in the philosophy of community health nursing.
5. **Changing Demography**: Shifting patterns in immigration, the number of births and deaths, and the rapidly increasing population of elderly persons affect community health nursing planning and programming efforts.
6. **Economic Forces**: Community nursing practices were impacted by economic factors such as rising healthcare costs, restricted access to healthcare, and shifting healthcare financing models. To address these forces, community nursing has launched new initiatives and programs.

2.2.4.3. Roles of Community Health Nursing

Seven major roles are:

- Clinician.
- Educator.
- Advocate.
- Managerial.
- Collaborator.
- Leader.
- Researcher.

The most familiar community health nurse role is that of clinician or provider of care. However, giving nursing care takes on new meaning in the context of community health.

1. **Clinician Role /Direct Care Provider**: As a clinician in community health, a nurse makes sure that health services are provided to populations and groups in addition to individuals and families. In contrast to basic nursing, the clinician role for community health nurses places more emphasis on skill development, health promotion, and holism.

- **Holism:** In community health, however, a holistic approach means considering the broad range of interacting needs that affect the collective health of the client as a larger system. The client is a composite of people whose relationships and interactions with each other must be considered in totality.
- **Health Promotion Focus on Wellness:** The community health nurse provides service along the entire range of the wellness–illness continuum but especially with an emphasis on the promotion of health and prevention of illness.
- **Expanded Skills:** the nurse uses many different skills in the community health clinician role skill. In addition to physical care skills, recent skills in observation, listening, communication, and counselling became integral to the clinician role with an increased emphasis on environmental and community-wide considerations such as problems with pollution, violence crime, drug abuse, unemployment, and limited funding for health programs.

2. **Educator Role:** Health education is one of the main responsibilities of a community health nurse and is widely acknowledged as a component of good nursing practice (Brown, 1988). There are two main reasons why the role of an educator is beneficial in promoting the health of the general public. The educator's role:

- Has the potential for finding greater receptivity and providing higher yield results.
- Is significant because a wider audience can be reached.

The emphases throughout the health teaching process continue to be placed on illness prevention and health promotion.

3. **Advocate Role**: In modern health care, the question of patients' rights is crucial. Every client or patient has the right to just, equitable, and compassionate care. However, the fragmented and depersonalized nature of our current healthcare system is a common feature. The underprivileged and destitute were notably impacted by this strategy. It is frequently necessary for the community health

nurse to represent the client group or plead the case on their behalf. Sometimes people receiving health care need someone to explain what services are appropriate for them and what they should anticipate.

4. **Managerial Role**: As a manager, the nurse provides administrative guidance to achieve predetermined objectives by determining the needs of the clients, organizing and planning to meet those needs, monitoring and controlling the process, and assessing the results to ensure that objectives are reached. When a nurse is in charge of patient care, manages caseloads, supervises support personnel, operates clinics, or leads community health needs assessments, they are acting in the capacity of managers.

5. **Case Management**: Case management is a methodical procedure wherein a nurse determines the needs of their clients, plans and organizes their services, directs them to other suitable providers, and tracks and assesses their progress to guarantee that their various service needs are satisfied.

6. **Collaborator Role**: It is rare for community health nurses to work alone. In addition to clients, other nurses, doctors, social workers, and community leaders, they also have to collaborate with therapists, nutritionists, occupational therapists, psychologists, epidemiologists, biostaticians, legislators, and others. As a part of the medical team (Williams, 1986; Fairly, 1993). The community health nurse takes on the role of collaborator, which entails cooperating as partners and working together on a shared project.

7. **Leader Role**: The role of community health nurses as leaders is growing in activity. In her role as a leader, the nurse guides, sways, or convinces others to take actions that will improve people's health. The main responsibility of a leadership role is to bring about change, and in this sense, the community health nurse acts as a change agent. Additionally, they aim to change people's perspectives and actions regarding health and the variables that affect it.

8. **Research Role:** In order to solve issues and improve community health practice, community health nurses who are also researchers conduct methodical research, data collection, and analysis. The literal definition of research is to look for, look into, find, and interpret facts. From the most basic investigation to the most extensive epidemiological study, all community health research follows the same basic methodology. The research process involves the following steps:

- Identifying an area of interest.
- Specify the research question or statement.
- Review of literature.
- Identifying the conceptual frame work.
- Select research design.
- Collect and analyze data.
- Interpret the result.
- Communicate the findings.

A problem or query is identified by the community health nurse, who then conducts an investigation by gathering and evaluating data, suggesting and assessing potential solutions before either accepting or rejecting each one and resuming the investigation. In a way, the nurse collects information for health planning and looks into health issues to create plans for the community that promote wellness and prevent disease.

2.2.4.4. Settings of Community Health Nursing Practice

Community health nursing practice occurs in a variety of settings, each tailored to meet the specific health needs of different populations. Here are some key settings:

- **Home Health Care**: Nurses provide medical care, education, and support to patients in their own homes. This setting is particularly important for individuals with chronic illnesses, disabilities, or those recovering from surgery who need continuous care but prefer to stay at home.
- **Schools**: School nurses address the health needs of students, providing first aid, managing chronic conditions, and promoting healthy behaviors. They also play a key role in health education and disease prevention programs.
- **Public Health Departments**: Nurses work within local or state health departments to conduct community assessments, develop and implement public health programs, and respond to health emergencies. They focus on population-level interventions to improve overall community health.
- **Community Clinics and Health Centers**: These facilities provide accessible healthcare services to underserved populations. Community health nurses offer primary care, preventive services, health education, and disease management.
- **Occupational Health Settings**: Nurses in this setting focus on the health and safety of workers. They conduct workplace health assessments, promote wellness programs, manage occupational injuries, and ensure compliance with health regulations.
- **Faith-Based Organizations**: Nurses collaborate with religious institutions to offer health screenings, education, and support services. These settings often reach populations that might not otherwise seek healthcare.
- **Correctional Facilities**: Nurses provide care to incarcerated individuals, addressing their physical and mental health needs, managing chronic conditions, and offering health education.
- **Homeless Shelters and Outreach Programs**: Nurses deliver care to homeless populations, offering medical services, health education, and support to access other healthcare resources.
- **Long-Term Care Facilities**: In settings like nursing homes and assisted living facilities, community health nurses care for elderly residents, managing chronic illnesses and promoting quality of life.
- **Mobile Health Units**: These units bring healthcare services directly to underserved or remote areas, offering screenings, vaccinations, and basic medical care.

By working in these varied settings, community health nurses play a critical role in improving public health outcomes and ensuring that all individuals have access to necessary health services. (Johnston et al., 2013; Weir et al., 2010).

2.3. Health Care Delivery System

The way that health care is provided to the public is commonly referred to as the "health care delivery system." The degree of professional specialization and the severity of the patient's illness are used to categorize the healthcare delivery system.

- Primary care level;
- Secondary care level;
- Tertiary care level.

1. **Primary Care Level**: is the usual entry point for clients of the health care delivery system. It is oriented towards the promotion and maintenance of health, the prevention of disease, the management of common episodic disease, and the monitoring of stable or chronic conditions. Primary care ordinarily occurs, in ambulatory settings. The client or the family manages treatment with health professionals providing diagnostic expertise and guidance.
2. **Secondary Care Level**: It entails a doctor or hospital providing specialized medical care after being referred by the primary care physician. A patient has manifested recognizable signs and symptoms that either need to be further investigated or are definitively diagnosed. It is designed for patients with more serious acute illnesses or worsening chronic illnesses. In most cases, hospitalization takes place in a community or district hospital. A primary care provider refers most patients to this level of care, though some patients choose to go there on their own. Typically, general practitioners and specialists work as secondary care physicians.
3. **Tertiary Care Level:** It is an extremely technical and specialized level of care for the diagnosis and treatment of complex or uncommon medical issues. Individuals in need of this level frequently have complex and extensive pathological conditions when they first present. This level of care is the most complicated. The condition is usually treated in a large hospital that is connected to a medical school, and it may be life-threatening. Workers in primary or secondary settings refer clients to them. Healthcare providers, such as doctors and nurses, are typically very specialized and concentrate on providing care in their particular field.

The other classification of health care delivery system is:

- **Preventive:** This is aimed at stopping the disease process before it starts or preventing further deterioration of a condition that already exists.
- **Curative:** This is aimed at restoring the client's health.
- **Rehabilitative**: This is aimed at lessening the pain and discomfort of illness and helping clients live with disease and disability. Some nurse theorists have conceptualized the nursing role as being focused on sustaining care and preventing disease. However, the work role of nurse practitioners and home health care nurses would probably span all three of these orientations. The nurse must understand and remember that the preventive services are also popularly categorized as primary, secondary, and tertiary preventive health care.

2.3.1. Factors Affecting the Delivery of Health Care Services

The healthcare delivery system has grown and becomes more complex due to several factors.

1. **Health Care as a Right:** The wealthy in this nation have the privilege of having access to healthcare. The impoverished must either forgo care altogether or accept care that is of lower quality. Today, in developed nations, universal health care is administered as a national health service (NHS) and is seen as a fundamental human right for all people, regardless of wealth.

i. Technological Advances

Today advances in technology has so far made an increasingly dramatic changes on health care.

Example

- Better diagnostic tools assist in recognizing conditions while they are treatable.
- Organ transplants e.g., Renal transplant, and bone marrow transplant are becoming common treatment procedures.
- Life can be maintained mechanically e.g., a mechanical ventilator.
- Changing technology alters the profile of hospital patients. e.g., after insulin was developed (1920s), people with diabetes could manage their disease at home instead of in the hospital.

2. **Rising Consumerisms:** The public's expectation that it will be able to influence the kind, standard, and price of healthcare is known as consumerism. The healthcare system used to function entirely under the presumption that doctors and nurses knew what was best for their patients and should make those decisions. However, these days, patient expectations and demands for involvement in healthcare decisions are steadily rising, leading to the development of new relationships between patients and healthcare providers.

3. **Changing Health Services**: Health services are now characterized by a comprehensive approach. Disease diagnosis and treatment are given equal weight with health promotion and disease prevention. Holistic care focuses on human integrity and stresses that the body, mind, and sprit are inter-dependent and inseparable holistic health care includes:

- Nutritional awareness;
- Environmental sensitively;
- Stress reduction;
- Spiritual health; and
- Self-responsibility.

Therefore, while organizing and providing care, all facets of the patient must be taken into account. In the absence or presence of co-morbid conditions, the healthcare provider predicts that the physical condition of the patient will progress predictably. The impact of psychosocial problems on the healing process is not as well understood. Care family focus, cultural diversity, sensitivity to openness, lifestyle, opinion, values, and beliefs, and inclusion of a support system. Therefore, to make an accurate assessment, nurses need to be knowledgeable about the bio-cultural, psychosocial, and linguistic differences in society.

2.4. Nursing Process in the Community

The nursing process is a methodical approach

to ascertaining the health status of a client, identifying health concerns and issues, creating plans to address them, starting actions to carry out the plan, and ultimately assessing how well the plan is working to promote wellness and solve issues. Whether the client system is an individual, a family, an integrated community, or something else entirely, the nursing process outlines interactions and interventions with that system.

The nursing process commonly consists of five phases:

- Community assessment;
- Community diagnosis;
- Planning;
- Implementation and;
- Evaluation.

When the community is the client, it is used to respond to and take care of its health needs. For this nursing service, the term "community as a client" refers to the wider notion of the community as a whole.

2.4.1. Community as a Client

Community health nurses have two primary goals when working with communities: (1) providing the most essential health services at the community level; and (2) recognizing that the community directly influences the health of the individuals, families, groups, and populations that may be a part of it.

2.4.2. Dimensions of the Community as Client

A community has three features

- Location;
- A population; and
- A social system.

It is useful to think of these dimensions of every community as a rough map to follow for assessing needs or planning for service provision.

1. **Location:** Every physical community lives out its days in a particular place on Earth. The location of health services, geographical characteristics, flora, animals, and man-made surroundings all have an impact on a community's overall health.

- **Community Boundaries:** To talk about community in any sense, one must first describe its boundaries. It serves as the basis for measuring the incidence of wellness and illness and for determining the spread of disease.
- **Location of Health Services:** When assessing a community, the community health nurse will want to identify the major health centers and know where they are located. The use of health services depends on availability and accessibility.
- **Geographic Features**: Communities have been constructed in every suitable physical environment and that environment certainly can affect the health of a community. Injury, death, and destruction may be caused by floods, cyclones, earthquakes volcanoes...etc., recreational activities at lakes, seashores, and mountains promote health and wellness.
- **Climate:** Climate has a direct effect on the health of a community e.g., extreme heat and cold).
- **Flora and Fauna:** Poisonous plants and disease-carrying animals can affect community health.
- **Human-Made Environment:** All human influences on the

environment (housing, dams, farming, types of industry, chemical wastes, air pollution...etc.) can influence levels of community wellness.

2. **Population:** The population is made up of all the different individuals who reside inside the limits of the community as well as a specific aggregate. Any community's population has a significant impact on its overall health. Various demographic characteristics point to the need for health care and serve as a foundation for health planning.

   - Population variables

- **Size:** The number and size of healthcare facilities are influenced by the size of the population. The size of the community offers crucial planning information.
- **Density:** Stress levels may rise with increased population density. In a similar vein, providing health care may become challenging when people are dispersed.
- **Composition:** The composition of the population often determines types of health needs. A health community takes full account of and provides for differences in age, sex, educational level, and occupation of its members, all of which may affect health concerns. Determining a community's composition is an important early step in determining its level of health.
- **Rate of Growth or Decline:** Rapidly growing communities may place extensive demands on health services. A marked population decline may be a signal of poorly functioning community.
- **Cultural Difference**: Health needs may vary among sub-cultural and ethnic populations. Cultural difference can create conflicting or competing demands for resources and services or create inter-group hostility.
- **Social Class and Educational Levels:** Social class refers to the ranking of groups within the society by income, education, occupation, prestige, or a combination of these factors. Educational level is a powerful determinant of health-related behavior. Health promotion and preventive health services are most needed for people with low income and educational levels.
- **Mobility:** Mobility of the population affects continuity of care and availability of services. Mobility has a direct effect on the health of a community.

3. **Social System:** Every community has a social system, which is a third dimension beyond population and location. Social system variables are the different components of the community social system that interact and have an impact on the system. The health, family, economic, educational, religious, welfare, legal, communication, recreational, and political systems are some of these variables. The health system is especially important to promote community health, even though community health nurses must look at all of the community's systems and how they work together.

2.4.3. Phases of Nursing Process in the Community

The nursing process in the community setting involves several interrelated phases aimed at promoting and maintaining the health of populations. The process begins with assessment, where nurses gather comprehensive data about the community's health status, resources, and needs through surveys, interviews, and observation. This is followed by the diagnosis phase, where collected data is analyzed to identify key health issues and prioritize them based on severity and the community's capacity to address them. In the planning phase, nurses collaborate with community members and stakeholders to develop specific, measurable, achievable, relevant, and time-bound (SMART) goals and interventions tailored to the identified health needs. The implementation phase involves executing the planned interventions through community education, health promotion activities, and direct care services, ensuring community engagement and participation. Finally, the evaluation phase assesses the outcomes of the interventions against the set goals, determining their effectiveness and making necessary adjustments. This cyclical process ensures continuous improvement in community health and enables nurses to adapt to changing health dynamics and emerging needs.

2.4.3.1. Assessment

The initial stage of the nursing process is assessment, which entails gathering and analyzing data and information regarding the health status of a community in order to identify any current or future needs that will serve as the foundation for planning.

2.4.3.1.1. Community Assessment

This is the process of looking for and verifying pertinent data from the community using a predetermined method in order to understand how people, resources, and the environment interact.

- Community assessment includes:
    - Collecting pertinent community data.
    - Analyzing and interpreting the collected data.

Community needs assessment: Is the process of determining the real or perceived needs of a defined community of people.

In some situations; an extensive community study becomes a priority. In others, all that is needed is a study of one system (e.g., health system, educational system, etc.) or organization (e.g., women association etc.).

1. Major Aspects of Community Assessment

i. **Physical Environment:** Physical examinations are crucial for individual patients, and the physical environment of the community should also be examined. In physical assessment, five senses are employed: laboratory studies, vital signs, auscultation, system review, and inspection.

- **Inspection:** inspection uses all sense organs and is done by walking survey in the community, or micro-assessment of housing, open spaces, boundaries, transportation service centers, markets places, meeting street people, signs of decay, ethnicity, religion, health and morbidity, and political media.
- **Auscultation:** listening to the community residents about the physical environment.
- **Vital Signs:** observe the climate, terrain, and natural boundaries such as rivers and hills.

- **Community Resources:** look for signs of life such as notices, posters, new housing, and buildings.
- **System Review**: hosing age, architecture, building materials used, signs of disrepair, running water, plumbing, sanitation, windows (glasses), etc. Also business facilities and churches.
- **Laboratory Studies:** census data or planning studies for community mapping.

ii. **Health and Social System:** Make a distinction between facilities that are inside the community and those that are outside. Health centers, clinics, or health posts; public health services; private clinics; pharmacies; dentistry; and other services; number of beds; staffing; and budget. indication of alcoholism or drug addiction. In addition to markets and stores, social services also include special needs, clothing, food, shelter, and counselling and support.

iii. **Economics:** Financial characteristics include the percentage of households with monthly incomes of less than 100 Birr in poverty and the median household income. Features of the labor force, including the employment situation of people in general who are older than eighteen. categories of occupations and the proportion of workers in government, agriculture, business and industry, and skilled and unskilled labor.

iv. **Safety and Transportation:** Services provided by police, fire, sewage, solid waste disposal, and water source sanitation. Walking, mule rides, taxis, buses, trains, private vehicles, and air travel are the main modes. The standard of roads, as well as the affordability and frequency of private and public transportation.

v. **Politics and Government:** Kebele, associations of peasants, religious organizations, business partnerships, associations for women and youth, professional associations, associations for ethics, political activism, etc., outline the goals and actions of the associations.

vi. **Communication:** Bulletin boards, posters, oral messages, radio, television, newspapers, postal services, telephone. Look for TV aeries, telephone wires, magazines, and satellite dishes.

vii. **Education:** Types of schools, colleges and universities. Note languages used, grades, courses offered, percentage of attendants (male, female), adequacy, accessibility, and acceptability of education. Average number of years completed by people at school.

viii. **Recreation:** Note facilities such as stadium, recreational areas, volley balls court, playground, picnic areas, museum, music/dancing, theatre/cinema. Who is going out during the evening and in the morning? Teenagers, mothers and children, the homeless?

2.4.3.2. Community Analysis and Nursing Diagnosis

Analyzing something is looking at and studying data. Analysis is required to ascertain the needs and strengths of community health as well as patterns of health responses and trends in the utilization of health care. Like a lot of the procedures we perform, community analysis can be seen as a multi-step process. The phases of analysis include:

- Data categorization (demographic, geographic, socioeconomic, health resource and services, etc.).
- Data summarization (rates, charts graphs, etc.).
- Comparing data (with similar data, identification of data gaps, incongruence, etc.).
- Draw inferences (draw logical conclusions from the evidence) that lead to a community diagnosis.

This is a declaration outlining the community's health risks, issues, and strengths. A true clinical judgment or conclusions about how people react to real or imagined problems are called nursing diagnoses (ANA). A community-based intervention starts with a community diagnosis. A nursing diagnosis has three parts

- Description of the problem (specific target or groups);
- Identification of factors/etiology related to (r/t) the problem; and
- The signs and symptoms (the manifestations) that characteristics of the problem.

2.4.3.2.1. Planning

Designing an organized, comprehensive plan of action to achieve particular goals and objectives based on community assessment and nursing diagnosis formulation is a rational, decision-making process.

1. **Setting Priorities Involves:** Putting the needs of the client in order of importance or rank and choosing which goals to tackle first. The objective may be short-term, medium-term, or long-term.
2. **Establishing Goals and Objectives:** A goal is a broad statement of desired end results. Objectives are specific statements of the desired outcomes. Characteristics of good objectives:
   - Specific- target specific population.
   - Measurable- when the results are stated.
   - Achievable- within the capacity of the available resources.
   - Relevant- fits with the general police.
   - Time bound- that is achieved within a specified time frame.

2.4.3.2.2. Implementation

The act of putting the plan into practice and having the nurse or other professionals carry out the tasks outlined in the plan is known as implementation. This stage of the nursing process is called action. Community interventions are therapeutic measures intended to treat and prevent health issues within the community, support the community as it evolves, and promote and safeguard the health of the community as a whole.

Key areas of nursing intervention in the community are:

- link the community members with the available resources
- pulls together information and resources to assist the community in addressing its health concerns and problems
- marinating its strength through facilitation, education, organization, consultation, and direct care.

2.4.3.2.3. Evaluation

It is an ongoing, methodical process that compares the community's response to the goal as specified by the care plan. Determining whether or not planned actions satisfied client needs, how well they were met, and, if not, why not, is the ultimate goal of evaluating interventions in community health nursing. Evaluation needs a clear goal, precise standards and criteria, and the ability to make judgment calls. (Mattson et al., 2012 & Bray et al., 2010).

2.5. Substance Abuse

Substance abuse, also known as substance use disorder, refers to the harmful or hazardous use of psychoactive substances, including alcohol and illicit drugs. This disorder is characterized by an inability to control the use of substances despite negative consequences on an individual's health, relationships, and responsibilities. Substance abuse leads to significant impairment or distress, manifesting in behaviors such as neglecting major obligations, using substances in physically dangerous situations, experiencing repeated legal issues, and continuing use despite persistent social or interpersonal problems. The causes of substance abuse are multifaceted, involving genetic, psychological, social, and environmental factors. Effective management and treatment require a comprehensive approach, including prevention, early intervention, behavioral therapies, medication-assisted treatment, and support systems. Community-based programs play a crucial role in addressing substance abuse by providing education, resources, and support to prevent initiation and facilitate recovery, ultimately aiming to reduce the social and health impacts associated with substance abuse.

2.5.1. Etiology of Substance Abuse

Substance abuse affects almost every facet of a person's life, both personally and socially, and it has been the subject of numerous studies and institutions. Numerous theories make an effort to address the problem's root causes, extent, and potential solutions. Certain theories focus on factors that are individual, physiological, spiritual, and psychological. Others address societal influences related to sex roles, politics, economics, family, ethnicity, race, and drug availability as well as environmental stressors and drug availability. The majority of theories propose that the root cause of substance abuse is a confluence of factors.

A growing body of research indicates that genetic variations may play a role like alcoholism within families, even though previous studies have suggested a link between genetics and alcoholism. There are environmental and individual factors that also raise the risk of alcohol abuse. Individually, the onset of alcohol abuse is predicted by an individual's inherited sensitivity to alcohol. There is also a correlation between two broad personality traits and a higher likelihood of alcohol abuse. Impulsivity and a lack of inhibition make substance abuse more likely. Other risks include a predisposition to anxiety and depression, and little is known about these comorbidities. Alcohol abuse is also predicted by alcohol expectancies, or views about the results of drinking. After using a medication, one is more likely to experience the desired effect—such as relief—if they are expecting it. Satisfied expectancies have the potential to establish neural pathways that are perceived as enjoyable.

It's possible that medical models of alcoholism and other substance abuse disorders don't explain the similarities between addictive behaviors (such as binge drinking, gambling, eating, drug use, and sexual behavior). Nowadays, there is a greater prevalence of cross-addiction, or multidrug use, and more research indicates that automatic and nonautomatic factors contribute to physiological and psychological dependence. Multicausal medical models are replacing specific biological models. According to the biopsychosocial model, an inclination toward drug or alcohol use develops as a result of the interaction between risk and protective factors. Substance exposure, availability, and the subjective interpretation of the drug experience (e.g., pleasant or unpleasant) all have an impact on this predisposition. It is also essential for the substances to remain accessible and for there to be a social support network that permits or encourages their use. The development and maintenance of addiction are determined by the combination of these factors.

2.5.2. Alcohol and Illicit Drug Use

Throughout the 20th century, changes in public tolerance as well as political and economic trends had an impact on swings in the use of alcohol and illegal drugs. Generally speaking, drinking has become more socially acceptable than using other drugs. In the US, alcohol consumption fell during Prohibition and the Great Depression and increased during World Wars I and II. When states lowered the drinking age to 18 in the 1980s, alcohol use peaked during that decade. Politicians changed their minds about the lowering of the drinking age because they were concerned about the rising rate of alcohol consumption and the higher number of alcohol-related deaths among 18 to 25-year-olds. After raising the legal drinking age to 21 in the late 1980s, there was a decrease in the consumption of alcohol. Reduced tolerance for alcohol consumption in the United States during the 1990s and into the twenty-first century, as well as more stringent social and legal restrictions and laws prohibiting drinking and driving, are all blamed for the decline in alcohol consumption. One example of a change in perspective from addiction as the main issue to other issues related to, say, alcohol use, is the recognition of and response to driving while impaired by alcohol or other drugs. These issues are therefore referred to as substance-related issues, and they are now a major community concern.

In addition to governmental policies, public attitudes have shaped the history of illicit drug use. Even though doctors in the nineteenth century used morphine to treat a wide range of illnesses, the early 1900s saw a rise in government regulation of cocaine and opiates due to their addictive qualities. The Harrison Narcotic Act of 1914 and later legislation limited the authority of the medical community to control the use of addictive drugs; doctors could only prescribe these drugs as part of their routine practice, not to feed an addiction. The supply of these drugs was restricted until the 1950s and 1960s due to restrictions on the importation of narcotics and limitations on the authority of physicians to prescribe and dispense addictive drugs. Heroin use was on the rise at the time due to an increase in illegal drug trafficking, especially in inner cities.

Drugs were becoming more widely available by the 1970s. Many members of the counterculture, who were mostly young people, saw drug use as a means of mental liberation during this time. They concentrated their efforts on improving social justice, ending the Vietnam War, and reducing "repressive" sexual norms. Adult use of marijuana occurred in social, communal settings, while alcohol use was less popular due to its association with the "establishment" that the youth were criticizing. As a result, the general public began using heroin, cannabis, and hallucinogens in addition to urban drug subcultures. The public became less accepting of drug use as a result of the social and personal issues raised by this shift, and prevention and treatment initiatives received increased funding. Most population segments saw a decline in illicit drug use in the 1980s, following a peak in 1979, and a low point in the early 1990s. Funding for treatment and rehabilitation was increased by the Anti-Drug Abuse Acts of 1986 and 1988; the 1988 act established the Office of National Drug Control Policy. The director, also known as the "drug czar," is in charge of directing the country's drug control strategy. Federal drug policy has placed a strong emphasis on law enforcement and interdiction—the War on Drugs—to cut down on the supply to address worries about the psychological, social, and physical effects of drug abuse and dependence.

A resurgence of interest has been observed in prevention and treatment initiatives aimed at reducing the prevalence of illicit drug use in society and mitigating its effects. Tackling drug control from a public health perspective, the Office of National Drug Control Policy (ONDCP) dedicated over $10 billion in 2012 to drug education initiatives and increased access to drug treatment for addicts. Nurses and other health care providers need to be aware of a plethora of federal resources. For example, the National Institute on Drug Abuse (NIDA) exists. Leading the country in drug abuse and addiction research is NIDA's mission. NIDA's strategic goals tackle substance abuse as a multifaceted illness with multiple underlying causes. Basic, clinical, and translational science research programs in genetics, functional neuroimaging, social neuroscience, medicine and behavioral therapies, prevention, and health services are all under the purview of the institute. There are four main goal areas: treatment, prevention, and reducing the transmission of AIDS and HIV. There are also other priority areas. Research is still in its early stages regarding pain and other compulsive disorders. Data on health disparities associated with drug addiction and its various effects are gathered by NIDA. The institute offers a wide range of educational programs covering the fields of medicine, education, and criminal justice. NIDA continues to support training and the distribution of factual, scientifically based information on drug abuse, in addition to research on HIV/AIDS, emerging trends, and nicotine addiction. The goal of the Substance Abuse and Mental Health Services Administration (SAMHSA) is to assist the country in acting upon knowledge that supports behavioral health treatment through all levels of prevention by developing and maintaining policies, programs, grants, contracts, and information and data. Programs that assist military families and the legal system are supported by SAMHSA.

2.5.3. Prevalence, Incidence, and Trends

Prevalence refers to the total number of cases of a particular condition, such as substance abuse, present in a population at a given time. It includes both newly diagnosed and pre-existing cases. High prevalence rates of substance abuse indicate that the issue is widespread within a community or population, which can strain healthcare systems and impact overall public health.

Incidence measures the number of new cases of substance abuse that develop in a specific population during a defined period, usually a year. This metric helps in understanding the rate at which new individuals are developing substance use disorders, providing insight into the emergence and spread of the problem. High incidence rates suggest that substance abuse is becoming more common, which can indicate the need for increased preventive measures and early intervention strategies.

Trends in substance abuse track changes in prevalence and incidence over time, helping to identify patterns and shifts in behavior. Trends can reveal whether substance abuse is increasing, decreasing, or remaining stable, and can be influenced by factors such as changes in law enforcement policies, availability of substances, economic conditions, and public health interventions. For instance, the opioid crisis in many countries has shown a significant upward trend in opioid abuse and related overdoses over recent decades, leading to increased public health efforts and policy changes aimed at addressing the epidemic.

Trends also help in forecasting future needs for healthcare resources and shaping effective public health strategies.

Understanding these aspects of substance abuse is crucial for developing targeted prevention and treatment programs, allocating resources effectively, and implementing policies that can mitigate the impact of substance abuse on individuals and communities.

2.5.3.1. Alcohol

Alcohol use is widespread across the globe, with a significant portion of the population consuming it regularly. The World Health Organization (WHO) reports that around 2.3 billion people are current drinkers. Prevalence varies by region, with higher rates often found in high-income countries. In the United States, for example, the National Institute on Alcohol Abuse and Alcoholism (NIAAA) estimates that about 85.6% of adults reported drinking alcohol at some point in their lives, with 69.5% drinking in the past year, and 54.9% in the past month.

The incidence of alcohol use disorders (AUDs) provides insight into how many new cases are emerging over a given period. According to the NIAAA, approximately 14.5 million adults aged 18 and older had an AUD in 2019. The incidence of underage drinking and the initiation of alcohol use among adolescents and young adults is also a significant concern, with early onset of drinking often linked to higher risks of developing AUDs later in life.

Trends in alcohol consumption and related disorders can fluctuate due to various factors, including cultural shifts, economic changes, and public health policies. Over recent decades, some countries have seen a decline in overall alcohol consumption, often attributed to increased awareness of health risks and stronger regulatory measures. Conversely, other regions have experienced rising trends in alcohol use, particularly in developing countries undergoing rapid social and economic changes.

Despite these fluctuations, alcohol remains one of the leading causes of preventable death and disease worldwide. The WHO reports that alcohol contributes to more than 3 million deaths each year, accounting for 5.3% of all deaths globally. This impact is seen in various health issues, including liver cirrhosis, cancers, cardiovascular diseases, and injuries from accidents and violence.

Efforts to address alcohol-related problems include public health campaigns, policy measures like taxation and advertising restrictions, and support services for those struggling with AUDs. The implementation of these strategies is crucial to reducing the harmful effects of alcohol on individuals and society as a whole.

2.5.3.2. Illicit Drug Use

Illicit drug use, encompassing the non-medical use of illegal substances and misused prescription medications, is a major global public health concern. According to the United Nations Office on Drugs and Crime (UNODC), around 275 million people used drugs at least once in 2020. In the United States, about 19.3% of people aged 12 or older reported using an illicit drug in the past year. The incidence of new users remains high, particularly among adolescents and young adults, underscoring the need for effective prevention and early intervention strategies. Recent trends highlight the opioid epidemic's devastating impact, marked by a significant increase in overdose deaths, and the rising use of synthetic drugs, which pose severe health risks due to their unpredictable effects. Concurrently, the legalization and decriminalization of cannabis in various regions have led to increased use and changing perceptions of its safety. Addressing the complexities of illicit drug use requires a comprehensive approach that integrates prevention programs, evidence-based treatment and rehabilitation, harm reduction strategies, and balanced policy enforcement to reduce supply and demand while supporting those affected.

2.5.3.2.1. Nonmedical Use of Prescription-Type Psychotherapeutics

Nonmedical use and abuse of prescription drugs constitute a serious public health problem in this country. An estimated 52 million people (20% of those aged 12 and older) have used prescription drugs for nonmedical reasons at least once in their lifetimes. The NIDA Monitoring the Future (MTF) survey found that about 1 in 12 high school seniors reported past-year nonmedical use of the prescription pain reliever hydrocodone (Vicodin) in 2010, and 1 in 20 reported abusing oxycodone (OxyContin)—making these medications among the drugs most commonly abused by adolescents. There are three classes of the most commonly abused prescription drugs: opioids, central nervous system depressants, and stimulants. There has been a significant increase in the lifetime nonmedical use of pain relievers (20.8% of individuals aged 12 years and older), specifically Percocet, Percodan, Vicodin, Lortab, Darvocet, Darvon or Tylenol with codeine, propoxyphene or codeine products, oxycodone, and hydrocodone.

2.5.3.2.2. Hallucinogen, Inhalant, and Heroin Use

Drugs classified as hallucinogens interfere with the way nerve cells and the neurotransmitter serotonin interact, which results in hallucinations. There are significant distortions in how people view the world. People can perceive sounds, see things, and feel things that are not real. Certain hallucinations can also cause emotional behavioral shifts. Mood, hunger, body temperature, sexual behavior, and muscle coordination may all change. Made from lysergic acid, LSD (D-lysergic acid diethylamide) was discovered in 1938 and is known for its unpredictable psychological effects, including 12-hour "trips." LSD can produce hallucinations and delusions at certain dosages. Since LSD can be purchased as tablets, capsules, or occasionally as liquid, it is typically taken orally. Usually, absorbent paper is mixed with LSD and cut into pieces that are adorned and represent one dose each. A person under the influence of LSD may behave psychotically. Additional symptoms include elevated body temperature, heart rate, and blood pressure, insomnia, and anorexia. Mescaline is the main active component of peyote, a tiny, spineless cactus. Native Americans in northern Mexico and the southwestern United States have long used the peyote cactus in religious rites. The peyote cactus's tops, or buttons, are removed from the roots, dried, and then consumed or soaked in water to create a potent liquid. The cacti can be boiled for several hours to prepare the bitter extracts into a tea. The effects of mescaline, which range from 0.3 to 0.5 grams, are hallucinogenic and last for approximately 12 hours.

There are specific kinds of mushrooms that grow naturally in tropical and subtropical areas of South America, Mexico, and the United States. These mushrooms contain psilocybin (4-phosphoryloxy-N, N-dimethyltryptamine). Psilocybin-containing mushrooms are usually consumed orally and can be found fresh or dried. They can be used to disguise the bitter taste of other foods or brewed as tea. Following ingestion, hallucinations may start to manifest within 20 minutes and last for up to 6 hours.

Phencyclidine, or PCP, was created as an intravenous anesthetic in the 1950s, but due to issues with clinical trials, including extremely detrimental psychological effects, it was never authorized for use in humans. PCP is a white, crystalline powder that dissolves easily in alcohol or water. PCP is frequently sold on the black market in a range of tablet, capsule, and colored powder forms that are typically snorted, smoked, or consumed orally. It is also easily combined with dyes. The taste of PCP is distinctly bitter and chemical. It is frequently applied to leafy plants like mint, parsley, oregano, or marijuana before being smoked. Its effects can last for four to six hours, depending on the concentration and mode of ingestion. After the age of 17, there is a noticeable increase in the use of PCP, LSD, psilocybin, and MDMA (methylenedioxymethamphetamine), popularly known as ecstasy. 2% of people between the ages of twelve and twenty-five abuse inhalants. The preferred inhalants are amyl nitrite, also known as "poppers," which are followed by glue, toluene, shoe polish, correction fluid, degreaser, or cleaning fluid, gasoline or lighter fluid, spray paints, and other aerosols. Numerous goods that are easily obtained for use at home or at work contain inhalants. Inhaled volatile substances possessing psychoactive properties can be found in spray paints, markers, glues, and cleaning fluids. Young children and adolescents can use them in particular, though not only. Usually, these drugs cause an abrupt high that mimics the effects of alcohol intoxication, which can lead to loss of feeling or even unconsciousness. Bone marrow damage, central nervous system or brain damage, limb spasms, and hearing loss are among the serious and irreversible effects. High concentrations of these substances can cause asphyxia or heart failure which can be fatal.

In 2011, 4.2 million Americans aged 12 or older (or 1.6%) said they had used heroin at least once in their lives. It is estimated that about 23% of individuals who use heroin become dependent on it. An opioid drug, heroin is synthesized from morphine. Heroin usually is a white or brown powder or as a black sticky substance, known as black tar heroin. Injection of drugs like heroin brings about the highest risk of contracting HIV and hepatitis C. These diseases are transmitted through contact with blood or other bodily fluids, which can occur with sharing of needles or other injection drug use equipment. Hepatitis C is the most common blood-borne infection in the United States. HIV can also be contracted during unprotected sex, which drug use makes more likely. There is a close association between drug abuse and the increase of infectious diseases.

2.5.3.3. Gender Differences

Prescription drug abuse is more common in men than in women overall, except those between the ages of 12 and 17. In this age group, more women than men use all psychotherapeutics—painkillers, tranquilizers, and stimulants—for non-medical purposes. Females between the ages of 12 and 17 who use prescription drugs for non-medical purposes are also more likely to meet the requirements for abuse or dependence on psychotherapy. There is little change in the use of illegal drugs by men, but there is an increase in the use of illicit drugs by women aged 12 and older.

2.5.3.4. Demographics

Regional, racial, and gender differences and changes over the past few years are indicated by demographic correlates. For instance, 12% of West Coast residents reported using drugs in the previous month, compared to 9.7% in the Midwest, 9% in the Northeast, and 9% in the South. Furthermore, there are notable differences in the prevalence of illicit drug use among the main racial/ethnic groups. The categories with the highest rates were American Indians or Alaska Natives (19.5%), then African Americans (16.9%), Whites (14.4%), and Hispanics (12.3%). With a rate of 7:4%, Asians had the lowest percentage.

2.5.4. Adolescent Substance Abuse

Adolescents are a group that is especially vulnerable to substance abuse. The largest percentage of people (65%) who have used illicit drugs at some point in their lives are those who are between the ages of 18 and 25. According to the 2012 MTF Survey, the percentage of youths between the ages of 12 and 17 who currently use marijuana climbed to 7.3% in 2009 and 7.3% in 2010 (Johnston et al., 2012).

The decrease in teen use of smokeless tobacco and cigarettes is a good development. In 2010, the percentage of adolescents between the ages of 12 and 17 who currently use alcohol was 13.6%, which was less than the rate in 2009 (14.7%). In comparison to 2009 (8.8% and 2.1%, respectively), youth binge and heavy drinking rates in 2010 (7.8% and 1.7%, respectively) were likewise lower (Johnston et al., 2012). Among tenth graders, it is noteworthy that the significant decline in adolescent smoking and use of smokeless tobacco has slowed down and appears to be about to stop. Young people still have easy access to cigarettes, and organizations that care about this issue keep an eye on advertisements that appeal to these groups of people as potential new smokers.

The percentage of young people reporting high risk associated with substance use was used to measure perceived risk in the 2010 National Survey on Drug Use and Health (NSDUH). There was a decline from 54.7% in 2007 to 47.5% in 2010 in the proportion of adolescents aged 12 to 17 who thought smoking marijuana once or twice a week posed a grave risk. Based on research conducted between 2002 and 2008, nearly 50% of participants aged 12 to 17 stated in 2010 that obtaining marijuana would be either very easy or fairly easy. In general, there has been a slight decline in teen substance use, but the trend has been mostly downward. To plan for the community's needs both now and in the future, the community health nurse needs to have access to the most recent comprehensive insight. There is a wealth of information on the Internet regarding the frequency, occurrence, and patterns of substance abuse at the local, state, and common levels. Community health nurses must gain a comprehensive understanding of drug culture, terminology, and the various signs and symptoms associated with the use of harmful, illicit substances, especially among youth.

2.5.5. Conceptualizations of Substance Abuse

The way that substance abuse and dependence are conceptualized has evolved, frequently due to social and political factors rather than scientific ones. The phenomenon of addiction, which is characterized by compulsive use patterns and the onset of withdrawal symptoms upon abrupt cessation of substance use, is the subject of some conceptualizations. Regardless of the existence of an addictive pattern, other perspectives center on the issues arising from substance use itself. Addiction to substances can lead to many problematic outcomes, such as intoxication, psychological dependence, relationship problems, problems finding work or money, legal issues, and health issues. For instance, the use of illegal drugs can have legal repercussions even in the absence of addiction, such as drunk driving or drug- or alcohol-related domestic violence. When it comes to substance use, it can be difficult to distinguish between the concepts of abuse, addiction, and dependence when there is evidence of problematic substance use. It could be misleading to categorize all repetitive or obsessive behavior patterns as addiction or dependence, since interventions may be necessary before addiction manifests itself, such as when use has turned into misuse and a problem is apparent. It is also becoming more and more clear that different kinds of interventions might be required for different types of addiction (such as gambling and overeating). Furthermore, a great deal of individual diversity exists within each particular group.

2.5.6. Sociocultural and Political Aspects of Substance Abuse

Substance abuse issues are not always simple to recognize in community settings. For instance, media coverage of the effects of crack cocaine use and sales in an African American inner-city neighborhood may be evident. Conversely, it's harder to identify when these drugs are being trafficked into the middle classes. It may come as a shock to some nurses that older people are becoming more and more dependent on alcohol and other drugs, including illegal ones. It can, however, be understood in a context-specific manner and could stem from a variety of factors, including anxiety, uncontrollable chronic pain, isolation, fears, and sleep disturbances. In providing community-based patient care, nurses need to consider sociocultural and political factors. To model a more comprehensive, multifaceted approach to substance abuse prevention and management, nurses must also possess knowledge that helps them refute stereotypes in the media.

Although there are subcultural and regional variations, the drinking norms of the dominant culture in the United States are relatively permissive. Traditional ethnic ceremonial and symbolic substance use patterns vary significantly. As acculturation occurs, however, cultural definitions of "appropriate" use of alcohol and drugs have been dulled, leaving a void regarding social expectations. Subcultural groups such as gay, lesbian, bisexual, and transgender persons have often had a social center that was a bar, and alcohol use was historically a way of demonstrating and celebrating differentiation from a more repressive majority. These cultural conditions create ambiguity in clearly determining when a substance abuse problem exists. Furthermore, each subculture may define abuse differently. It can be theorized that stigmatized minorities might be under more stress, and perhaps more likely to use substances, but this cannot be assumed in any individual case.

In a range of social contexts, both legal and illicit, substances are valued economically and traded like commodities. Economic, cultural, and political factors have a significant influence on the production and distribution of drugs, including nicotine, prescription drugs, and alcohol, among different groups in society. The dynamics of drug distribution can have numerous other effects as different subgroups achieve and preserve status. A group experiencing conflicting or nonexistent cultural values is chaotic and disorganized. Conflicting value systems cause cultures to break apart and people to feel helpless and hopeless. The gang becomes vulnerable to elements that put its survival at even greater risk. When divergent values prevent the group from coming together or from agreeing on a common course, the members become disenfranchised and isolated. People of color's history of cocaine abuse and dependence serves as an illustration of the connections between these disorders. Although crack cocaine was most common in impoverished areas, cocaine use was epidemic in the 1980s and early 1990s. However, in recent years, the use of cocaine has significantly decreased. (Stanhop et al., 2000; Sheila et al., 2000).

A Closer Look

Maternal/Child Health Programs

Maternal and child health programs are vital components of public health initiatives aimed at improving the well-being of mothers and children. These programs encompass a range of services designed to address the unique health needs of women during pregnancy, childbirth, and the postpartum period, as well as the health and development of children from infancy through adolescence. Key components of maternal and child health programs include prenatal care, which ensures early and regular monitoring of the health of the mother and fetus, helps manage pre-existing conditions, and screens for potential complications. Prenatal care is critical for preventing adverse outcomes such as preterm birth, low birth weight, and maternal mortality. Additionally, maternal health programs often provide education on nutrition, exercise, and lifestyle choices that promote a healthy pregnancy and prepare mothers for childbirth and parenting.

Child health services within these programs are equally comprehensive, focusing on essential aspects such as immunizations, growth monitoring, and developmental screenings. Immunizations protect children from preventable diseases like measles, polio, and whooping cough, which can have severe or fatal consequences. Regular health check-ups allow for the early detection of growth or developmental issues, ensuring timely interventions that can significantly improve long-term outcomes. Maternal and child health programs also emphasize the importance of breastfeeding, offering support and education to mothers to encourage breastfeeding, which provides optimal nutrition and strengthens the immune system of infants.

Nutrition programs are a critical component, addressing both maternal and child malnutrition, which remains a significant global health challenge. These programs provide access to essential vitamins and minerals, fortified foods, and education on balanced diets. They also address the specific nutritional needs of pregnant and lactating women to support healthy pregnancies and breastfeeding.

Mental health services are increasingly integrated into maternal and child health programs, recognizing the profound impact of mental well-being on physical health. For mothers, screening for and treating conditions such as postpartum depression is essential, as untreated maternal mental health issues can adversely affect both mother and child. Child mental health services focus on identifying and addressing behavioral and emotional problems early, supporting healthy psychological development.

Community-based interventions play a crucial role in the success of maternal and child health programs. By engaging local health workers and volunteers, these programs can reach underserved populations, providing education and services in culturally appropriate ways. Community health workers often serve as vital links between healthcare providers and families, ensuring adherence to health recommendations and facilitating access to healthcare services.

Policy and advocacy are integral to the sustainability and effectiveness of maternal and child health programs. Governments and international organizations work to create supportive policies, allocate funding, and promote practices that enhance the health of mothers and children. This includes advocating for paid maternity leave, access to quality healthcare, and education for girls, which are all factors that contribute to improved maternal and child health outcomes.

Overall, maternal and child health programs are essential for building healthy societies. They reduce mortality and morbidity rates, promote healthy development, and contribute to the overall well-being of communities. By providing comprehensive, accessible, and culturally sensitive healthcare services, these programs ensure that mothers and children receive the care and support they need to thrive. Effective maternal and child health programs are characterized by their holistic approach, addressing physical, nutritional, and mental health needs, and by their ability to adapt to the unique challenges of different populations.

Summary

- Community health nursing revolves around promoting and preserving the health of populations within specific communities. Unlike other nursing specialties that primarily focus on individual patient care, community health nursing adopts a broader perspective, targeting entire communities or populations.
- Community health nurses fill health system gaps for underserved populations. They go to organizations, schools, and businesses to offer health education, medical services, and rehabilitation.
- The responsibilities of these nurses differ in each career path, but all community health nurses promote healthy living, disease prevention, and necessary medical treatment. Additionally, community health nurses create programs that promote community health and collect data to identify community needs. Careers can be pursued in public health, faith community nursing, and school nursing.
- Community health nursing is a multifaceted discipline that requires professionals to assume various roles and responsibilities to foster community well-being.
- Faith community nurses, often known as parish nurses, provide health education for a specific church parish. They also counsel their faith communities on health issues and perform medical evaluations for congregation members like administering blood pressure screenings in their place of worship or at a hospital.
- The nursing process is defined as a systematic, rational method of planning that guides all nursing actions in delivering holistic and patient-focused care. The nursing process is a form of scientific reasoning and requires the nurse's critical thinking to provide the best care possible to the client.
- The unique approach of the nursing process requires care respectful of and responsive to the individual patient's needs, preferences, and values. The nurse functions as a patient advocate by keeping the patient's right to practice informed decision-making and maintaining patient-centered engagement in the health care setting.

References

1. Allender, J. A., & Walton, B. (2001). *Community Health Nursing: Concept and Practice* (5th ed.). Lippincott Williams & Wilkins.
2. Barbara, W., & Judith, A. (1996). *Community Health Nursing: Concept & Practice* (4th ed.). Lippincott Williams & Wilkins.
3. Bray, R. M., Pemberton, M. R., Lane, M. E., & Hoggatt, K. J. (2010). Substance use and mental health trends among U.S. military active-duty personnel: Key findings from the 2008 DoD health behavior survey. *Military Medicine, 175*(6), 390–399. https://doi.org/10.7205/MILMED-D-09-00128.
4. Bullough, B., & Bullough, R. (1990). *Nursing in the Community*. CV Mosby Company.
5. Center for Substance Abuse Treatment. (2005). *Medication-Assisted Treatment for Opioid Addiction in Opioid Treatment Programs* (Treatment Improvement Protocol [TIP] Series

43, DHHS Publication No. [SMA] 05-4048). Substance Abuse and Mental Health Services Administration.

6. Center for Substance Abuse Treatment. (2009). *Substance Abuse Treatment: Addressing the Specific Needs of Women* (Treatment Improvement Protocol [TIP] Series 51, HHS Publication No. [SMA] 09-4426). Substance Abuse and Mental Health Services Administration.
7. Cole, D. C., Davison, C., Hanson, L., Jackson, S. F., Page, A., Lencucha, R., & Kakuma, R. (2011). Being global in public health practice and research: Complementary competencies are needed. *Canadian Journal of Public Health, 102*(5), 394–397. https://doi.org/10.1007/BF03404255.
8. Edmonds, J. K., Campbell, L. A., & Gilder, R. E. (2017). Public health nursing practice in the Affordable Care Act era: A national survey. *Public Health Nursing, 34*(1), 50–58. https://doi.org/10.1111/phn.12275.
9. Johnston, L. D., O'Malley, P. M., Bachman, J. G., & Schulenberg, J. E. (2013). *Monitoring the Future National Results on Drug Use: 2012 Overview, Key Findings on Adolescent Drug Use.* Institute for Social Research, The University of Michigan.
10. Kunyk, D., & Austin, W. (2012). Nursing under the influence: A relational ethics perspective. *Nursing Ethics, 19*(3), 380–389. https://doi.org/10.1177/0969733011426596.
11. Lane, D. C., & Simmons, J. (2011). American Indian youth substance abuse: Community-driven interventions. *Mount Sinai Journal of Medicine, 78*(3), 362–372. https://doi.org/10.1002/msj.20261.
12. Mattson, R. E., O'Ferrell, T. J., Lofgreen, A. M., & Fink, E. E. (2012). The role of substance uses in a conceptual model of inmate partner violence in men undergoing treatment for alcoholism. *Psychology of Addictive Behaviors, 26*(2), 255–262. https://doi.org/10.1037/a0026657.
13. National Institute on Drug Abuse. (2010a). *Drugs, Brains, and Behavior: The Science of Addiction* (NIH Publication No. 10-5605). National Institutes of Health.
14. Sheila, T., Barhana, R., & Sarah, A. (2000). *Community Health Care Nursing: Principles & Practice.* HarperCollins.
15. Stanhope, M., & Knollmiller, M. (2000). *Community & Public Health Nursing* (5th ed.). Mosby.
16. Stanhope, M., & Knollmiller, M. (2000). *Handbook of Community-Based & Home Health Nursing Practice* (3rd ed.). Mosby.
17. Weir, E., Schabas, R., Wilson, K., & Mackie, C. (2010). A Canadian framework for applying the precautionary principle to public health issues. *Canadian Journal of Public Health, 101*(5), 396–398. https://doi.org/10.1007/BF03404095.

Chapter 3

ROLE OF SOCIAL AND BEHAVIORAL SCIENCE IN PUBLIC HEALTH

Contents

Introduction

Today, smoking, eating poorly, exercising infrequently, abusing drugs or alcohol, engaging in sexual activity, and not having access to healthcare are the main behavioral and social factors that contribute to mortality. Studies conducted in the past ten years have shown how successful interventions based on social and behavioral science theory are in preventing HIV, heart disease, alcohol-related issues, cancer, homelessness, and mental health issues. The importance of behavioral and social sciences to the practice of public health is demonstrated by these studies. Multilevel interventions that take into account the interactions between social, environmental, biological, and behavioral factors are more likely to be successful in promoting community health, according to mounting evidence.

Disease surveillance, safeguarding the public from health risks like tainted food and water, putting policies in place to stop and manage epidemics, and offering restricted clinical services (like STI and maternity care) have historically been the top priorities of state and local public health departments. Activities aimed at preventing disease and promoting health have become part of the health department's expanded mandate in recent years. The application of social and behavioral sciences in public health, especially in the areas of health promotion and disease prevention, has been supported by the National Institutes of Health, the Centers for Disease Control and Prevention, and other federal agencies. The Committee on Capitalizing on Social Science and Behavioral Research to Improve the Public's Health was established by the Institute of Medicine in 2000.

Orientation and Directional Terms

Term	Definition	Illustration
Clinical services	Clinical services means counselling, assessment, group therapy, family therapy, medication management, or other services that require specialized knowledge and training in the assessment and treatment of mental health and substance use disorders.	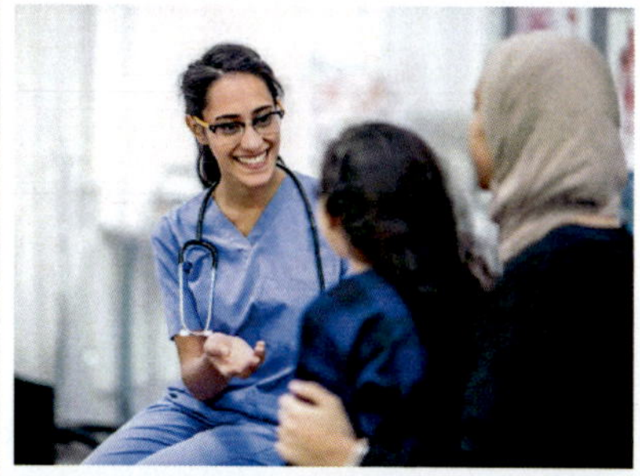
Community Health	Community health refers to non-treatment-based health services that are delivered outside hospitals and clinics. Community health is a subset of public health that is taught to and practiced by clinicians as part of their normal duties.	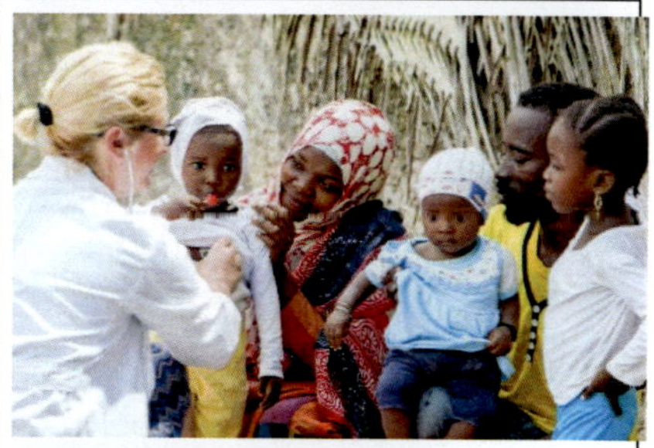
Epidemic	An epidemic is the rapid spread of disease to a large number of hosts in a given population within a short period.	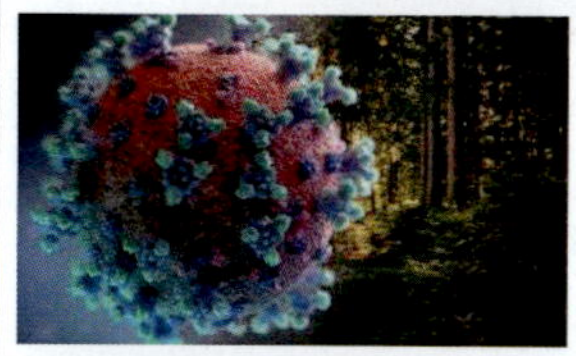
Infectious diseases	Infectious diseases are disorders caused by organisms — such as bacteria, viruses, fungi or parasites. Many organisms live in and on our bodies. They're normally harmless or even helpful. But under certain conditions, some organisms may cause disease.	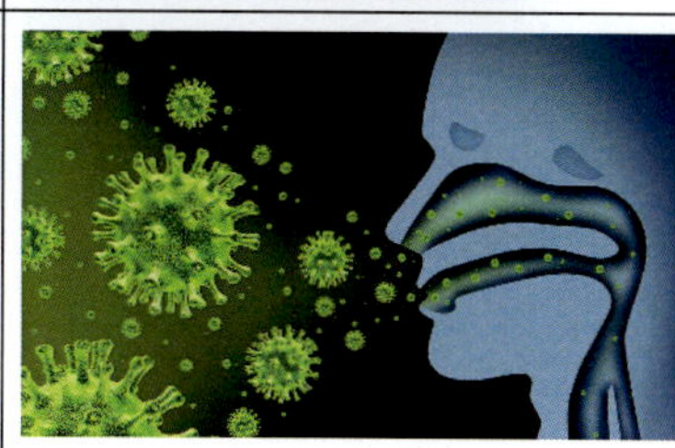
Health promotion	Health promotion is the process of enabling people to increase control over, and to improve, their health. It moves beyond a focus on individual behavior towards a wide range of social and environmental interventions.	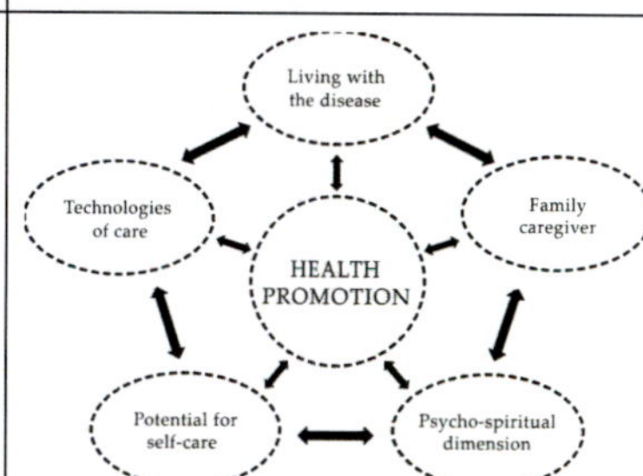

3.1. Social Science In Public Health

Discovering the characteristics of human behavior has been the primary goal of social scientists for several decades, and one of their main concerns has been the comparative study of communities. Public health professionals are especially interested in learning about these attributes since they typically focus on the social rather than the individual organism. To put it another way, social organisms have unique physiologies and anatomy. Even though a community is made up of unique individuals, as a whole it is far more than the sum of its parts; it possesses unique qualities.

Every community has its own social structure—the way individuals relate to one another—as well as a corresponding cultural pattern made up of common beliefs, attitudes, and values. Communities also have their habitats. Any group's sociocultural structure is an integral part of their environment, just like the actual physical surroundings they live in. As a result, it has a significant impact on how health and illness are portrayed as well as how community health initiatives perform. Sociocultural system analysts can make a valuable contribution to basic health research, particularly in cases where social factors are important for the etiology of a disease, such as chronic and psychiatric disorders. They can also help advance the cause of better program execution, especially by supporting the challenging undertaking of program evaluation.

3.1.1. Evaluating Health Programs

In public health work, the term "evaluation" frequently has specific technical connotations, so for current purposes, the word "assessment" might be more appropriate. Program performance can generally be evaluated using criteria related to effort, effect, or process, or any combination of these. The effort criterion gauges the health team's vigor and productivity. Using this approach, progress is recorded in terms of distance traveled, meetings attended, speeches delivered, leaflets distributed, films screened, questions answered, visits made, interviews conducted, and patients seen. Effort outcomes are measured by the effect criterion, not the effort itself. Program objectives must typically be stated clearly in order to use the effect method. The project outlines its goals and attempts to bring about the changes in behavior, mindset, or organization. It then evaluates the extent to which its goals have been met. The process criterion evaluates how the effect was attained; even in the absence of notable changes, it may be helpful to examine why the program cycled back and forth.

3.1.1.1. Assessment of Effort

There are several reasons why the first of these three, the effort yardstick, is useful. Maintaining administrative statistics is typically simpler than understanding or quantifying the true state of the community. Listing the things one has done and the people one has seen has a certain objectivity and concreteness to it; these can be quantified and added up, making them facts rather than conjectures. Additionally, it appears that American culture values effort highly for its own sake—that is, that if one stays busy, good things will eventually happen. Many middle-class Americans believe that gauging one's level of busyness is akin to gauging one's morality and productivity.

The program assessment effort yardstick has actual value in addition to being somewhat of a magic trick to lift our spirits. Effort statistics can be, at most, inconclusive in a negative way. Statistics indicating an agency's inactivity suggest that not much progress is being made in terms of health promotion. Even though not all effort yields positive outcomes, it does require effort to get anything done.

3.1.1.2. Assessment of Effect

Suppose a health agency is dedicated to changing a community's health habits or attitudes. After a period of effort the agency wants to know: Did any change occur? Was the change the one intended? Was the program the cause of the change? There are fairly standardized techniques for supplying the answers. The classical experimental design is simple in principle for this use. The health habits of a community are measured before and after the campaign, for example, using questionnaires or interviews and appropriate sampling techniques.

A few years ago, Dodd implemented a design in several Syrian villages and discovered that hygienic practices had improved by approximately 20% over time. This improvement might have occurred independently of the health campaign. To investigate further, Dodd also collected data from other Syrian communities where no health initiatives were implemented, expecting to see less improvement compared to the experimental villages. Surprisingly, the control villages also showed a 20% improvement, casting doubt on the impact of the health program. The reason for this outcome remains unknown in the Syrian case, highlighting a limitation in measuring effects. To truly understand the cause, we need to evaluate the process. Another example can help illustrate this concept.

In a relatively wealthy Canadian prairie town, a group of social workers, sociologists, and psychiatrists recently launched a rigorous six-month campaign to change public perceptions of people with mental illnesses. They reasoned that the high rate of readmission to overcrowded hospitals and relapse was influenced by an unfavorable attitude toward mentally ill patients who were discharged. They made a name for themselves in the experimental community, won over editors, civic leaders, and other powerful people, and employed a variety of strategies and tools, including radio broadcasts, movies, pamphlets, unique books kept in the library, newspaper notices, public speakers, small-group discussions, and so on.

Before and after the campaign, hundreds of questionnaires were revealing to reveal attitudes toward mental illness, including beliefs about its causes, curability, the extent of one's responsibility for supporting a sick relative, and willingness to interact with someone who had been released from a mental health facility. Similar to Dodd's experience in Syria, they conducted the same tests twice in a different town without attempting to launch a health education campaign. As anticipated, there was no discernible shift in the attitudes of the residents of this control town during the course of the six months. Regretfully, though, neither did the locals in the area where the comprehensive awareness campaign had been implemented. The project staff possessed nearly zero effect in good measure. This disappointing result had instructive reasons. But to comprehend the need for their investigation process. It should be mentioned, incidentally, that program success is not always a prerequisite for useful program assessment in terms of process. Looking for the mechanisms underlying failure can be just as insightful.

3.1.1.3. Assessment of Process

Three conditions in the Canadian experiment allowed for an understanding of the working mechanisms. Project staff members, for example, conducted a series of in-depth interviews both prior to and following the educational campaign; this data allowed them to examine the dynamics of the public's perceptions regarding mental illness. For another, they observed the shift in the response they got; formerly friendly, the tone gradually shifted to indifference and finally turned hostile. In addition, they made sense of the data they gathered and examined using a social science framework.

They came to the following conclusion regarding the procedure that rendered their efforts useless. One of the concepts they had worked so hard to instill was that personality types ranged from completely normal to fully abnormal, and that most patients who were released from hospitals were not fundamentally different from other people and should be treated as such. There was also no clear-cut boundary between the sane and the insane. Relapse rates were to be decreased by increasing comprehension and tolerance through the use of this kind of information.

However, the community's members obstinately held onto their binary understanding of normalcy and abnormality. It appeared that they had built a psychological wall at the bottom, separating the insane from the sane, never sure about their sanity. The hospitalized minority suffered as a result of this attitude, but the majority felt somewhat reassured and kept within the norm. By questioning this prevalent mindset, the educators were igniting long-suppressed fears. It was preferred by the populace to let sleeping dogs lie. With no prepared rational defenses and subjected to reasonable educational efforts, they responded as most people would in similar circumstances. Following a brief period of willing cooperation, they eventually displayed open hostility toward the program staff.

In this Canadian case, the practical lesson is rather obvious. It is wise to assess the established habits and ideas and, more importantly, the psychological and social roles these beliefs and practices serve before attempting to replace outdated health habits and ideas, whether they relate to sanitation or sanity. It is important to comprehend both the overt and covert goals of a community's customs. Social science can be particularly helpful in determining the implicit purposes of a group's beliefs and behavioral patterns. Social scientists can help measure the effects of programs, but their bigger contribution to program evaluation will likely come from looking deeper to uncover the implicit processes that are always at play in the community beneath successful and unsuccessful cases.

It should be clear that social scientists can assist program operations in other ways as well, provided they are carefully chosen and employed. In addition to helping to maintain programs' effectiveness and vitality by serving as a liaison between project staff and the community, they can perform social mapping in advance of program planning. This isn't to say that social scientists should take on the roles of health educators or social workers, who are the operational members of the public health team. Social scientists are frequently best served by monitoring public opinion to determine the effects of health action, as opposed to actively taking part in the program's action phase. Understanding the various subfields of social research and their standard methods of inquiry is necessary for the wise application and selection of social scientists.

3.1.2. Social Science Disciplines

In this day and age, universal social scientists are as rare as universal natural scientists. In actuality, men are educated to be economists, political scientists, psychologists, sociologists, or anthropologists; they typically do not hold doctorates in social science per se. Health professionals should take note of this fact because it can be more advantageous to use a certain social science discipline in a given teaching or service scenario than another.

Every social science discipline has its strong points, and even though there may be more similarities than differences between them, it may still be helpful to take into account the methodological quirks that set some of the social sciences apart. All three disciplines—psychology, sociology, and anthropology—have a propensity to generate their own data, which sets them apart from the fields of government and economics, which primarily rely on statistical compilations and library materials. However, there are differences between psychology, sociology, and anthropology in terms of the types of primary data that they typically generate. Experimental data involving humans or animals as subjects is a major source of information for social psychology. Sociology makes extensive use of questionnaires and interviews, typically one-on-one conversations with numerous participants. Field notes, which are based on their own firsthand observations of behavior, and in-depth interviews with a small number of relatively well-known informants are typically the main sources of information used by anthropologists.

Because anthropologists typically work in environments where little is known and where less can be taken for granted, there is a chance that the methodological differences between anthropology and sociology reflect differences in the populations that each discipline has traditionally studied as well as differences in the stages of inquiry. Sociologists have therefore examined the variations between American parents who agreed to let their kids participate in experimental polio vaccination trials and those who declined to give their consent. To identify systematic differences between the two subpopulations, the issue was formulated, the population was divided into some-do and some-do-not categories, and many questions were asked that were successfully pretested.

Anthropologist Edward Wellin was also intrigued by a some-do and some-do-not criterion when he tried to explain why many other women in a Peruvian town did not alter their habits despite being persuaded to do so by the health department to boil tainted drinking water. But he didn't prepare a list of questions to ask methodically or set up two populations that were starkly different from one another beforehand. He spent several months talking to housewives, having conversations with the local hygiene worker, and observing both in their daily routines while working in an environment where he was unable to predict ahead of time which questions would prove to be pertinent. At last, he discovered that he could divide his population into six categories based on how they handled the boiling water problem. Even before the health department arrived, two groups of women had formed the habit of boiling their water, though they did so for very different reasons. Though the reasons for persuasion were different, two other groups of housewives submitted to influence. For different reasons, two sizable groups remained unconverted.

Important information that came to light gradually was that boiling drinking water was something that was always done in the brief time that followed making breakfast, if it was done at all, and for whatever reason. For a variety of pragmatic and cultural reasons, including the widespread notion that water that boiled in the afternoon or evening and was stored overnight would need to be reboiled the next day, all other times of the day were excluded. This idea was connected to the widespread perceptions of "hot" and "cold" substances found throughout much of Latin America. However, they emphasize the importance of direct observation, developing close relationships with a small number of informants, and mastering the local vernacular more than they do. Various social scientists can contribute to public health practice in different ways, depending on the nature of the problem, the target population, and the research stage.

It is unrealistic to expect public health professionals to fully utilize social science theories and practices unless they are given the chance to become knowledgeable about social science methodology. Integrating social science education into the curricula of public health schools is one method of disseminating this knowledge.

3.2. A Framework for Social Science in Epidemics

Social science plays a crucial role in guiding action when it comes to epidemic preparedness and response. Anthropologists were included in response teams during the Ebola outbreak in West Africa, and social scientists with subject-matter and regional expertise, emergency responders, public health professionals, and local communities were able to share ideas on these platforms. Epidemic response organizations have since realized that knowing the social dynamics and contexts in a community can help avoid the unnecessary expenses and harm associated with "context-blind" interventions.

Regretfully, social science has been mostly excluded from RCCE initiatives. Although they are important for highlighting contextual factors that need to be addressed to enhance messaging and alter behaviors that raise the risk of infection, social science applications to all facets of epidemic response are overlooked. Researchers and practitioners in the field of public health find it challenging to interact with social science research, and they would benefit from resources that allow them to utilize social science insights.

To rethink social science's role in epidemic response and make it more approachable for public health and practitioner communities, we offer a new framework that builds on the experience of the Social Science and Humanitarian Action Platform (SSHAP) and research funded by the Office of US Disaster Assistance (OFDA) at USAID that examines entry points for social science in epidemics. The framework does more than just break down the social, political, economic, and cultural aspects of context; it also places disease in its proper context and examines how the response to it is dynamic. It also looks at how various people, social groups, and organizations change their knowledge and behaviors during an epidemic through dialogue and learning processes that are laden with power, or even by marginalizing and silencing one another.

3.2.1. The Framework

The framework consists of the three key dimensions of an epidemic, which are illustrated below in Figure 3.1 as the points of a triangle: disease, context, and response. The framework also explores three different types of interactions between each of these dimensions (captured in the sides of the triangles): between disease and context, between context and the response, and between the response and the disease. Lastly, the framework shows an emergent dimension as a result of these interactions: dialogue and learning.

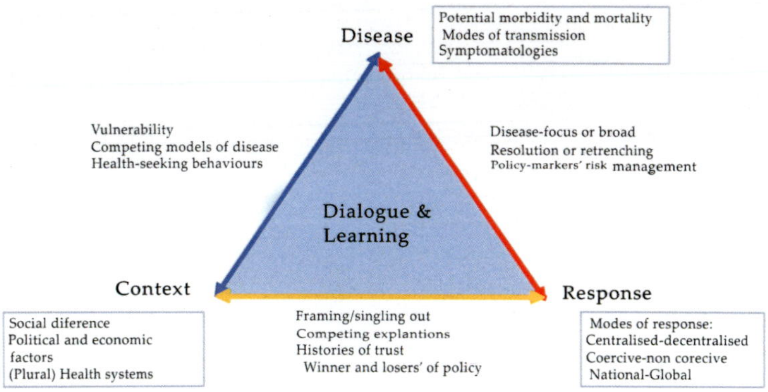

Figure 3.1. *The social science in epidemics framework.*

Source: *https://www.berghahnjournals.com/view/journals/aia/29/1/aia290102.xm.*

3.2.1.1. Disease

The severity of a disease is influenced by the socio-biological traits of a microorganism that (re) emerges in that particular setting. Its pathogenic features will determine the disease's potential rates of morbidity and mortality, specific populations' biological susceptibility, and its ability to spread across species. It also establishes the symptoms and mechanisms of transmission of the latter. The epidemic disease might exhibit synergistic traits that amplify its negative effects on health when it coexists with other illnesses.

For example, SARS-CoV-2 variants and their transmissibility, morbidity, and ability to evade immune response are always a concern in the ongoing COVID-19 pandemic. Due to its syndemic potential, SARS-CoV-2 is far more dangerous for elderly individuals, those with heart problems, obesity, diabetes, and other medical conditions. These "pre-existing" conditions are influenced by the social and political factors that determine a context's health. (Williamson et al., 2020).

3.2.1.2. Context

There are specific social, political, economic, and cultural settings in which infectious diseases arise. The emergence of the disease and its course among various vulnerable groups are shaped by this context. Three main dimensions can be identified within context: political economy, social difference, and cultural logic. Political economy examines politics and power among various stakeholders in the context of the pandemic. Depending on the social and political histories of the impacted communities, different social groups will have different levels of trust for particular individuals and organizations. Social difference illustrates how, as a result of social roles and practices, different social groups are more or less susceptible to infection, disease, and death. Cultural logic describes how communities understand health and illness, how they explain the emergence of epidemics, and how they can respond locally. Health systems frequently have a variety of health providers, both conventional and alternative (such as faith-based and traditional healers, and drug dealers), and various communities have varied disease models and etymologies that may or may not coincide with conventional models.

3.2.1.3. Response

Governments and international aid organizations may present a disease as an "outbreak," label it as endemic, or choose to ignore it completely. Framings of outbreak diseases lead to interventions that extend beyond the standard operations of health systems, involving a range of initiatives implemented at various levels and by various institutions and response organizations. Relationships between these responders and the impacted local populations grow out of the local politics and history as well as the type of intervention—local or global actors leading, decentralized or centralized, coercive or participatory, etc.

Resentment and mistrust are caused by coercive government responses to epidemics. For instance, when the Ebola outbreak struck Monrovia in 2014, the city's mandatory cremation policy sparked mistrust in the response and an increase in covert burials. While coordination may be aided by centralizing response efforts, trust can be built and service uptake increased through decentralizing response efforts carried out by impacted communities and supported by neighborhood trusted actors. Successful instances of the devolution of activities include the establishment of Community Care Centers for Ebola in Sierra Leone and the hiring of local teams for the distribution of vaccines. Epidemic response has the potential to grow into a complex web of national and international public, nonprofit, and private sector organizations. It is essential to comprehend the political dynamics of a response and to recognize the ways in which various response actors and activities are viewed by various social groups within a given context.

3.2.2. Interactions Between Disease and Context

People in affected communities have varying susceptibilities to disease because these communities are diverse. For instance, women who perform unpaid caregiving are more likely to contract Ebola than men. Healers and caregivers are also more vulnerable to infection. When there is an epidemic, people's (in)ability to follow public health measures is frequently greatly influenced by their low-wage or informal employment. Low-paid "frontline" workers have been more vulnerable to respiratory illnesses like influenza and COVID-19 because they are unable to work remotely, must use public transportation, and are more likely to live in impoverished and crowded environments. Social groups that have historically experienced material disadvantage and marginalization at the national level (migrants, Indigenous peoples, nomadic populations, etc.) are more likely to have poorer access to health services and underlying health conditions that increase their susceptibility (such as undernutrition and measles vulnerability). For example, in the United Kingdom, COVID-19 has disproportionately affected Black and Asian ethnic minority communities, who have historically experienced systemic discrimination that has led to poor health and high exposure.

Biomedical models may not align with regional disease models, alternative health providers' methods, or patient behaviors when it comes to seeking medical attention. Overlaps are possible, though, and local models are flexible and dynamic. An excellent illustration of this adaptability is the change to modified "safe and dignified burials" during the Ebola response in West Africa that satisfied public health objectives as well as symbolic, social, and emotional priorities.

3.2.3. Interactions Between Context and Response

Focusing on specific groups without understanding the context can have unintended negative outcomes. In the 1990s, targeted Cholera interventions in Latin America led to victim-blaming and stigmatization of the most affected populations: the poor and Indigenous groups lacking access to proper water, sanitation, and healthcare. Similarly, public health measures like transport bans and culling animals in response to diseases like Avian Influenza have disproportionately harmed small-scale farmers and pastoralists economically.

Causal interpretations of disease are invariably shaped by socio-political fault lines and historical grievances. For instance, when epidemics strike historically underprivileged populations, people often have misgivings about the response and see the government as either the disease's source or a careless responder. A common phrase in post-colonial states where resource extraction has occurred in the past and continues now is "Ebola business." In the DRC, the Ebola outbreak was perceived as an additional revenue stream for the government.

3.2.4. Interactions Between Response and Disease

Focusing on specific diseases during epidemics can attract resources but may not align with local priorities. For instance, during the Ebola response in North Kivu, DRC from 2018–2020, affected communities were more concerned about safety from violence and receiving proper support for issues like malaria and undernutrition. COVID-19 responses in lower- and middle-income countries have negatively impacted other health outcomes in the short and long term. Setting up disease-specific treatment centers can also result in stigmatization. In the case of Cholera, providing services through comprehensive programs for diarrheal diseases and promoting universal messaging helped decrease stigma, rather than targeting already marginalized populations.

When cholera outbreaks are treated with symptomatic treatment and emergency vaccination, they are likely to recur unless states provide the necessary WASH infrastructure. In the case of COVID-19, vaccine disparities will probably result in the virus's almost complete eradication in the Global North, but the illness will continue to pose an endemic threat in developing nations. The unpredictable nature of many diseases' emergence is another cause for concern. Policymakers, for instance, have little incentive to address animal cases of Rift Valley Fever in Kenya since doing so would be expensive both politically and economically and there's no guarantee that the disease would spread to humans. To reduce these disincentives, consensus policy mechanisms that define response strategies based on ambiguous evidence should be established.

3.2.5. Dialogue and Learning

The dynamic interactions between pathogens, context, and response lead to the emergence of various knowledge within diverse communities and social groups. Each group may have different perspectives on defining problems, relevant questions, what constitutes good evidence, and reasons for changing practices. The competition over which knowledge is valued in an epidemic is filled with power struggles. Groups may compete, ignore, or cooperate, either engaging in dialogue and learning or attempting to dominate and silence others.

3.2.6. Framings of the Disease

Disease will be portrayed differently by different social groups with varying levels of power. For example, it may be framed as an individual or structural issue, as a medical or political phenomenon, or as an outbreak emergency or not. For instance, the Ethiopian government preserved its face as the ruling party but failed to communicate the urgency of the cholera outbreak to communities when they referred to it as "Acute Watery Diarrhea" instead of the illness's local name. Strong nations in the Global

North may ignore chronic infectious diseases in favor of responding to outbreaks with significant funding, especially if the spread is expected to cross national borders.

3.2.7. Dialogues Between Different Types of Expertise and Evidence

Based on varying ideas of what constitutes "good evidence," various social groups develop conflicting explanations of illness and the necessary course of action. The preponderance of "expert" evidence in the fields of biomedicine and epidemiology may be at odds with information from non-experts, other disciplines, and local communities' models of disease. Because biomedical and epidemiological knowledge dominated the COVID-19 response in the UK, assumptions about people's behavior were frequently off, which resulted in inappropriate contact tracing, delayed lockdowns, and a failure to build on pre-existing community initiatives. The Ugandan response occurred in the context of recent and controversial elections in January 2021, even though it was primarily led by biomedical experts and was layered on top of pre-existing socio-political realities. The harshness of the response and its military implementation were frequently seen as more political than scientific, especially in the disenfranchised communities on the outskirts of the nation. However, these perceptions are context-dependent and vary over time.

3.2.7.1. Learning Processes

As epidemics and responses develop within a context, communities, organizations, and the response as a whole learn and adapt accordingly. There are various ways to learn; for example, learning from direct empirical observations might be more significant than learning through traditional communication techniques. The perception of risk and adherence to public health recommendations may rise as more people become aware of those who have fallen ill or passed away. A response's ability to recognize uncertainty and iteratively incorporate community feedback may determine how successful it is. A review and collection of social data from radio, hotlines, SMS, and in-person meetings has informed UNICEF's Eastern and Southern Africa Regional Office (ESARO)'s RCCE activities during COVID-19. These observations guarantee that COVID-19 communication is in line with the needs and concerns of the community. As demonstrated by the West African Ebola pandemic, communities, and other local actors can offer solutions to an epidemic locally even before the official response is launched. The 2018 DRC Ebola outbreak provides yet another illustration of a response shaped by learning. Teams were able to adjust quickly because Oxfam field workers routinely asked community members about their perspectives. For example, upon discovering that the community members were uneasy interacting with outside responders, they assisted in the establishment of comité cellules, which are groups of trusted, locally elected community members who facilitated local communication and action plan implementation.

3.2.7.2. Openings

The framework highlights some of the "openings" for operations and policy that result from integrating social science intelligence in attempts to comprehend the relationships between illness, context, and response as well as how specific knowledge, skills, and learning processes develop throughout an epidemic. These "openings," which need to be modified for particular epidemic contexts, include the following elements.

3.2.7.3. Advocating for the Devolution and/or Decentralization of the Response and the Need for Multi-Scalar and Multi-Sectorial Coordination

Effectiveness and trust are increased when impacted populations take ownership of response efforts. It is essential to coordinate efforts across sectors (human and animal health, WASH, education, livelihoods) and at various scales (international, national, regional, and local).

3.2.7.4. Leveraging Existing Community Mechanisms

One can build upon communities, their social structures, movements, and initiatives. Having said that, it's critical to recognize potential rifts within local communities and to recognize both formal and informal sources of locally dependable public authority.

3.2.7.5. Framing of the Response as a Dialogue of Different Forms of Expertise

A more comprehensive picture will be obtained by incorporating a variety of knowledge sources, such as big data technologies, social science inputs, first-hand community knowledge and feedback, local and frontline health providers' insights (including those from alternative health providers), epidemiological and medical knowledge, etc. Being truthful about what is and is not known as the epidemic develops is essential.

3.2.7.6. Addressing the 'Behavioral' and the Structural

To respond to an epidemic, people must alter risky behaviors. There are valid and logical justifications for the actions that people take. This can include situations where the new behavior is not "resisted," but rather is not adopted due to a lack of the necessary infrastructure, as in the Horn of Africa's case with sufficient WASH infrastructure, or the vulnerability of West African health systems before the Ebola outbreak.

3.2.7.7. Incorporating Social Science Intelligence in Epidemic Preparedness and Response in a Systematic Way

Social science evidence applies to all sectors and pillars of epidemic response, despite its typical relegation to RCCE. It should be integrated into the systems of preparedness and response architecture that are already in place. One excellent example is the Social Science Analysis Cell, which carried out social science research in North Kivu that was operationally relevant for all response sectors and pillars.

3.2.7.8. Embracing Uncertainty: Balancing Preparedness with Nimbleness and Adaptability of Response

During epidemics, there is a great deal of biological, epidemiological, and social uncertainty. To address new and emerging biological threats, unpredictable epidemiological trajectories, and social reactions of various communities and institutions, the response must be quick, sensitive, and adaptable. It also needs to build on local ideas and innovations. (Carleton et al., 1995; Heubner et al., 1991).

3.3. The Future of the Social Sciences in Public Health

The field of social sciences has significantly improved population health. The value of the social sciences stems in part from their shared emphasis on recognizing and addressing enduring social realities and inequalities as well as their shared interest in expanding knowledge of the social forces that influence population health, even though the precise theories and methodologies used by each discipline differ. The health effects of stigma, prejudice, and discrimination; the influence of socioeconomic status, stress, social networks, social support, and place on shaping health and health inequalities; the role of policy, power, and politics in structuring population health; and the taking of social context into account when developing and implementing multilevel interventions that improve population health are just a few of the contributions made by social science research to population health (Sorensen et al., 2007).

There are plenty of chances for the social sciences to keep improving population health in revolutionary ways, but maintaining and growing these contributions will also present formidable obstacles. Obstacles arise from both the academy's internal and external sources. Recent congressional calls for drastically cutting, or even eliminating, funding for the social sciences present an external challenge. These calls may stem from beliefs that the social sciences are too "soft" and "liberal." Parts of the American public are becoming more and more hostile to science and experts, which is contributing to these dangers. Given the recent political upheavals, social scientists are increasingly uncertain about how the social sciences will be regarded and supported, which makes this an important moment to assess the social sciences' worth and role in public health.

The social sciences present their own set of difficulties. Nicholas Christakis, a sociologist and physician at Yale, criticized the social sciences in a widely read OpEd in The New York Times, saying that the field's continued stagnation is "counterproductive, constraining engagement with the scientific cutting edge and stifling the creation of new and useful knowledge." Christakis stated that it could "result in having the natural sciences co-opt topics rightly and beneficially in the purview of the social sciences" if the "basic DNA of the social sciences" were not changed. The significant financial investments being made in biomedicine (e.g., precision medicine, clinical healthcare) overpopulation health are further instances of the devaluation of the social sciences.

We contend that the field needs to address several critical tensions that we and others have identified to successfully navigate these difficulties. The balance between disciplinary and interdisciplinary structures; the social sciences' role in framing questions to advance public health; the dissemination of research beyond academia to impact population health; and the financial and institutional sustainability of the social sciences in public health are the four areas in which we highlight these tensions. This is by no means a comprehensive list, but it does highlight some of the tensions the field is currently facing and how they directly affect the way that the next generation of social scientists studying public health is trained. We also bring up other issues that the field needs to address outside of training, especially in light of the rapidly shifting political landscape that could diminish the importance of the social sciences. As academics from a variety of social science specialties within public health—including psychology, sociology, political science, and behavioral science—we address the issues discussed below from this point of view.

3.3.1. Consideration of Discipline Versus Interdisciplinary Structures and Foundations

The first major conflict concerns the motivations behind interdisciplinary work in public health as opposed to disciplinary work, as well as the proper place of conventional social science disciplines in organizations engaged in interdisciplinary public health research and training. There are currently many different institutional approaches to addressing the lack of structures in place to support and sustain traditional social science disciplines in public health. For instance, social science departments house certain programs related to population health, while public health schools house other social science programs related to public health.

Even though there seem to be a variety of approaches to integrating the social sciences with public health within academic institutions, many departments and schools have not invested as much in hiring different social scientists with specialized training (such as historians or anthropologists); instead, they have hired a comparatively higher number of behavioral scientists, some of whom may have received general training in social and behavioral science and do not possess specialized training in social science. Additionally, our experience has shown that there are occasionally ambiguities between the kind of training someone receives and the department in which they work (for example, a sociologist may be employed by a department of epidemiology with a strong focus on social epidemiology or by a department of social/ behavioral sciences).

The best way to educate the upcoming generation of social scientists in the field of public health will be significantly impacted by this tension. Right now, there are two primary strategies. One adopts the viewpoint of furthering social science discipline scholarship. This school of thought holds that maintaining disciplinary ties and providing social scientists with initial training and mentoring in their respective departments is crucial. Departments of social science offer a foundation in the ideas and practices that characterize their fields. Social scientists may be able to address significant public health issues with greater insight thanks to this disciplinary foundation, all the while advancing their fields.

This strategy has advantages, but it may also have disadvantages. For example, traditional social science departments might not see public health research as advancing discipline-specific theory or methods, or as answering the central questions these disciplines are pursuing. Keeping ties with the field can sometimes make it more difficult to address problems that are most pertinent to public health. The social sciences that are not related to public health, for instance, might concentrate on more specialized, disciplinary-specific issues, diverting attention from the problems that are most important to public health. Returning to the social sciences' original focus of addressing enduring, basic social issues like poverty and inequality may be necessary to solve this problem.

The second strategy is for public health researchers to go beyond social science departments and pursue training through an interdisciplinary degree. Proponents of this model contend that to effectively address public health issues and foster innovation, rigorous interdisciplinary work incorporating theories, methods, and approaches from across the social sciences is essential. The next generation is trained in this interdisciplinary science approach through a variety of programs. The Health and Society Scholars training program, for instance, was created by the Robert Wood Johnson Foundation and is the first postdoctoral program specifically focused on population health. Through weekly seminars led by interdisciplinary faculty, scholars from a variety of social science disciplines gained training in developing collaborative competencies, broadening their cross-disciplinary thinking, and acquiring a shared language across disciplines. One of the program's most significant legacy, despite its demise, was transforming the institutional culture and structure of the locations where it was based; new interdisciplinary research teams were formed, disciplinary silos were gradually dismantled, and the importance of interdisciplinarity was institutionalized.

However, there are many obstacles that could prevent this kind of training. For instance, multidisciplinary studies on public health are frequently conducted in settings that do not always support the social sciences. In addition, structural conditions within disciplines and institutions (e.g., expectations for tenure/promotion; funding structures; administrative or physical space barriers); and time constraints to foster such relationships can all make interdisciplinary work challenging. Language, values, and methods can all be obstacles to interdisciplinary work.

3.3.2. Content and Scope of Social Science Research in Public Health

The question of how the social sciences should frame questions to advance public health and whether social science research should concentrate on problems deemed to have high policy relevance represents a second major source of conflict. The "strategic science" approach aims to support evidence-based policymaking by methodically directing scholarship to have a more timely and purposeful impact on policy. According to its definition, strategic science is "research aimed at filling in knowledge gaps crucial to policy decisions, originating from the mutual exchange of information between researchers and policymakers, and disseminated not only through scholarly publications but also in formats pertinent to policymakers." As an illustration of this strategy, Roberto et al., examined the efficacy of including the total recommended calorie intake (2,000 calories) on menu labels—a topic that policymakers are currently debating. The researchers presented their findings to decision-makers, who incorporated them into the Affordable Care Act and the country's menu-labeling regulations.

Research that may not directly address policy issues but advances theory, scholarship, and the body of knowledge on a given topic or discipline is an alternative approach to strategic science. Meyer's research on minority stress theory serves as an illustration of this strategy. His stated objective when he began this work in the 1990s was knowledge production or the development of a theory explaining how social stressors shape health disparities related to sexual orientation. When or if this work would be used to influence policy was unclear.

The way that training is approached will be significantly impacted by these two strategies. Practitioners with doctorates and MPHs frequently lack the abilities to convert their research into evidence-based policy because formal public health training usually places little emphasis on policy-related competencies. In the future, a crucial choice will be whether to offer a foundation in training related to policy, which would include creating multi-sectoral teams, translating policies, writing policy briefs, and presenting research findings to policy-makers. A cross-university seminar to teach doctorate students how to translate policies using an apprenticeship model is one possible remedy.

3.3.3. Dissemination and Communication of Social Science Research in Public Health

The function of social scientists in interpreting and communicating research outside of academic settings is a further area of conflict. "An active approach of spreading evidence-based information to the target audience via determined channels using planned strategies" is the definition of dissemination. The scientific community cannot agree on what the proper roles of researchers should be in translating knowledge or where the lines should be drawn between advocacy, policy-making, and research. It is argued by some that social scientists shouldn't translate and distribute the work because it is perceived by some as overly advocative. In the past, there have been worries in academia that sharing research with decision-makers, important stakeholders, and the general public compromises the idea of scientific objectivity. In addition, social scientists are frequently unprepared to communicate outside of academia, and some argue that this is not their job.

An alternative perspective holds that social scientists have a fundamental duty to convey novel ideas in a way that upholds social science within broader networks, contexts, and systems. In recent years, a science of dissemination and implementation has emerged to address this responsibility. Brownson along with others, for example, have identified a variety of structural strategies and systems to promote the dissemination of research, such as requiring a dissemination plan in funding announcements and offering academic incentives (e.g., related to tenure). There is a spectrum of activities that researchers can undertake to varying degrees to translate their research: from bringing attention to a problem (e.g., publishing scientific articles, giving presentations at meetings, creating a press release or popular piece) to informing policymakers of findings (e.g., creating brief policy summaries, testifying at hearings) to actively advocating for a cause (e.g., media advocacy, writing letters to the editor, meeting with elected officials).

As the field considers the types of training offered to MPH and PhD students and whether to develop competencies to enhance dissemination and communication of research (e.g., media training, writing for popular press, social media dissemination, communicating with stakeholders, engaging with knowledge brokers), it will be crucial to more formally decide how to resolve this tension going forward. Training in group dynamics, conflict resolution, and stakeholder communication are possible extra competencies to support interdisciplinary collaboration and team science. These are critical abilities for carrying out interdisciplinary research and communicating findings to important stakeholders outside of academia. Knowledge translation training affects not only how scientists communicate with the public, policymakers, and media, but also how well researchers translate knowledge and communicate with one another. (Neta et al., 2015).

3.3.4. Institutional Sustainability and Funding of the Social Sciences in Public Health

The last point of contention concerns the social sciences' potential contribution to and role in "soft-money" settings, a tension that is especially apparent in the current political and financial landscape. Public health schools rely on outside grant support because they are soft-money institutions. This presents a significant challenge for the social sciences. History and anthropology are particularly vulnerable because they typically receive fewer NIH grants than other academic fields. Political science, history, and anthropology may receive funding from private foundations, but these programs lack the institutional overhead necessary for long-term institutional viability. In the social sciences, the current funding landscape remains dangerous for those with access to NIH support. Many public health schools are starting to think about the possibility of corporate support for research projects due to the current funding prospects. Even when conflicts of interest are taken into account, this still raises serious ethical questions about how corporations shape research agendas, the viability of research projects without corporate support, and the evident issues of reputational risk. All of these concerns are raised even though it may help to resolve financial difficulties. This conflict has implications for the way grant writing is taught in formal education, training programs, and mentorship programs.

3.3.5. Future Directions for Social Sciences in Public Health

We've talked about important issues that are pertinent to educating the upcoming cohort of social scientists studying public health. Concerns about interdisciplinarity and disciplinary structures and foundations, research focused on advancing social science theory and knowledge versus research with high policy relevance, the path social scientists take for research dissemination and translation for wider consumption, and institutional sustainability are a few of these tensions that social scientists must deal with. The richness of the social sciences in public health has been enhanced by the diversity of viewpoints we have represented throughout these conflicts. For instance, the field of public health benefits from both knowledge production aimed at filling in knowledge gaps and strategic science that specifically aims to address policy-relevant questions. As such, we are not endorsing one strategy over another. Rather, we want to draw attention to these conflicts and different points of view so that we can identify them and the effects they have on various institutional and departmental choices more clearly.

The conflicts that we have brought to light here have significant ramifications for the curriculum and organization of public health schools, the path that the upcoming generation of social scientists in public health will take in their research, the distribution and scope of their findings, and our capacity to encourage and finance them. As mentioned at the outset, we focus on training-related issues because decisions about how best to address these tensions will directly affect how the next generation of social scientists studying public health is trained. The Council on Education for Public Health (CEPH) Accreditation for Schools of Public Health recently updated its criteria to place more emphasis on skill-building (as opposed to topical areas) in its coursework, making training issues especially pertinent at this time.

3.4. The Role of Behavioral Science Theory in the Development and Implementation of Public Health Interventions

In the US and around the world, behavioral factors—most notably, alcohol consumption, diet and exercise habits, tobacco use, sexual behavior, and preventable injuries—are the leading causes of death and disease. Changes in behavior at multiple levels are typically necessary for public health programs to be effective in helping people manage illness, lower the risk of disease, and maintain and improve their health (e.g., individual, organizational, and community). The foundation of the most effective public health initiatives and programs is knowledge of health behaviors and the environments in which they take place. Models of strategic planning offer an organized framework for creating, overseeing, and refining public health interventions via assessment. Health behavior theory can help with research to test novel intervention strategies as well as program planning and evaluation.

The best way to design interventions to improve health behavior is to have a solid understanding of pertinent behavior change theories and the ability to apply them effectively. A increasing amount of research indicates that certain strategies that integrate several theories and concepts have greater effects than others, and that interventions developed with an explicit theoretical foundation or foundations are more effective than those without a theoretical basis. The application of health behavior theories is both a science and an art that combines techniques, methods, and strategies from the social and health sciences. Throughout this article, the term "behavioral science theory" refers to a wide range of viewpoints from the social, behavioral, and health sciences. Prominent scholarship incorporates ideas, findings, and methods from a variety of social and behavioral science fields, including psychology, sociology, social psychology, anthropology, nursing, economics, and marketing. The evidence base must be made available to researchers and practitioners alike as the body of research literature expands.

1. **Multiple Determinants and Multiple Levels of Health Behavior:** The emergence, preservation, and modification of health-related behavioral patterns are influenced by a wide range of social, cultural, and economic factors. There is no one factor or combination of factors that can fully explain why people eat the way they do, smoke or not, and engage in active or sedentary lifestyles. Individual factors such as motivation, knowledge, attitudes, and stress-related responses are significant predictors of health behavior. Other significant factors include social relationships, families, geography, socioeconomic status, and culture. In addition to helping identify the most influential factors for a given individual or population, having a broad understanding of some of the key factors and models for understanding behaviors and behavior change can serve as a foundation for well-informed public health programs and allow program developers to concentrate on the most important issues.

Interventions in the fields of public health and health promotion that adopt an ecological perspective are most likely to be successful. Interventions should address interpersonal, organizational, and environmental factors that influence health behavior in addition to focusing on individuals. When one considers the setting of groups of employees buying food and dining during the workday, this mindset is amply demonstrated. Workers can purchase food from vending machines and workplace cafeterias or bring food from home. Availability, pricing, location, habits, nutrition facts, availability, and personal preferences are some of the factors that affect their decision-making. The process is intricate and influenced by several variables that operate at different levels.

Prior to the 1970s, training programs placed a strong emphasis on community organization skills and promoted a broad understanding of the social determinants of health in public health education. Health educators and practitioners concentrated more on intra-individual elements like a person's beliefs, knowledge, and skills over the following 20 years. These priorities are still present in a lot of behavior-change initiatives aimed at lowering risk factors. Present perspectives indicate a return to the earlier roots of public health and propose that promoting health can be more successful if it considers factors other than the individual, such as the environment and social milieu. Planners of programs can and should endeavor to comprehend the different levels of influence that impact the health and behaviors of individuals and populations.

3.4.1. Important Theories and Their Key Constructs

A discipline's recognized theories help define the field, the parameters of practice, and the professional development and socialization of its members. Research and practice in health promotion and education are not dominated by a single theory or conceptual framework these days. Nonetheless, the most popular theories and patterns in theory application have been identified through reviews of journal articles covering a wide range of health behavior topics that were published in the last 20 years.

3.4.1.1. Health Belief Model

One of the earliest theories of health behavior, the HBM is still regarded as one of the most important in the field. It was created in the 1950s to help understand why people used or did not use the preventive services provided by public health departments. Over time, it has changed to address more contemporary issues with prevention and detection (such as mammography screening and influenza vaccinations) as well as lifestyle choices like avoiding injuries and taking risks with sexual activity. According to the HBM, people's readiness to take action is influenced by their beliefs about whether they are at risk for a disease or health issue, as well as their opinions about the advantages of acting to prevent it. The fundamental ideas of the HBM are perceived vulnerability and severity, perceived advantages and barriers, cues to action, and the more recent addition of self-efficacy. When it comes to preventive and asymptomatic health issues, like early cancer detection and hypertension screening, where beliefs are just as important as or even more significant than overt symptoms, the HBM has been used most frequently. It is also evident that the HBM has relevance for programs aimed at lowering cardiovascular disease risk factors.

3.4.1.2. Transtheoretical Model/Stages of Change

Long-term behavioral changes related to health entail a variety of actions and gradual adaptations. While some people might not be prepared to try changes, others might have started making adjustments to their diet, activity level, smoking habits, etc. One of the main components of the TTM of behavior change is the stage of change construct, which postulates that individuals are at varying stages of preparedness to adopt healthy behaviors. In health behavior research, the idea of readiness to change, or stage of change, has been investigated and found to help explain and forecast changes for a range of behaviors, such as eating habits, physical activity, and smoking. The TTM has also been used in a variety of contexts.

A heuristic model called "Stages of Change" outlines the steps involved in successfully altering behavior: pre-contemplation (not realizing the need for change or showing interest in it), contemplation (thinking about it), preparation (making plans for it), action (forming new habits), and maintenance (continually engaging in the new, healthier behavior). People frequently recycle and repeat particular stages rather than going through the stages of change linearly (e.g., depending on their levels of motivation and self-efficacy, individuals may relapse and go back to an earlier stage).

The stages of change model can be used to increase the effectiveness of health counselling as well as to help explain why individuals who are at high risk for diabetes might not be prepared to try behavioral change. Organizing groups along the stages-of-change continuum based on the leaders' and members' (e.g., employees') readiness for change is another way to apply the stages of change model in communities and organizations.

3.4.1.3. Social Cognitive Theory

Social cognitive theory (SCT), which Bandura has best articulated, is a cognitive formulation of social learning theory that describes human behavior in terms of a three-way, dynamic, reciprocal model in which behavior, environmental influences, and personal factors interact continuously. SCT is easily applicable to counselling interventions for disease prevention and management because it integrates ideas and procedures from behavioristic, cognitive, and emotional models of behavior modification. A fundamental tenet of SCT is that learning occurs not only from personal experience but also from witnessing other people's actions and the outcomes of those actions. Important SCT concepts that apply to interventions aimed at changing health-related behavior include self-efficacy, self-control, reinforcement, and observational learning. Goal-setting, self-monitoring, and behavioral contracting are a few components of behavior modification based on SCT constructs of self-control, reinforcement, and self efficacy.

The ability to take action and stick with it in the face of setbacks or difficulties is known as self-efficacy, and it plays a significant role in health behavior change initiatives. Three types of strategies are available for health providers to intentionally work toward increasing patients' self-efficacy: (a) setting small, incremental, and achievable goals; (b) utilizing formalized behavioral contracting to set goals and specify rewards; and (c) monitoring and reinforcement, which includes patient self-monitoring through record-keeping.

A person can be both an agent of change and a responder to change, according to the fundamental SCT concept of reciprocal determinism. Therefore, it is possible to encourage healthier behavior through modifying the surroundings, providing role models with examples, and using rewards. This fundamental idea is more significant than ever and is at the heart of social ecology models as well.

3.4.1.4. Social Ecological Model

The social ecology model offers direction for creating effective programs that use social environments in addition to assisting users in understanding factors that influence behavior. Social ecological models place special emphasis on the idea that behaviors both shape and are shaped by the social environment, as well as various levels of influence, including individual, interpersonal, organizational, community, and public policy. Social cognitive theory (SCT) concepts align with the tenets of social-ecological models, which have been proposed in multiple ways. These models suggest that fostering a change-friendly environment is crucial in encouraging the adoption of healthy behaviors. For instance, more attention is being paid to assessing and enhancing the health-promoting aspects of communities and neighborhoods as well as lowering the prevalence of high-calorie, high-fat food options in light of the rising obesity epidemic in the United States and other developed nations. (Adams, Breen, & Joski, 2007).

3.4.2. Applications of Theory in Public Health Interventions

Large-scale women's health interventions and a statewide health improvement program are two recent examples of programs that highlight the potential and difficulties associated with creating, implementing, sharing, and assessing theory-based and theory-informed public health initiatives.

3.4.2.1. Women's Health Programs

Behavioral science theories have been widely applied in large, widely distributed women's health programs to help develop core interventions and to train managers and interventionists to conduct programs for a variety of women in a variety of settings. To improve access to breast and cervical cancer screening services for medically underserved women, the National Breast and Cervical Cancer Early Detection Program (NBCCEDP) was founded in

1991 as a comprehensive national public health program. In many states, the NBCCEDP works in tandem with the WISEWOMAN project (Well-Integrated Screening and Evaluation for Women Across the Nation) to offer lifestyle interventions and risk factor screening for cardiovascular disease to underinsured and uninsured women.

3.4.2.1.1. Analysis of Theory Use in Recruitment and Professional Development in the NBCCEDP

With expansion and continuous operation spanning nearly two decades, the National Breast and Cervical Cancer Early Detection Program (NBCCEDP) is currently available in all 50 states, five U.S. territories, as well as twelve American Indian/Alaska Native tribal organizations, to offer breast and cervical cancer screening services. Every year, hundreds of thousands of women are screened by the program. The initiative has reduced the disparity in early detection of breast and cervical cancers between African American and White women, but not between Hispanic and White women.

The National Breast and Cervical Cancer Early Detection Program (NBCCEDP) has been growing and running continuously for almost 20 years. It currently offers breast and cervical cancer screening services in all 50 states, five US territories, and 12 American Indian/Alaska Native tribal organizations. Each year, hundreds of thousands of women participate in the program. This initiative has helped reduce the gap in early detection of breast and cervical cancers between African American and White women, although the disparity between Hispanic and White women remains.

The NBCCEDP consists of two main components: interventions to recruit or enroll eligible women in breast and cervical cancer screening services, and interventions to enhance the professional development of healthcare professionals. These program elements are similar to the "provider-directed" and "client-directed" screening interventions that the Task Force on Community Preventive Services thoroughly examined. Behavioral science theory is frequently the basis for these kinds of interventions, and experts have found that applying theory can enhance their efficacy.

Escoffery recently finished interviewing 61 coordinators of recruitment and 59 coordinators of program development for NBCCEDP programs. The study's primary objectives were to list the recruitment and professional development initiatives undertaken by NBCCEDP grantees, evaluate the degree to which evidence-based cancer prevention strategies were applied, and comprehend the rationale and assessment of these tactics.

Interviewers questioned participants about whether intervention strategies were based on one or more theories. Two separate coders coded the answers to open-ended questions. Less than half of those surveyed said that the professional development (provider-directed) strategies were created using one or more theories. The theories of adult learning, social influence, diffusion of innovations, and stages of change were the ones that were most frequently brought up. Of the coordinators who responded, 27% mentioned one or more theories related to recruitment or client-directed strategies. These theories included social marketing, stages of change/TTM, HBM, social influence theory, social networks, and peer-to-peer theory. Some responded by simply listing terms or concepts rather than theories, while others stated they believed a theory had been applied in the design of the system or strategy but were unsure of its name. When asked why specific recruitment or professional-development activities were selected, the organization's backing, the activity's inexpensive cost, and its simplicity of execution were among the most frequently cited explanations.

These results offer insight into the world of public health practice, showing that program coordinators have a moderate understanding of the theoretical constructs used in their interventions. In the NBCCEDP, theory plays a secondary role in program planning and evaluation, with practical considerations taking precedence. This raises the issue of how practitioners can effectively incorporate theory into large-scale public health initiatives.

3.4.2.1.2. The Role of Theory in the WISEWOMAN Program: Lifestyle Interventions, Community Linkages, and Environment and Organizational Change

Phase I of the WISEWOMAN program ran from 1995 to 1998 in three states. Phase II ran from 1999 to 2007 and covered sixteen state and tribal health agencies. Phase III, which has been funding 21 programs since June 2008, is currently underway. At NBCCEDP cancer screening locations, the program provides low-income and uninsured women with assessments of their cardiovascular disease (CVD) risk factors, which include blood pressure, cholesterol, smoking, weight, diet, and physical activity. Over 80% of women have at least one risk factor, and over three-fourths are overweight or obese, according to data from these screening assessments, which consistently show high rates of risk factors among program participants. (Besculides et al., 2008).

Since the program's inception, WISEWOMAN program sites have carried out and assessed lifestyle modification initiatives to lower the risk of CVD by promoting better diet and more exercise. The "enhanced interventions" must be supported by behavioral science theory, culturally appropriate for the local population, and based on evidence, even though they differ amongst project sites. The socio-ecological model, SCT, stages of change/TTM, social support, lay health advisors, and the HBM was the basis for the strategies employed at the first project sites. The standard intermediate measures comprise readiness to change and barriers to behavior change, two fundamental constructs. One of the main ideas of the TTM is readiness to change, and obstacles to change can be understood in terms of the HBM, the TTM, social cognitive theory, and other theories.

Numerous studies, including randomized controlled trials, quasi-experiments, case studies, and mixed-method evaluations, have assessed the locally customized, variable-intensity lifestyle change interventions. The data unequivocally demonstrate that WISEWOMAN's lifestyle interventions are a workable and appropriate means of reaching women who are medically and socially vulnerable. When different types of enhanced interventions were compared to minimal interventions, it was found that the enhanced interventions led to slightly larger but still incremental changes in physical activity, nutrition, and certain risk factors.

Analyzing the benefits and drawbacks of WISEWOMAN, which is by all measures an excellent public health intervention that has expanded to be widely disseminated for more than ten years, requires a close examination of the theoretical underpinnings of the interventions as well as published program evaluations. In counselling sessions, the focal theoretical constructs that are most frequently employed are self-monitoring, self-efficacy, social support, readiness to change, goal-setting with monitoring and reinforcement, and overcoming obstacles. Cross-cutting themes, which are not theories at all but are frequently grouped together with "theory," include multiculturalism and individual tailoring.

Important insights about these interventions were gleaned from case studies involving managers and program leaders from the first three WISEWOMAN states. First, the need to alter provider practices and organizational culture at the clinical sites was noted by the respondents. They also mentioned that one of the main challenges is to go beyond an individual-focused approach. Jilcott and colleagues surveyed program counselors, and the results indicated that counselors who led enhanced intervention sessions spent more time with participants and had higher self-efficacy for their effectiveness. They frequently reported issues with the program's sustainability and cited a lack of time as a barrier. The results imply that environmental and organizational issues could potentially interfere with or even interact with the efficacy of individual counselling.

3.4.2.1.3. Minnesota Statewide Health Improvement Program

To address the rising costs of health and healthcare, the Minnesota Legislature requested in 2007 that a plan for statewide health promotion be developed. This request led to the creation of the Statewide Health Improvement Program (SHIP). By lowering the proportion of obese or overweight Minnesotans and those who use or are exposed to tobacco, SHIP aims to lessen the burden of chronic illness. Steps to a Healthier US, a federal program evaluated in four Minnesota communities, served as the inspiration for SHIP. Building on Steps' achievements, SHIP was created to use practical, research-based methods to modify systems, environments, and policies to encourage healthy behavior in Minnesotan communities.

The strategy used by SHIP communities is based on an ecological model and supports several levels of behavioral influence, including intrapersonal, interpersonal, organizational, community, and governmental. A community's social and physical environments, as well as individuals and families, can all be included in healthy community initiatives by using an ecological model as a framework. The New Spectrum of Prevention, initially created in 1982 by a county public health agency, is implemented by SHIP.

This framework reflects the core tenets of the ecological model through seven levels:

i. strengthening individual knowledge and skills;
ii. promoting community education;
iii. educating providers;
iv. fostering coalitions and networks;
v. changing organizational practices;
vi. mobilizing neighborhoods and communities; and
vii. influencing policy and legislation.

In Minnesota, local public health has long relied on the first three levels of practice. Lately, the emphasis has widened to encompass the final four levels, particularly concerning tobacco. To reinforce this pattern and bring about significant modifications in settings that are likely to encourage and maintain healthy habits, the SHIP community grantees will primarily concentrate on these more expansive ranges. The recent request for proposals includes a Menu of Interventions from which the SHIP communities will choose their interventions to help achieve this shift in focus.

Every intervention in the menu(s) satisfies several requirements. Interventions should focus on prevention over individual treatment, be population-based rather than individual-based, address policy, systems, or environmental change, be evidence-based or use practice-based evidence, and have associated evaluation outcomes. They should also address at least one SHIP risk factor (tobacco, physical activity, nutrition), occur in at least one SHIP setting (school, community, work site, or health care), and be supported by evidence.

The Minnesota Department of Health (MDH) and several stakeholders, including representatives from the Centers for Disease Control and Prevention (CDC), healthcare providers, nonprofit organizations, legal organizations, cultural groups, the University of Minnesota and Extension Services, local public health agencies, tribal governments, and other state government agencies, rigorously reviewed each intervention before it was chosen to be included in the Menu.

The CDC's "Best Practices for Comprehensive Tobacco Control Programs" or its Guide to Community Preventive Services serve as the foundation for most of the physical activity and tobacco interventions found on the Menu of Interventions. These articles and the materials that support them are regarded as the gold standards for choosing evidence-based tactics. As a course of action, programmatic interventions were either incorporated into larger policy, system, and environmental interventions or left out.

Even though community-based health promotion is becoming more and more important, the majority of these programs have only had a little effect, which is partly because of shortcomings in the way the available theoretical models have been applied. Although ecological models offer a valuable framework, they typically lack sufficient detail to accurately conceptualize the interplay between various interventions and multiple levels of influence that encompass the broader community. Better articulation is required for behavior-specific ecological models.

According to Merzel and D'Afflitti, the most advanced theories are grounded in behavioral psychology and frequently lead to interventions that emphasize individual change while failing to sufficiently take into account the contextual elements that affect behavior. For instance, while SCT recognizes the impact of social influence, it makes minimal mention of how the physical environment or local problems—like high unemployment rates—affect behavior.

Program processes and outcomes are frequently difficult to evaluate effectively due to the lack of proper recognition, measurement, or reporting of mediating influences within the context of communities. Few community-based programs have shown significant effects on behavioral or health status outcomes, despite the fact that many of them stress community involvement and collaboration. This lack of significant impact highlights the need for interventions grounded in an integrated theory of ecological change, which goes well beyond holding quarterly community advisory board meetings and targets social and policy influences through an "intensive process of community mobilization."

Important community decision-makers frequently operate under tight deadlines, particularly when funding is linked to planning. Because social norms and a community's physical environment can take years to show significant change, ecological models that take into account a protracted, frequently slow chain of events are essential for program design as well as for assisting decision makers in realizing the need of persistence and patience. This strategy must be used in conjunction with continued, focused efforts to change the environment, systems, and policies.

3.4.3. Constructs and Issues Across Theories

The most often used models for comprehending behavior and behavior change are divided along several important dimensions, including the effects of the environment, behavior change as a multistage process, intention versus action, and altering behavior versus maintaining it.

3.4.3.1. Environmental Influences

The idea that social, organizational, and physical environments play a significant role in shaping behavior is becoming more and more common. Even highly motivated individuals may find their behavior constrained by their surroundings and their perceptions of them. Health disparities are frequently rooted in environmental and policy issues. Communities of color frequently have less access to these resources in their neighborhoods, even though having access to safe parks, walkable communities, and recreational facilities is linked to higher levels of physical activity and a lower risk of obesity. Such disparities in environmental health have a great deal of potential to be reduced or eliminated with the help of well-designed interventions grounded in an ecological model. Furthermore, as was already mentioned, the idea of environment is crucial to several prominent theoretical frameworks and should be kept in mind when implementing individually oriented theories.

3.4.3.2. Behavior Change as a Process

Over the last three decades, research has demonstrated the complexity of the relationships between knowledge, awareness of the need for change, intention to change, and actual behavior change. Changing behaviors for health in a sustained way requires a variety of actions and long-term adjustments.

The fundamental idea that behavior modification is a process rather than an event has become widely accepted in recent years. It's not as simple as someone deciding to give up smoking one day and stick with it for the rest of their life. Although this concept is not new, it has recently received more attention. While the stages of change construct is well known for addressing a range of individual circumstances on change, these processes are also covered by other theories. The cognitive stages of readiness and decision-making for action are also clearly identified by the TPB and the Precaution Adoption Process Model.

3.4.3.3. Intentions Versus Action

The stages of preparation and contemplation and overt action are distinguished clearly by the TTM. The TPB offers an additional use for this distinction. According to the TPB, intentions are the most accurate indicators of behavior. Even closer to the action and potentially a more accurate indicator of behavior and behavior change are "implementation intentions."

3.4.3.4. Changing Behaviors Versus Maintaining Behavior Change

Relapse is common, even in cases where a lifestyle change program—such as stopping smoking or starting an exercise regimen—is initially well-complied with. For instance, a lot of people give up smoking only to pick it back up a year later. Different kinds of strategies are needed for starting and maintaining behavior changes. This phenomenon is implicitly addressed by the TTM division between the action and maintenance stages. Relapse prevention is particularly concerned with maintenance of a recently altered behavior. It entails creating new behavioral patterns that prioritize enhanced self-efficacy, environmental management, and perceived control in addition to learning coping mechanisms and self-management techniques. These tactics combine elements of applied behavioral analysis, the TPB, SCT, and the early stages of the stages of change model.

3.4.4. Challenges and Unresolved Issues

3.4.4.1. Selecting the Right Theory or Theories

Using the most appropriate theory and practice strategies for a particular situation is essential for effective public health and health promotion. Instead of picking a theoretical framework just because it is interesting, well-known, or trendy, the process of choosing an appropriate theory should start with determining the issue, objective, and practice units. As Green and Kreuter have suggested the best approach is to identify possible solutions by working backwards from a logic model of the problem. Theories can be evaluated differently depending on how practitioners and researchers use them. But rather than being distinct problems, theory, research, and practice are interconnected phenomena. When evaluating a theory, practitioners can apply the pragmatic criterion of usefulness and focus primarily on how well it aligns with real-world observations. When a theory or a theoretically based intervention is empirically tested, researchers might be more interested in whether the findings support the theory. We must repeatedly test our theories in both more controlled and real-world environments. Theory, research, and practice are more likely to converge when we do this.

3.4.4.2. Population-Focused Programs and Individual-Focused Strategies

Adopting a program that is only focused on changing an individual's behavior (e.g., teaching a patient low-fat food cooking techniques) has limited value in population-focused programs. A more fruitful approach would also involve altering the environment, such as increasing the accessibility and cost of healthier food options. Longer-lasting and significant changes can be attained when this step is combined with individualized skill training. Although they are underutilized, many theories of organizational and policy change serve as a complement to individually oriented theories. They ought to be distributed, tested, and operationalized further. (Sorensen et al., 2007; Neta et al., 2015).

A Closer Look

Marxist Approach Towards Health and Capitalism

Engels first presented the Marxist perspective on capitalism and health in 1845, when he described the living and working conditions of industrial workers in the early nineteenth century. He linked the working class conditions to the industrial policy of high productivity in a shorter amount of time. According to a Black report from the UK, lower classes had greater rates of illness and death depending on their occupation. A high number of accidents and suicides also occurred in the majority of disadvantaged occupational groups.

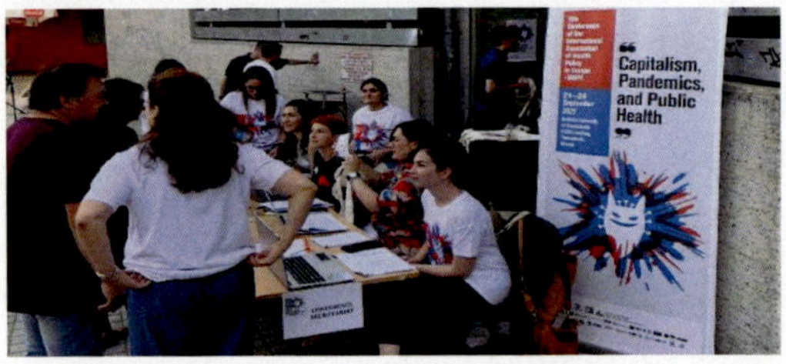

Additionally, Marxists examined lifestyle or chronic diseases like diabetes, heart disease, and cancer and concluded that these conditions were the result of biological maladjustment brought on by ecological contradictions created by industrial capitalism. For instance, the prevalence of these illnesses is higher among Black Americans than it is among Native Black Africans. This is due to the fact that migration brought about dietary changes, a lack of social support, a demanding work environment, low-paying jobs, and devalued working conditions. The population explosion, according to Marxists, is a myth that draws attention away from the real reasons why third-world countries' poor health status exists. Marxists contend that the primary offender is the capitalist system, which exploits workers' arduous physical labor and profits by selling the goods these workers produce while providing the workers with meager benefits. The system maintains all the wealth in a small number of hands in this way.

Under capitalism, medicine looks for personal factors that contribute to illness, and interventions also emphasize changing behavior. The social causes of risk that individuals face are not taken into consideration by the medical profession. Marxists criticize the capitalist system for reducing medicine to a biological level and pushing for the earliest possible return of sick people to the workforce in order to maximize profits, which do not benefit the sick people but instead go into the pockets of a select few wealthy individuals. Some Marxist academics, such as Doyal and Pennell, believe that under a socialist system, logical and pure medical knowledge that has been cleansed of the capitalist motive can be applied to social needs. One of the key ideas in Marxist's theory of health is that the state has an obligation to ensure that the underprivileged have access to affordable medical care. The biotechnology industry is one of the recent developments that can be explained using Marx's analysis of capitalism.

Summary

- The major contributors to mortality today are linked to behavioral and social factors such as tobacco use, poor diet, lack of physical exercise, use of drugs and alcohol, sexual behavior, and lack of access to medical care.
- For several decades the comparative study of communities has been a central concern of the social scientist, whose primary aim is to discover the "properties" of human behavior.
- Each of the social science disciplines has its strong points, and although the similarities among the several social sciences may be greater than the differences between them, it may be useful to consider the peculiarities of methods that distinguish several of the social disciplines.
- In epidemic preparedness and response, it is now commonly accepted that social science is important in shaping action.
- Infectious disease occurs in a particular social, political, economic, and cultural context. This context shapes both disease emergence and its trajectory across different vulnerable groups.
- Outbreak disease framings generate interventions that go beyond the routine running of health systems, with a series of activities rolled out at different levels and scales by diverse response organizations and institutions.
- Cholera outbreaks addressed through emergency vaccination and symptomatic treatment are likely to recur, unless states deliver appropriate WASH infrastructure.
- Different competing explanations of disease and what actions are necessary to emerge from different social groups, based on different notions of what is 'good evidence.'
- The first key tension relates to what drives interdisciplinary versus disciplinary work within public health, and the appropriate role of traditional social science disciplines within institutions that conduct interdisciplinary research and training in public health.
- The most prominent contributors to death and disease in the United States and globally are behavioral factors, particularly tobacco use, diet and activity patterns, alcohol consumption, sexual behavior, and avoidable injuries.
- Interventions to improve health behavior can be best designed with an understanding of relevant theories of behavior change and the ability to use them skillfully.
- The social ecological model helps users to understand factors affecting behavior and also provides guidance for developing successful programs through social environments.
- Several key constructs cut across the most often cited models for understanding behavior and behavior change: environmental influences, behavior change as a multistage process, intention versus action, and changing of behavior versus maintenance of behavior change.

References

1. Adams, E. K., Breen, N., & Joski, P. J. (2007). Impact of the National Breast and Cervical Cancer Early Detection Program on mammography and Pap test utilization among white, Hispanic, and African American women: 1996–2000. *Cancer, 109*(2), 348–358. https://doi.org/10.1002/cncr.22555.
2. Ammerman, A. S., Lindquist, C. H., Lohr, K. N., & Hersey, J. (2002). The efficacy of behavioral interventions to modify dietary fat and fruit and vegetable intake: A review of the evidence. *Preventive Medicine, 35*(1), 25–41. https://doi.org/10.1006/pmed.2001.0999.
3. Barnett, E., Anderson, T., Blosnich, J., Halverson, J., & Novak, J. (2005). Promoting cardiovascular health: From individual goals to social environmental change. *American Journal of Preventive Medicine, 29*(5 Suppl. 1), 107–112. https://doi.org/10.1016/j.amepre.2005.08.020.
4. Baron, R. C., Rimer, B. K., Breslow, R. A., Coates, R. J., Kerner, J., ... & the Client-Directed Interventions to Increase Community Demand for Cancer Screening Workgroup. (2008). Client-directed interventions to increase community demand for breast, cervical, and colorectal cancer screening: A systematic review. *American Journal of Preventive Medicine, 35*(S34–S55). https://doi.org/10.1016/j.amepre.2008.06.001.
5. Berry, T. R., Plotnikoff, R. C., Raine, K., Anderson, D., & Naylor, P. J. (2007). An examination of the stages of change construct for health promotion within organizations. *Journal of Health Organization and Management, 21*(2), 121–135. https://doi.org/10.1108/14777260710758205.
6. Besculides, M., Zaveri, H., Hanson, C., Farris, R., Gregory-Mercado, K., & Will, J. (2008). Best practices in implementing lifestyle interventions in the WISEWOMAN program: Adaptable strategies for public health programs. *American Journal of Health Promotion, 22*(5), 322–328. https://doi.org/10.4278/ajhp.22.5.322.
7. Brownson, R. C., Jacobs, J. A., Tabak, R. G., Hoehner, C. M., & Stamatakis, K. A. (2013). Designing for dissemination among public health researchers: Findings from a national survey in the United States. *American Journal of Public Health, 103*(9), 1693–1699. https://doi.org/10.2105/AJPH.2012.300936.
8. Carleton, R. A., Lasater, T. M., Assaf, A., Feldman, A., McKinley, S. M., & Pawtucket Heart Health Program Writing Group. (1995). The Pawtucket Heart Health Program: Community changes in cardiovascular risk factors and projected disease risk. *American Journal of Public Health, 85*(6), 777–785. https://doi.org/10.2105/AJPH.85.6.777.
9. Drury, J., Reicher, S., & Stott, C. (2020). COVID-19 in context: Why do people die in emergencies? It's probably not because of collective psychology. *British Journal of Social Psychology, 59*(3), 686–693. https://doi.org/10.1111/bjso.12393.
10. Heubner, R. B., & Crosse, S. B. (1991). Challenges in evaluating a national demonstration program for homeless persons with alcohol and other drug problems. In R. Rog (Ed.), *Evaluating Programs for The Homeless: New Directions in Program Evaluation* (Vol. 52, pp. 33–46). Jossey-Bass.
11. Mutua, E. N., Bukachi, S. A., Bett, B. K., Estambale, B. A., & Nyamongo, I. K. (2017). "We do not bury dead livestock like human beings": Community behaviors and risk of Rift Valley Fever virus infection in Baringo County, Kenya. *PLOS Neglected Tropical Diseases, 11*(5), e0005582. https://doi.org/10.1371/journal.pntd.0005582.

12. Neta, G., Sanchez, M. A., Chambers, D. A., Phillips, S. M., Leyva, B., Cynkin, L., & Oh, A. (2015). Implementation science in cancer prevention and control: A decade of grant funding by the National Cancer Institute and future directions. *Implementation Science, 10*(1), 1. https://doi.org/10.1186/s13012-014-0200-2.

13. Parker, R. (2002). The global HIV/AIDS pandemic, structural inequalities, and the politics of international health. *American Journal of Public Health, 92*(3), 343–347. https://doi.org/10.2105/AJPH.92.3.343.

14. Sorensen, G., Stoddard, A. M., Dubowitz, T., Barbeau, E. M., Bigby, J., Emmons, K. M., & Wallace, L. (2007). The influence of social context on changes in fruit and vegetable consumption: Results of the Healthy Directions studies. *American Journal of Public Health, 97*(7), 1216–1227. https://doi.org/10.2105/AJPH.2006.087577.

15. St. Lawrence, J. S., Brasfield, T. L., Jefferson, K. W., Alleyne, E., O'Bannon, R. E. III, & Shirley, A. (1995). Cognitive-behavioral intervention to reduce African-American adolescents' risk for HIV infection. *Journal of Consulting and Clinical Psychology, 63*(2), 221–237. https://doi.org/10.1037/0022-006X.63.2.221.

16. Warner, K. E. (2000). The need for, and value of, a multi-level approach to disease prevention: The case of tobacco control. In B. D. Smedley & S. L. Syme (Eds.), *Promoting Health: Intervention Strategies from Social and Behavioral Research* (pp. 35–50). Institute of Medicine. National Academy Press.

17. Williamson, E. J., Walker, A. J., Bhaskaran, K., Bacon, S., Bates, C., Morton, C. E., ... & Goldacre, B. (2020). Factors associated with COVID-19-related death using OpenSAFELY. *Nature, 584*(7821), 430–436. https://doi.org/10.1038/s41586-020-2521-4.

18. Wingood, G. M., & DiClemente, R. J. (2000). Application of the theory of gender and power to examine HIV-related exposures, risk factors, and effective interventions for women. *Health Education & Behavior, 27*(5), 539–565. https://doi.org/10.1177/109019810002700502.

Chapter

HEALTH COMMUNICATION

4

Contents

Introduction

Health communication encompasses both written and spoken tactics to empower and encourage people to make healthier decisions as individuals, groups, and communities. It is common for health communication to incorporate elements from several theories and models to encourage constructive modifications in attitudes and behaviors. Social marketing, which entails creating initiatives and activities intended to modify behavior positively, is connected to health communication.

Effective health communication and social marketing strategies include the following components:

- Forming products and materials according to research-based methodologies and choosing the best distribution channels to reach the target market.
- Comprehension of prevailing beliefs, ideas, terminology, and priorities in various contexts and cultures.
- The audience's cultural competency, media exposure, internet access, and health literacy are all taken into account.
- Creation of content for a variety of media platforms, including social media posts, workbooks, billboards, newspaper articles, radio and television commercials, public service announcements, newsletters, films, digital tools, group discussions, health fairs, field trips, and case studies.

Health messages can influence campaigns at the community, small-group, interpersonal, and mass media levels by utilizing a range of communication channels. The goal of health communication strategies is to alter people's beliefs, attitudes, and/or actions. A few examples are as follows:

- Increase risk perception;
- Reinforce positive behaviors;
- Influence social norms;
- Increase availability of support and needed services;
- Empower individuals to change or improve their health conditions.

Examples of media strategies to convey health messages include the following components:

- Radio.
- Television.
- Newspaper.
- Flyers and brochures.
- Websites.
- Social media (for example Facebook, Instagram, and YouTube).

Orientation and Directional Terms

Term	Definition	Illustration
Social marketing	Social marketing is an approach used to develop activities aimed at changing or maintaining people's behavior for the benefit of individuals and society as a whole.	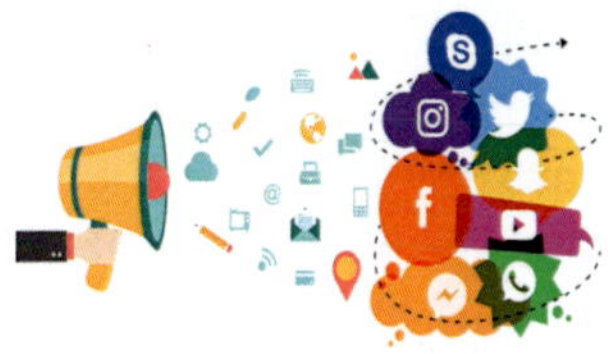
Cross-cultural communications	Cross-cultural communication is a field of study investigating how people from differing cultural backgrounds communicate, in similar and different ways among themselves, and how they endeavor to communicate across cultures. Intercultural communication is a related field of study.	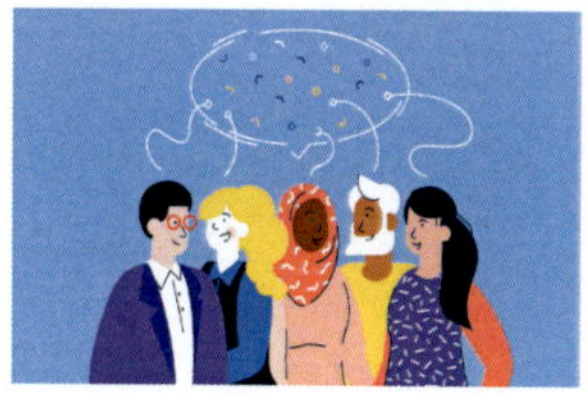
Medication	A medication is a drug used to diagnose, cure, treat, or prevent disease.	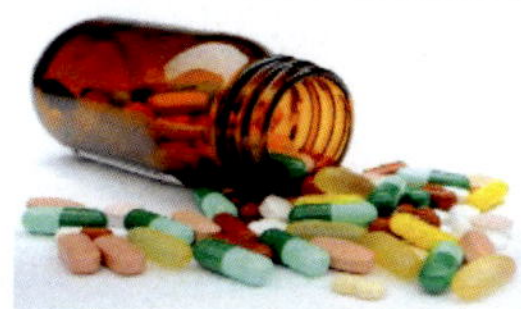
Text messaging	Text messaging is the act of sending electronic messages between two or more devices. Learn more about how it works, the history of texting and more.	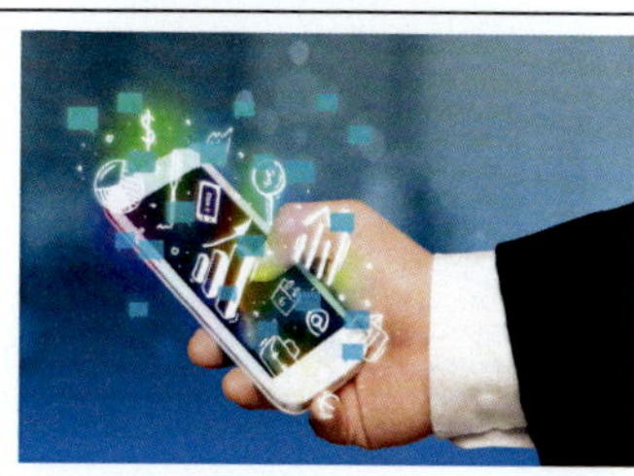
Health campaign	A health campaign is a type of media campaign which attempts to promote public health by making new health interventions available.	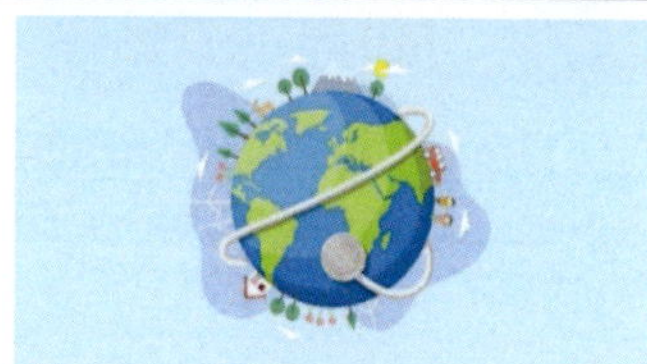

4.1. Basics of Healthcare Communication

In the game telephone, participants move from person to person while sitting in a circle and whispering a brief message. When the final player repeats what they heard and discovers that the original message has been misinterpreted due to a sequence of misunderstandings, the game usually ends with the entire room erupting in laughter.

Unlike telephone communication, effective healthcare communication is not a game. A lot is on the line:

- To receive effective treatments, patients must feel comfortable enough to be open and honest in their communication with their healthcare providers.
- For patients to receive the best care possible, providers must communicate treatment plans and health education in a clear, understandable, and compassionate manner.
- To preserve patient confidentiality, administrators and providers must exchange information ethically and responsibly.
- To close the communication gaps amongst stakeholders, healthcare organizations must implement culturally sensitive strategies.

In the medical field, good communication can mean the difference between life and death. Understanding more about the various forms of healthcare communication, the obstacles to healthcare communication, and the evidence-based tactics for modern, successful healthcare communication can be beneficial to health administrators and other healthcare professionals.

4.1.1. Barriers to Communication in Health Care

Effective communication is essential in all aspects of the healthcare system; however, it is frequently challenging. Thankfully, individuals in this field can implement strategies to address common obstacles and improve communication in healthcare.

4.1.1.1. Patient Distrust and Discomfort

Patients may not feel comfortable sharing private information with their healthcare providers, such as substance abuse or sexual dysfunction, at the patient-provider level.

Patients withhold medical information for many reasons:

- They feel intimidated by their provider.
- They believe their provider won't listen to them.
- They feel disrespected by the request to disclose.
- They question medical advice in general.
- They struggle with physical or psychological trauma.

4.1.1.2. Common Language Barriers

When a patient's healthcare provider is non-English speaking or the organization has not provided an interpreter, patients frequently experience difficulty expressing their needs or symptoms.

Healthcare organizations are unable to provide their communities with the necessary support if they do not place a high priority on providing culturally competent care, which includes using interpreters to help patients and providers communicate more effectively.

4.1.1.3. Providers Stretched Too Thin

Effective communication is essential for healthcare providers to build relationships with patients, gather important health information, and collaborate effectively with colleagues and the community. However, the busy nature of a typical day in a medical clinic can lead to rushed interactions and communication breakdowns. Healthcare professionals who appear detached or indifferent risk harming the patient-provider bond, potentially eroding patient trust and cooperation. Utilizing evidence-based communication techniques can help streamline interactions and improve the overall efficiency of care delivery. Taking just a few additional minutes to communicate can lead to more effective healthcare outcomes for everyone involved.

4.1.1.4. Mismanaged Healthcare Files

The number and reach of care teams have increased in tandem with the growing volume of healthcare data. A single patient file may need to be read by dozens of physicians, nurses, administrators, and other medical staff members at a hospital, which could lead to misunderstandings that could compromise care. Healthcare information must be kept private and available to only the members of a care team who require access, thus providers and administrators must put forth a lot of effort to guarantee this. Limiting the number of people who have access to private patient data promotes accurate and clear communication among healthcare teams and reduces miscommunication.

4.1.2. Importance of Communication in Health Care

Healthcare executives are aware that listening to one another is crucial to having effective communication within their organizations. Medical professionals possess a vast amount of knowledge and expertise collectively. This resource is not used when healthcare professionals rush through appointments without taking the time to listen to their patients and communicate effectively, when patients feel unsafe, when care teams mishandle the storage of medical records, or when health organizations neglect to hire interpreters for cross-cultural communications.

Effective communication is crucial to providing healthcare. Accurate diagnosis and treatment choices are made possible by open, sincere communication between the patient and the healthcare provider. Similar to this, prompt, morally responsible care is provided without jeopardizing confidentiality when members of a care team—which frequently consists of patients and numerous providers—communicate openly and honestly with one another. In addition to easing patients' anxieties and encouraging them to divulge pertinent information, providers can help patients feel heard. For instance, a patient who is self-conscious about a pubic rash will probably feel more comfortable discussing it with a doctor they trust to handle it professionally and compassionately.

Furthermore, everyone has a right to comprehend the medical care they get. This implies that in order for patients to give their informed consent to treatment, healthcare organizations may need to improve the way they train and employ interpreters.

4.1.3. Types of Communication in Health Care

Since technology is always changing, it's critical for healthcare providers to consistently improve communication in order to meet patient expectations. Healthcare providers can stay ahead of the curve in the current landscape by using a variety of communication methods.

4.1.3.1. Patient Portals Provide Access to Health Information

Health care facilities have the option to create patient portals, where patients can enroll and securely access their personal health information. These portals can house educational resources tailored to the patient's specific health concerns, as well as provide clinical summaries of recent appointments and test results with explanations. Recommendations, like scheduling follow-up appointments, can also be included in these summaries.

4.1.3.2. Emailing Can Improve the Patient-Provider Connection

Previously hesitant to use email for communication, medical professionals are now discovering that it saves them a ton of time. It takes far less time to reply to emails from patients during outages than it does to answer calls. Emails can be used as reminders to send orders to other providers, or they can include common questions that can be quickly answered. Emails are a more efficient way to review and handle medication requests than phone calls because they save time.

4.1.3.3. Texting Can Keep the Patient Informed

Health care providers may find that text messaging is a useful tool for quickly communicating vital information to patients. Prescription reminders, patient portal messages, and appointment delays can all be communicated directly through texting. Being an essential part of patient security measures like two-factor login authentication, it can also aid in maintaining the security of a patient's portal information.

4.1.3.4. Social Media Can Reach a Large Audience

One of the most affordable methods of reaching a wide audience with information is through social media. Answers to general inquiries and information are available. It is possible to respond to critical remarks posted on social media, which may change the perception that the public has of your medical center. It can also advertise special health-related events held by the facility. Information that provides people with accurate facts and guidance during public health emergencies can be disseminated, assisting in the containment of panic and the spread of false information.

4.1.3.5. Apps and Websites Can Target Different People

Apps can be used by healthcare providers to target and communicate with various populations. For those who are interested in learning more, they might have a website with instructive health information. They might also provide videos of actual patients to demonstrate how a treatment operates. An app that can remind users to follow certain healthy habits, like exercising or monitoring their blood sugar, could be developed by healthcare providers. Patients experiencing comparable problems may also be able to support one another through online forums. Patients may also be offered live chat.

4.1.4. Strategies and Methods

A persuasive health communication tactic is to customize a health message. Health communication professionals need to compile a superior and audience-appropriate collection of information that targets population segments for health communication messages to reach specific audiences accurately and quickly. For information to be delivered effectively, it is essential to understand who the audience is.

The healthcare industry and a patient's subsequent health suffer from the enigma of communication. Oral speech, voice, tone, nonverbal body language, listening, and other skills are all part of communication. It is a process through which interpersonal connections lead to a shared understanding. The way a patient communicates with their medical team and vice versa influences how their health turns out. A patient's condition can be continuously improved and improved upon by having strong, transparent, and positive relationships with their physicians. This can be effectively accomplished using two methods: the biopsychosocial model and the biomedical model. There is evidence that communication and its customs have changed over time. Thanks to numerous discoveries and developments in the technology industry, communication has significantly improved and is now instantaneous.

Communicators must constantly integrate information from a variety of other academic fields, such as psychology, behavioral sciences, and marketing. Professionals can select from a range of communication techniques and strategies to determine which would best deliver their message after gathering this data. Campaigns, media advocacy, entertainment advocacy, new technologies, and interpersonal communication are some of these strategies.

4.1.4.1. Campaigns

A health campaign is an effort by an organization to persuade someone to adopt new habits or see things from a different angle. Empirical studies demonstrate the efficaciousness of campaigns in motivating individuals to modify unhealthy lifestyle choices that may exacerbate their health conditions. Health communication has been used to address health issues or behaviors that hurt mortality. A mediated campaign uses the media to reach a large audience, disseminate knowledge, or persuade people of a specific viewpoint based on research that has helped the behavior change campaign succeed. a massive media campaign with the main goal of showing people a sign that includes the precise recommendation on eating fruit and vegetables. This campaign includes bus signs, panel street signs, radio ads, television ads, and other advertisements. Calling random numbers was another technique used to get people's thoughts on maintaining a healthy diet and getting regular exercise. "The proportion of participants who deemed walking to be highly significant rose. The results of the recall show that people's opinions about eating fruits and vegetables and going for walks were generally more favorable. The campaign's perspective on these two essential behavioral shifts related to health has improved thanks to the media. The findings substantiate the notion that campaigns for healthy lifestyles can be supported by media coverage.

Perhaps the most popular and successful way to disseminate public health messages is through health communication campaigns, particularly when it comes to supporting illness prevention (e.g., cancer, HIV/AIDS), as well as in promoting overall wellness and health (e.g., contraception and reproductive health). According to the Institute of Medicine, there are three main ways that health communication campaigns structure their messaging for a wide range of audiences:

- By catering to the common denominator within the audience.
- By creating one central message and then later making systematic alterations to better reach a certain audience segment, while retaining the same central message.
- By creating distinctly different messages for different audience segments.

The significance of strategic planning during a campaign is emphasized by both health communication experts and the Centers for Disease Control and Prevention. This involves taking many actions to guarantee that a well-crafted message is conveyed:

- Reviewing background data to identify the nature of the issue and those it affects.
- Establishing communication goals and putting forth a strategy to achieve the desired result.
- Examine the target audience's interests, attitudes, behaviors, advantages, and disadvantages.
- Choose communication channels and materials based on what will reach audiences the most effectively.
- Create and pretest message concepts to gauge comprehension, acceptability, and response.
- Communicate with the targeted audience, keeping an eye on exposures and responses to the message.
- Make sure the information is available in the languages that the target audiences understand.
- Determine whether any adjustments are necessary after assessing the campaign's impact and effectiveness.

1. Historical Campaigns

i. **2014 African Ebola Outbreak:** In 2018, four years after the first significant Ebola outbreak in Western Africa, UNICEF and the Democratic Republic of the Congo collaborated to spread awareness of the deadly virus to approximately 800,000 people in affected areas through a multi-national campaign. Nurse home visits, market and city campaigns, and mass media broadcasts were among the methods used to spread the word about safe practices and preventive measures regarding the virus.

ii. **China's 2019 "Zero-COVID" Policy:** The "Zero-COVID" policy was a significant health communication campaign launched by the Chinese government under Xi Jinping in the wake of the COVID-19 pandemic that struck the entire world in 2019. The goal of this new set of regulations was to try and stop the spread of Covid-19. They included lockdowns, more stringent contact-tracing procedures, and more testing for Chinese nationals. The program did result in significant food shortages and other issues, but it was largely successful in slowing the virus's spread.

iii. **World Health Organization's (WHO) Heatwave Initiative:** To inform people in South and Central America about the risks associated with heatwaves, the World Health Organization and the Pan American Health Organization jointly launched the "Heatwave and Health" campaign in 2021. Webinars, educational YouTube videos, and online articles were used to spread awareness of heatwaves, including what to do before and during them. The campaign also emphasized creating public safety plans for when heatwaves are expected and expanding or enhancing local governments' awareness of the issue.

2. **The Prevention of Cigarette Smoking:** Student smoking at grade schools has decreased as a result of cigarette prevention programs offered to students in grades 6 through 8. According to the study, when smoking prevention was paired with other elements in a specific youth-influencing channel, there was a long-term impact. The results of quitting smoking differed, though. The results of the study show that youth-focused media programs are

implemented more successfully. The study comprised two student groups: one group participated in the school program and received extensive media production, while the other group only participated in the program for four years. By highlighting the advantages of stopping smoking, specifically the ability to refuse cigarettes and the belief that people their age shouldn't smoke, the program aimed to modify the smoking habits of its participants. An end-of-year survey of the students had a long-lasting impact on how they felt about smoking. Moreover, studies show that extensive anti-tobacco media campaigns combined with other anti-tobacco control initiatives are linked to a decline in smoking rates and a rise in the rate of smoking cessation. According to the study, "over the past 40 years, the prevalence of smokers in the United States has declined." The success of smoking cessation is the main focus of the media campaign. The campaign gives those who are trying to stop the opportunity to maintain self-restraint from smoking and advances the notion that those who are "exposed to the message have the motivation to seek additional information for quitting."

i. **American Smallpox Epidemic:** Health communication played a role in reducing the smallpox outbreak in Boston in 1721. Politician Cotton Mather advocated smallpox vaccination through speeches and pamphlets.

ii. **Alcohol Abuse:** For as long as there has been alcohol, there has been an issue with alcohol abuse in society. The Women's Christian Temperance Union spearheaded an anti-alcohol abuse campaign in the 1800s. They disseminated the intended message through mass media. The anti-alcohol movement was made possible by the promotion of newspapers and magazines.

iii. **Cardiovascular Disease:** Two experimental campaigns aimed at educating middle-aged men about the causes of cardiovascular disease were the five-city project and the three-community study. Television, radio, newspapers, cookbooks, booklets, and bus cards were all used to spread health-related messages. The three "communities" consisted of three trial communication tactics: a media-only campaign, a media campaign enhanced by in-person interactions, and a control group that received no intervention. Following a year, the experiment demonstrated that the most knowledgeable at-risk men were those in the second experimental group, who had both attended by a healthcare provider and consumed the media campaign.

4.1.4.2. Communication Channels

1. **Entertainment Media***:* A communication tactic that is gaining popularity is using the entertainment sector as a platform to promote health education and information. The most common tactic used by health communication specialists to include public health information into television show plots is to form alliances with writers of storylines. To continue creating fresh television and movie plots that support public health education, the Centers for Disease Control and Prevention has forged a solid alliance with Hollywood, Health, and Society at the University of Southern California Norman Lear Center. A few of the resources made

available through this collaboration are thorough "tip sheets" that give writers reliable, easily accessible information on health-related topics, as well as panels and meetings to talk about fresh data and resources. NBC's series Parenthood, which focused on Asperger's syndrome, the CW's 90210, which raised awareness of cancer, and the movies Contagion and I Am Legend are a few of the most noteworthy examples of this kind of communication in recent years. The American Public Health Association, the International Health Film Festival, the Global Health Film Initiative of the Royal Society of Medicine, and the Public Health Film Society have all recently organized film festivals and competitions that are especially focused on health films.

The establishment of the Sentinel for Health Awards in 2000 provided writers and storyline developers with even more incentive to keep including public health information in their scripts. These awards recognize storylines that successfully raise audience awareness of public health issues and health-related topics. A 2001 survey by Porter Novelli revealed a wealth of intriguing data regarding the efficacy of this tactic, including the fact that more than half of regular viewers of daytime drama and prime-time television said they had gained knowledge about illness prevention or health promotion from a TV program. Minority groups are well-represented in this data; more than half of African American and Hispanic viewers reported that they had either taken preventative action after learning about a health issue on TV or that a TV storyline had assisted them in giving important health information to a friend or close relative.

2. **Direct Marketing:** Media advocacy is the strategic use of mass media tools in conjunction with broad organization to promote public policies or lifestyles that are healthful. This can involve sending messages from person to person via email and text messaging, as well as promoting health information to a broad audience through social networking sites. The platforms for media advocacy-based health communication will surely grow along with technological advancements.
3. **Social Media:** Social media refers to websites and applications that let users exchange and produce content, including health-related communications. Health information is now more widely accessible thanks to technological advancements. Millions of people can receive real-time health information through social media platforms. Due to this instantaneous communication, social media use as a platform for global health connections has dramatically increased. It is possible to follow the growing trend of using social media to share public health concerns during times of crisis and disaster in recent years. Misinformation can spread quickly when health communication-related content is posted on social media. A lot of these platforms have fact-checking statements in place to help make sure the material being shared is reliable.
4. **Interpersonal Communication:** Strong interpersonal communication is essential for health communication to have an impact on behaviors and decisions related to health. These relationships are most crucial when they involve the exchange and communication between a patient and their healthcare provider (e.g., doctor, therapist, and pharmacist) as well as a person's network of social support (friends, family, and

the community). These relationships may have a favorable impact on the person's decision to make healthful decisions. When patients experience emotional investment in the situation, they are more likely to pay attention. They are more likely to base their decisions objectively on what they hear if they believe they understand what is being said. Two of the most well-known fields of research in interpersonal health communication are the relationship- and patient-centered care models.

4.1.5. Tips for Effective Health Communication

To overcome the many barriers to effective health communication, consider the following recommendations.

4.1.5.1. Sit Down and Be Humble

Research indicates that during office visits and hospital check-ins, trust can be established more easily between patients and providers when they are seated. A patient feels that their visit with a provider is longer and more personal when they sit down to talk. This helps reduce a patient's communication anxiety.

4.1.5.2. Ask Open-Ended Questions

Even after a few minutes of sympathetic conversation, patients frequently feel uncomfortable sharing their concerns. Physicians and other healthcare professionals ought to inquire if patients have additional input. Asking patients a question along the lines of "Is there something else you'd like to talk about today?" can help them think things through and express worries they might not have otherwise.

The "BATHE" technique guides providers to ask patients questions that solicit more information and develop rapport.

- **Background:** Ask a patient about their present situation. "What is going on in your life?"
- **Affect:** Ask your patient how they are emotionally relating to their health concern. "How is it affecting you?"
- **Trouble:** Ask your patient about what they are worried about or what they foresee as obstacles. "What troubles you most about the situation?"
- **Handling:** Ask your patient about how they are dealing with their situation. "How have you been handling this so far?"
- **Empathy:** Show patients you are listening; reflect on what you hear them saying about their feelings. "That sounds [frustrating, confusing, difficult, satisfying, etc.]."

Communication in health care gets easier when we all ask questions and prepare to listen.

4.1.5.3. Speak in Plain Language

Whenever feasible, healthcare providers should steer clear of medical jargon and stick to using plain language when speaking with patients. When using medical jargon, healthcare professionals should always define the terms precisely (e.g., "This stethoscope is a heartbeat measurement tool.") Instead of just giving a monologue, using simple language shows patients that providers are interested in engaging in a two-way conversation with them.

4.1.5.4. Keep Communications Confidential

Only the patient's care team should have access to individual case files, not an entire hospital wing. It is important to refrain from discussing patient issues with anyone outside the team.

4.1.5.5. Hire Interpreters and Culturally Competent Staff at Every Level

Healthcare facilities should be safe havens for those in need of care, not places where racism, xenophobia, classism, homophobia, transphobia, sexism, or other forms of discrimination are condoned. To guarantee that all patients can communicate effectively, healthcare organizations should employ interpreters as needed. Hearing and being heard by medical professionals is a fundamental right for all patients and is necessary for providing effective, culturally sensitive care. Interpreters assist in ensuring that healthcare institutions acknowledge and uphold this right.

4.2. Interpersonal Communication: Patient-Provider Communication

Over the past few decades, the level of interaction between patients and healthcare providers has evolved. Effective communication is a fundamental skill in the healthcare industry, as it fosters a strong therapeutic relationship based on trust. Not only do medical staff and facilities need to be capable, but patients also value friendly, open, and attentive interactions. How healthcare professionals address the needs and preferences of their patients plays a significant role in enhancing the reputation of the healthcare sector and attracting more patients and clients.

There are various ways to communicate and various contexts in which it can be observed. Since it provides a large portion of the information required for diagnosis, communication between the patient and the physician is arguably the most crucial of these. Linguistic (oral and written), non-verbal (gestures, facial expressions, postures, movements, appearances), and para lingual (intonations, tones, rhythms, linguistic flows) are the three forms of interpersonal communication. The emphasis is on verbal communication in the medical system because of the significance of the information content of patient-doctor communication (diagnostic process, treatment). Nonverbal and paralinguistic forms play a significant role in the formation of credible capital, emotional impact, and the necessary empathy between them. This is due to the lack of logical and semantic significance of these forms.

The relationship between the patient and the healthcare provider is much more complicated in the medical field and entails a higher degree of existential therapeutic communication through the foundational level of care. The most significant therapeutic communication that has ever occurred is incorporated into health communication (Chichirez & Purcărea, 2018) since medical practice intertwines elements of personal instability and uncertainty with the patient's destiny. Patient and healthcare professional communication occurs in the field of healthcare research. Research has demonstrated that effective communication improves the performance of the medical unit and has a positive impact on patient satisfaction and the perceived quality of the medical care received (AlQarni, Alsharqi, Qalai & Kadi, 2013; Boudreaux, Mandry & Wood, 2003). In health law, communication entails the active exchange of information between two parties, at least one of whom actively listens, comprehends the message, and can interpret nonverbal cues to encourage the speaker. Must respond to the query. Support for conversations starts (Van Servellen, 2009).

Within the medical domain, effective communication is an essential clinical competency that encompasses establishing therapeutic alliances, comprehending the patient's viewpoint, investigating ideas and feelings, and offering direction on enhancing well-being. The level of communication between a physician and a patient is directly linked to the quality of information obtained during a medical examination. The literature suggests that a patient's health and function, as well as their satisfaction with medical care at a medical facility, can be greatly impacted by a physician's ability to listen, explain, and empathize with them (Brock, et al., 2013; Matusitz & Spear, 2014).

Regardless of the patient's emotional state, the method of cognitive manipulation in patient communication depends on listening and time (availability). The first dialogue rule is "knowing to hear" (Athanasiu, 1998). To be effective and helpful to the doctor, there are numerous guidelines that need to be adhered to. It must be constructive, comprehensive, sympathetic, open-minded, and critical (Chichirez and Purcărea, 2018). Positive listening is necessary first. This involves both mental engagement (attention and concentration) and physical mobilization. An excessively relaxed posture, for instance, can be hard to remember and comprehend, but a somewhat uncomfortable posture fosters a wakefulness that is appropriate for listening. However, listening needs to be a comprehensive process.

Not only should linguistic messages be received and understood, but non-verbal cues like gestures also require close attention. It's important to keep an eye on the patient's facial expressions to prevent them from becoming agitated, upset, or demoralized. An empathic listener is required. Doctors can gain an open and unrestricted understanding of the patient's thoughts and feelings by following this cognitive and emotional process, which begins with self-awareness and progresses to other sightings. stimulates expression. According to Larson & Yao (2005), empathy encompasses not only identification with the patient's feelings, biological and psychological states, but compassion and intuition for the patient's emotions. Healthcare providers must be accessible to patients to allow them to schedule and receive the best possible care for their priorities and goals. This will facilitate effective communication in the health sector. To set themselves apart from other departments within the medical facility, the doctor's response during the examination, the staff's candor, attentiveness, and utility to the patient and their family, as well as the overall performance of all healthcare professionals, must be upheld (Oliver, 2014).

Speakers anticipate verbal cues to clarify unclear situations or meet expectations. Keep in mind that this message should be truthful, impartial, suitable, instructive, timely, courteous, and unduly informal. It's also important to consider the tone of voice in this particular communication scenario. (Chichirez & Purcărea, 2018) Must be. As a result, the patient receives information that clarifies some of the uncertainty and is indicative of respectful behavior and an acceptance of responsibility. Relationships are impacted by unclear answers. In front of patients, doctors attempt to define the illness and arrange every step of the diagnosis and treatment process. Reaction is a necessary precondition for its efficacy, and hesitation, vibration, or undue delay in offering a solution negatively impacts those relationships.

Identification and treatment planning should be tailored to the patient's information needs regarding crucial clinical aspects. This is essential for the physician-patient relationship, as misinformation can lead to patient noncompliance, confusion, dissatisfaction, and stress. Effective communication with the patient should be based on the patient's condition, understanding, and support for a positive relationship. Building strong communication skills, including medical knowledge, information gathering, emotional support, and interpersonal skills, is crucial for developing a professional therapeutic alliance. Therapeutic communication involves providing specific information and education to patients (Van Servellen, 2009).

Communication that takes place face-to-face or virtually between communicators is referred to as interpersonal communication. Because both parties can exchange information during the communication process and receive direct feedback from one another by their respective functions, interpersonal communication is thought to be more effective than other forms of communication (Cangara, 2011). A key component of clinical practice is interpersonal communication, which enables information sharing between patients and medical staff via both verbal and nonverbal cues. The interpersonal communication process is seen as a crucial component between medical professionals and patients who are ill or in need of care from the perspective of healthcare. Furthermore, the improvement of health outcomes in interactions between healthcare professionals and patients is influenced by interpersonal communication in the healthcare setting. A positive tone can help solve diagnostic puzzles, interpersonal communication is frequently continuous through verbal communication, and counselling sessions can offer patient-related health information (Vimala, 2017).

Speaking and writing are two forms of verbal communication that people use to express their ideas. The language choices made by patients and healthcare professionals greatly influence how well they can communicate with one another. In addition, patients frequently speak in slang, dialects, and accents that make it challenging for medical professionals from different areas to comprehend them. Additionally, patients frequently use bizarre explanations for health issues, which often reflect their own opinions about the origin and seriousness of the illness. Research has shown that cancer patients can more effectively adjust to their condition when they have positive interpersonal relationships with their doctors that are marked by kindness, empathy, respect, and trust (Bakker et al., 2001). (Fogarty et al., 1999; McWilliam, 2000; Finset, Smedstad, & Ogar, 1997). According to Koutsosimou (2013), there are notable disparities in the scientific perspectives regarding the therapeutic relationship between physicians and patients, which contributes to the complexity of doctor-patient relationships.

4.2.1. Types of Interpersonal Health Communication Model

4.2.1.1. Patient-Centered Model

The understanding of the patient as seen by the patient is the main focus of the patient-centered model. Healthcare providers listen intently to the concerns, emotions, and opinions of their patients. The patient is seen as a member of the healthcare team in the patient care-centered model because they are involved in the development, planning, and management of their care. It also demonstrates how the medical team sees the patient as a fellow team member who can be assisted in sharing information to accomplish a particular goal with a clear vision.

Interruptions in health communication are studied because they are crucial to patient-centered communication and connection. Since disruptions could reduce the effectiveness of the patient-centered model, guidelines are provided for healthcare professionals to follow. According to research, patients take two to three minutes to communicate their needs when speaking with a healthcare provider about their care, particularly when the provider asks a question that necessitates clarity and specificity (Naughton). After, on average, twenty-three seconds, the patient is interrupted by the healthcare provider. Cooperative and disruptive interruptions were distinguished in a study. In the study 84 natural interactions between the physicians and the patient, the primary goal of classifying the interruption as cooperative or intrusive was conducted. This suggests that interruptions don't always have to be intrusive; they can also be cooperative, which means that the interruptions can be constitutive and, thus, can result in a continuance of the conversion process. According to the data, 82.9% of the 2,405, interruptions were helpful rather than obtrusive. In general, the patient-centered model aims to reduce disturbances. The patient-centered model of health communication, which is the basis for training programs for medical professionals, emphasizes interruptions, with the main recommendation for practice being that doctors refrain from interjecting too soon into the interview.

4.2.1.2. Relationship-Centered Model

The contributions of cooperation, mutual understanding, and the physicians' and patients' respective assessments of the worth of their relationships are what define relationship-centered care. The relationship between the patient and the medical professional is still vital. When making decisions under the relationship-centered care paradigm, the clinical provider should consult with the patient, family, and other clinicians for the patient to receive relationship-based assistance. The relationship care center's methodology starts with the implementation of a patient care center that centralizes the patient, unlike a relationship-based center that evolved to understand the patient. Medical personnel are encouraged to sympathize with patients through relationship care. Because patients can express their emotions, relationship-centered care places a greater emphasis on developing empathy for them. In terms of the health professional's comprehension of the patient and ability to meet their needs, it is beneficial when the patient communicates their emotions. Medical practitioners focus on the concept of the relationship center in the cognitive domain, emphasizing patient education and the provision of medical information. Mutual respect, acceptance, and trust in the emotional sphere are all part of care.

4.2.2. Verbal and Nonverbal Communication in Healthcare

4.2.2.1. Verbal Communication Used by the Doctors

Speaking and writing are two forms of verbal communication that people use to express their ideas. How well patients and healthcare professionals understand one another during interactions has a big influence on the language they use. Medical terminology facilitates accurate and clear communication between healthcare professionals, but when speaking with patients, scientific and clinical terminology can be imprecise and inappropriate (Hull, 2016). Patients frequently use their dialect, accent, and colloquialisms when speaking with a doctor. This can make it challenging to comprehend service providers in different regions of the nation. Additionally, patients' descriptions of health issues are distinct and frequently reflect how they perceive the illness, its cause, or its severity. A patient's perception of their illness or symptoms may be influenced by local conditions. For instance, a patient may wait to report symptoms until they are extremely unwell because they believe the symptoms to be commonplace. Nonetheless, to correctly diagnose a patient and create a treatment plan that works, physicians must recognize early and even mild symptoms (Women, Yawn, & Yawnand Uden, 1992). Healthcare professionals can frequently calm patients and enhance interpersonal relationships by extending cordial greetings and asking insightful questions. These activities don't take much work, but they can have important repercussions. Information that cannot be expressed with words alone is communicated through nonverbal communication.

One cue that has been utilized in speaking and talking is verbal communication. When it comes to providing health care information, verbal communication is crucial. When providing medical information, medication advice, and treatment process guidance based on diagnosis, healthcare providers converse verbally with their patients. Patients have always occasionally received excellent care as well as bad care. Inadequate service leaves customers wondering why they ever went there in the first place, while excellent service encourages customers to return. One term that has been used in speaking and speaking is verbal communication. Verbal communication is a vital tool for sharing health information in the healthcare industry. Oral communication is a tool used by health professionals to communicate with patients about diagnosis, treatment plans, and medication advice. Patients have consistently received both good and bad care.

4.2.2.2. Language Used by the Doctors

When interacting with patients, doctors use verbal communication. To determine the verbal communication that the doctor uses to communicate with the patient, the researcher's language is closely related to the doctor's interpersonal communication skills with the patient. In this phenomenon, the physician initially discusses his ideas, then works to allay the patient's concerns and persuade them of the advantages of a different course of treatment (Swinglehurst et al., 2014). It was believed that speaking more than one language would help to establish a close bond with the patient. Physicians are multilingual and will tailor their consultations to the patient's condition, course of treatment, and dosage regimen. Verbal communication conveys information about the multilingual nature and is reflected as a significant factor. Scientist Lisa Sparks (2010) states that medical personnel can communicate in both the patient's native tongue and English. Typically, family members lack the expertise to explain options or medication protocols, or to use specific medical terminology. According to McGorry (1999), family members who are supported by this statement accompany their parents to a doctor's appointment and act as interpreters. In this sense, multilingualism in doctors has been found by researchers. Observations indicate that the majority of patients bring their families to IJN appointments. Clinical assistants support the doctor-patient interaction in multiple languages in the majority of cases. The patient's interpreters in this case are their family members or friends.

4.2.2.3. Clear Information by the Doctors

Physicians are frequently questioned about the patient. the encounter of a medical professional who upheld the doctor-patient relationship and gave the patient's parents or spouse clear information about their health. To help the patient make an educated treatment decision, the doctor first educates them about all pertinent options, including the pros and cons. This claim, supported by Travaline (2005), will be gradually made clearer by doctors during conversations without their prior knowledge of the patient. They will also incorporate and communicate the information clearly and understandably. A key component of a doctor's daily job is verbal communication. Doctors can help patients understand their illness and health issues by making clear statements. Physicians communicate verbally to patients in a way that is understandable to them. According to Silverman (2010), oral communication in medical consultation is generally acknowledged as being crucial for medical care, occurs at a specific point, only occurs in one mode, is primarily controlled voluntarily, and more. Since it communicates a lot of concepts cognitively, it is usually simple to understand.

4.2.2.4. Positive Environment Created by the Doctors

By helping the patient comprehend their condition, oral communication at the appropriate time can have a positive impact on their health. In the medical field, a doctor's verbal communication with a patient transmits health information, and the patient and doctor develop a positive relationship as a result of the communication and sense of participation. Doctors and staff must verbally convey important information to avoid providing too much information, as Graham (2008) pointed out. The majority of patients forget what they were told. Speaking slowly and avoiding medical attention is crucial, as the author made clear in the oral communication information. It is clear from this study's oral communication that the patient and doctor engage in an interactive process to exchange pertinent health information while trying to persuade, explain, motivate, advise, or guide. This method of developing interpersonal communication skills focuses on verbal exchanges and the relationships that exist between medical professionals and their patients. To empower patients to accept and control their disease, supportive strategies are used. Verbal communication offers support and encouragement during a patient-doctor visit, which helps patients better understand their health communication and achieve positive medical outcomes. By acknowledging the toll that illness takes on patients and their families, the literature promoting compassionate associations can be strengthened (Balaban, 2000). For patients and their families to comprehend the medical issue, scholars also underlined that they supported and assisted them in growing accustomed to the explanations. Getting the right health information to patients and their families is facilitated by efficient and cooperative communication. Patients are urged to think about participating in clinical trials when choosing their treatment regimens.

During the examination, the doctor's words of support and encouragement to the patient and his family members are effective treatments for this illness. According to scientists, using supportive dialogues, such as a doctor verbally validating a patient's emotional or motivational state, is one of the styles that define patient-centric care. The patient's positive perception increases with the strength of the supportive conversation (Denio, 2013). When it comes to patients' queries, worries, opinions, and preferences, doctors should always be more perceptive, understanding, and encouraging. Comparably, in the event of a severe illness, the physician is required to accompany the patient and provide support by sharing thoughts, worries, and words of encouragement. According to research, some clinicians give more information daily—including reassurance and encouragement—to foster partnerships through cooperative communication (Roter, 1997 & Street, 1992).

4.2.2.5. Nonverbal Communication Used by the Doctors

Another crucial component of healthy behaviors is nonverbal communication. Nonverbal communication is defined by scientists as a component of communication in which signals such as gestures, touches, facial expressions, eye contact, clothes, and hairstyles are the only means of exchanging information (Hall & Montague, 2013). Physicians frequently react to a patient's facial expressions because they can often reveal signs of fear, anxiety, or melancholy. Ambady (2002) linked the therapeutic effects of physicians' nonverbal communication patterns. Nonverbal communication by doctors and patient outcomes. The most researched is patient satisfaction.

Nonverbal cues include posture, body language, gestures, and even quiet. A physician who pays close attention keeps his or her eyes off other things, smiles, and sits at the same level as the patient sends a powerful message of empathy, compassion, and listening. Numerous nonverbal communication aspects are ingrained in cultural norms and practices. For instance, making direct eye contact may be seen as disrespectful or improper in some cultures, especially when done by people of the opposite gender, but it can also be a sign of positive gratitude and respect in others. In certain cultures, making physical contact during a conversation—touching the patient's hand or arm—is interpreted as a show of affection.

1. **Touch:** Another crucial interpersonal communication signal in the medical field for fostering empathy between a physician and a patient is touch. The literature suggests that physicians may touch their patients as a way to express concern and empathy (Horton, Clance, Sterk-Elifson, & Emshoff, 1995). Doctors' interpersonal communication skills are influenced by two different types of touches: i) social touch, which involves social behaviors like handshakes and back pats, and ii) physical touch, which is a touch used for clinical purposes during an examination. In their daily work, physicians use social touch as an adjunct to verbal communication. In their practice of medicine, doctors only make physical contact.

Touch is generally a very effective way to convey happy emotions. But how much social interaction keeps a person in close proximity to significant others, manages interpersonal interactions, and preserves social bonds like affection and trust between dyads? Whether it will be established is still up in the air (Ainsworth, 1989; Hazan, 1987). A gentle touch on the patient's hand, arm, or shoulder that expresses concern is known as a social touch. In this phenomenon, social interaction facilitates better patient-doctor communication. The majority of patients believed that expressive touch was appropriate, particularly under pressure. Patients anticipate concerns from doctors who use touch to offer support and encouragement during consultations, such as shaking hands and tapping backs, even though the majority of doctors are aware of their touch. When it comes to social contact, doctors touch their patients to convey their concerns. Research demonstrates the connection between social interaction and empathy, as well as how sharing emotional experiences between doctors and patients can strengthen empathy (Adolphs, 2009). The literature also asserts the importance of interactions for a variety of reasons. According to Howard & Friedman (2010), healthcare providers must win patients' cooperation during treatment, instill positive expectations, and offer emotional support. Hirsch (2007) concurred that doctors are far more likely to feel empathy, express it, and treat patients and illnesses successfully when they have a personal understanding of each patient. Patients want their doctors to be understanding.

Physical contact indicates interindividual variation. Simply put, physical touch is when two people come into contact with each other and set off a series of chemical reactions in the body that reduce stress and pain. It fosters a feeling of contentment, safety, and warmth. Additionally, physical contact boosts immunity, reduces blood pressure, and raises blood sugar levels. Physical contact is employed in medical procedures from a healthcare perspective. Physicians have been observed to use the physical touch effects of social support on patients' cardiovascular responses to their behavior, including blood sugar content, heart rate, and diastolic blood pressure, in the medical setting. Patients typically rely on doctors to use physical touches for diagnostic purposes, and from a healthcare perspective, examination-based touches are seen as a promising aspect of the patient-physician relationship (Blair & Wasson, 2015).

One of the most important forms of nonverbal communication in the doctor-patient relationship is physical touch during the examination. When providing care for a patient, highly skilled doctors with years of experience always prioritize the kind of contact. According to the literature, a doctor's touch can be used to diagnose, treat, and—possibly most importantly—show that the patient feels that the doctor is acutely aware of their needs, concerns, and problems (Masu, Roter, & Hall, 2006). Touch and hold the patient's hand or arm until the examination is through, paying special attention to elderly patients. Touching the patient's arm or hand, particularly to convey that the doctor plans to stay in the patient's corner, offering support and caring guidance through the medical procedure. By allowing the doctor to touch him, the patient affirms his trust, and the doctor gradually learns to see, hear, and feel what the patient's body communicates while also demonstrating his commitment to the partnership (Olson & Roth, 2007).

2. **Body Language:** Nonverbal communication is a key aspect of linguistic communication, with body language playing a crucial role in expressing thoughts, intentions, and emotions. Physical behaviors such as facial expressions, postures, gestures, eye movements, and the use of space all contribute to nonverbal communication. In the field of health care, body language is essential for effective counselling, as it helps to convey empathy and understanding to patients. Physicians use different body language techniques to maintain strong relationships with their patients, as research shows that a physician's body language can have a powerful positive effect on patients. By displaying open and receptive body language, health providers can gather important information from patients that can aid in diagnosis and treatment.

The research indicates that open body language, tactful and unhurried hand gestures, upright head posture, a relaxed chin, and firmness are all indicators of good body language that respects the patient and makes a positive first impression. Patients typically seek out encouraging nonverbal cues that convey optimism. Patients believe that comforting remarks are more effective when they are accompanied by consistent facial and vocal attention. Nonverbal communication always yields answers. Researchers have also shown that doctors can partially or accurately correlate an individual's body position—that is, how their body reflects them—with the type and speed of their movements and gestures.

3. **Tone of Voice**: Voice tones are a key component of nonverbal communication in healthcare, along with gestures, body language, and facial expressions. Research has shown that displaying empathy through voice tones can lead to improved outcomes, such as decreased error complaints in the workplace. How words are spoken, the language used, and the organization of sentences all play a role in communication. Different voice tones can convey friendliness, anger, frustration, and more. Studies have shown that the tone of a healthcare provider's voice can impact the patient's experience and perception of care.

To facilitate better reconciliation, tone of voice plays a crucial role in doctor-patient communication by instructing the doctor to listen. Concurrently, the doctor's voice concerning patient consultation in terms of volume, tone, rhythm, pace, and pause (Mackenzie, Farah, & Savage, 2002). Patients who communicate with their doctor in tones that are characterized as "warm and supportive" or "possible and worried" suggest that they were given more "choice and/or management." The outcomes were comparable but also positively correlated with medication adherence if the doctor spoke in a "more enthusiastic" manner (Joyce, 2015).

To establish trusting relationships with their patients, doctors use tones in their voices. Research has indicated that the most unfavorable voice tones—hostility and rudeness—are linked to severe, ongoing pain and poor patient outcomes. It seems that the doctor's satisfaction with different aspects of his experience with the patient was reflected in the tone of his voice (Hall, Stein, Roter, & Rieser, 1999). Positive communication with patients tends to elicit fewer controversial emotions than negative communication, such as abrupt or impatient voices from doctors. Research has demonstrated that the tone of a doctor's voice can significantly influence the mood and result of a procedure (Ambady et al., 2002).

One more nonverbal communication tool used in healthcare is voice tones, along with gestures, body language, and facial expressions. It has to do with how words sound, how sentences are put together, and how uniquely they convey ideas. Voice tone refers to how one speaks in three different tones: friendly and pleasant, angry and angry, or frustrated and frustrated. According to the literature, a clinician's conversation with a patient will mirror the effects of the doctor's voice when discussing the patient, and the patient will respond differently to a doctor's tone of voice (Roter & Hall, 1989). Since it instructs the doctor to listen, the tone of voice is a crucial component of doctor-patient communication and helps to promote better reconciliation. To establish trust, doctors use their voices to communicate with their patients. Patients will trust their doctors more if they speak in a tone that demonstrates their ability to treat their illness. The most hostile and disrespectful tone of voice has been linked to significant and persistent pain as well as worse physical health in patients, according to the literature.

4. **Eye Contact**: Another nonverbal component of interpersonal communication that is crucial since it lacks language is eye contact. Similar to other nonverbal cues like body language, facial expressions, and body gestures, eye contact is a behavior. Linguistic and nonverbal communication are combined when making eye contact. According to McDonald, Marshall, Johnson, & Polkinghorne (2009), maintaining academic eye contact is a crucial nonverbal behavior that is necessary for fostering positive relationships with senior citizens. The healthcare system is influenced by eye contact, and the patient's sense of empathy is influenced by eye contact as well. Furthermore, according to a different study, it was primarily seen as an indication of the doctor's consideration, respect, and attentiveness (Marcinowicz, 2010). In a doctor-patient consultation, eye contact influences the flow of the conversation. Research in the field of literature highlights the importance of a doctor's eye contact being paired with appropriate verbal cues and focused attention. This not only shows that the doctor is listening to the patient while jotting down notes, but also gives the

patient a sense of being heard. Studies have revealed that a skilled doctor's care for a patient begins the moment they make eye contact. It has been found that patients value the doctor's attention through eye contact, and even subtle expressions like frowning can positively impact patient satisfaction. Regular but brief visual interactions have been proven to be more effective for patients in enhancing their overall experience with the doctor.

Doctors practice interpersonal communication skills with their patients, which involve verbal and nonverbal aspects. Scholars define these skills as the way communication affects others, and they are crucial in achieving positive patient outcomes. (Adolphs et al., 2009; Ainsworth et al., 2021).

4.3. Crisis Communication and Management

Strong leadership is essential during any crisis, especially in healthcare. In times of a healthcare crisis, leaders must carefully balance patient-centered care with limited resources. This highlights the need for wise guidance and robust leadership. For instance, providing healthcare during the COVID-19 pandemic has required careful consideration of what is best for each patient, while also taking into account the overall availability of treatment. Crisis management in the healthcare industry is not limited to pandemics. The ability to navigate a wide range of disasters, including fires, chemical emergencies, terrorist attacks, and weather-related events like floods or tornadoes, is essential for healthcare leaders

4.3.1. Crisis Management

The main objective of crisis management is to minimize the negative effects of a crisis by organizing several factors that harm the establishment. To put it succinctly, crisis management aims to shield the organization, its stakeholders, and the entire sector in which it works from potential harm by preventing or minimizing the negative effects of a crisis. It is feasible to take a different tack when defining crisis management and emphasize the opposite of what it is. To begin with, poor management is not the same as crisis management. Organizations frequently find themselves forced to respond to crises only after they worsen as a result of their own improper, insufficient, or nonexistent planning, or the total lack of a planning approach. However, managers of organizations rarely know which situations demand their increased and urgent attention and which do not in the absence of clearly defined priorities. It is not crisis management, but rather a classic case of poor management when there is an inability of the management to respond appropriately in such circumstances. Thus, true and effective crisis management necessitates a methodical approach to handling crises that permits the business to continue operating normally. The public views organizational crises very differently from public crises, viewing them as either an opportunity or a problem for organizations. This illustrates the significance of organizational crisis management. Organizational managers ought to address this issue internally. At the same time, crises present a chance for each organization's stakeholders to evaluate the management teams' qualifications. Some theorists and public relations specialists (Fink, 2002) distinguish crisis management as the art of eliminating risk and uncertainty in order to attain a greater degree of control over one's own destiny. They also compare crisis management to crisis planning. As a rule, organizations view crises as completely isolated events that can be analyzed through a total of four elements:

1. Causes - The presence of immediate mistakes that trigger the causes of the crisis and exacerbate existing problems

and deficiencies that facilitated the mistakes in the first place.

2. Consequences - can have immediate and long-term effects.
3. Caution - imply the inclusion of measures taken to prevent or minimize the effect of a potential crisis.
4. Response - implies measures taken to suppress a crisis that has already occurred.

Essentially, crisis management helps the business to develop a methodical and structured reaction to emergency situations. The foundation for the organization's ability to manage the crisis and carry out regular business is that response. On the other hand, the implementation of an early crisis detection system is what sets apart an effective and methodical crisis management system from an ineffective one. Specifically, by planning, which it is desirable to include, i.e., it is possible to prevent many crises or create a more favorable position for mitigating their negative effects by employing the skills of people from relevant organizational management sectors.

4.3.2. Crisis Communication

Crisis communication is the interaction between an organization and its audience prior to, during, and following a detrimental event. It involves developing strategies and tactics to lessen harm to the organization's reputation. Understanding the correlation between crisis management and crisis communication is crucial as effective crisis management involves effective communication. This not only helps to reduce and resolve the crisis but can also improve the organization's reputation in some cases.

While public relations deals with specific audiences such as employees, clients, shareholders, local community members, board members, unions, and retired employees of the company, crisis communication and public relations are closely intertwined. In this situation, proactive public relations initiatives can both make audiences an organization's ally in times of need and greatly strengthen the bond between them and the public, thereby preventing crises.

Crisis communication managers must comprehend, develop, and distribute messages to both internal and external recipients while simultaneously getting ready to receive feedback from these groups. Crisis communication entails identifying internal and external recipients who must receive information during a crisis.

Effective crisis communication is essential to successfully resolving crises. Rapid communication is a critical component of crisis management. It was typical for organizations to wait 24 hours following a crisis event before making a public statement in the "old days" of crisis communication. 24 hours is just too long to wait these days. Any crisis, no matter how big or small, is also an information crisis. Such an information crisis eventually becomes out of control, making control of the crisis itself impossible.

"A continuous process of creating shared meaning between groups, communities, individuals, and organizations, all to prepare, limit, and responding to risks and possible damage" is another definition of crisis communication. According to this definition, communication in a crisis involves a variety of communicators, message senders, and recipients, as well as instrumental and functional components. Communication processes imply a sense-making methodology that allows individuals, groups, communities, and organizations to co-create frameworks for understanding activities in situations that imply a high level of uncertainty, demands, and threats. This definition should be viewed in the context of this reality. The basic sense of stability and predictability that the majority of people rely on in their daily lives is severely shaken by such occurrences. In this context, the diversity of the public, their cultures, experiences, and background events, as well as the impact of new technologies on the forms of crisis situations, emphasize how much more complex crisis communication processes have become. In these situations, knowing how to communicate effectively can mean the difference between life and death, so it's important to grasp the process.

Without a doubt, crisis communication necessitates the quick creation of a communication team and includes it in the communication process. This process calls for an early start to communication with the public and the stakeholders involved, which enhances the organization's reputation and fosters trust. All relevant stakeholder groups and the general public must have their needs met by the communication's content, or the messages that the organization sends out, while also giving them access to the tone and context of each message. Simultaneously, it is important to consider that the objective and primary messages need to be consistent, and the specifics of their communication strategy may change based on the public groups and stakeholders (Crandall, Parnell, & Spillan, 2014).

4.3.2.1. Developmental-Situational Crises

A system that facilitates quick identification, action, prevention, and dissemination of health risk information to the larger community is necessary to effectively address public health threats. In crisis public health situations, it is imperative to enhance both vertical and horizontal communication channels by utilizing a shared platform that triggers pertinent factors automatically. Transitive processes in the world, such as a strong epidemiological transition (change in disease patterns), pandemics and the emergence of new infectious diseases (new viruses), the migrant crisis, followed by natural disasters (fires, earthquakes, floods), etc., are what condition crisis public health situations. Healthcare developmental crises are persistent, ingrained issues that have a big impact on the effectiveness and stability of healthcare systems.

Financial pressure is a major contributing factor to the crises in health systems. Insufficient funding limits the ability to keep up with technological advancements, upgrade infrastructure, and provide adequate salaries for health personnel. This lack of investment leads to a decrease in quality of service and difficulty accessing healthcare. The global shortage of health professionals exacerbates these challenges. By investing in education and training for health personnel, and implementing policy and management changes, long-term improvements in healthcare quality and accessibility can be achieved.

Unexpected and extraordinary events that have a major impact on the delivery of healthcare are known as situational crises in the healthcare industry. These emergencies frequently call for quick decisions and changes to the way health systems operate. Such situational health crises include, but are not limited to, pandemics, natural disasters, mass casualties, shortages of supplies and equipment, biological threats, and technological malfunctions. Effective preparation, coordination among various healthcare system levels, prompt decision-making, and collaboration with other sectors are essential for managing situational crises in the healthcare industry. It is imperative to consistently practice and revise emergency plans to guarantee that systems are prepared to handle unforeseen circumstances. Every crisis plan's primary purpose is to outline protocols, allocate personnel and material resources, and inform and direct participants toward the plan's execution. While acknowledging that no crisis manager can fully prepare us for every scenario that could arise, their significance in the healthcare system cannot be overstated as it gives us insight into the variety of emergencies and crises that can arise in healthcare facilities and help us hone our analytical abilities.

4.3.2.2. Communication Models During Times of Crisis

Healthcare institutions, like any other organization, engage in daily communication with both their internal and external audiences. Some of these organizations have a structured communication strategy in place, often outlined in formal documents known as Communication Strategies. These strategies often include communication models and are implemented by highly skilled communication professionals who can facilitate two-way, symmetric communication. The most successful organizations prioritize two-way symmetrical communication with both internal and external audiences as a key component of their overall communication strategy.

With their strategic public, many organizations use two-way communication, although this communication is more asymmetrical. It's looking like the most popular model of communication between organizations and their stakeholders is the asymmetrical two-way model. This model is not perfect. When a crisis arises, organizations that only communicate in one direction with the public—including the media—find themselves in a challenging position. Such an organization lacks the manpower and resources necessary to set up quick two-way symmetrical communication. The media and other audiences will not support taking such a turn, even during emergencies. Given the foregoing, it makes sense that healthcare organizations prefer a two-way, symmetrical communication model. When communicating the organization's crisis, this kind of model will yield the greatest outcomes.

4.3.3. Target Audiences (Stakeholders) in Crisis

Identifying the audience during a crisis is yet another crucial management responsibility. A homogeneous group of people known as an audience exerts influence over a corporation through their actions and vice versa. The degree to which the corporation can effectively and efficiently manage its relations with the public will determine its eventual success and survival. To effectively communicate in a crisis, a company must identify ahead of time the major audiences that may be directly or indirectly impacted by the crisis. Depending on the kind of crisis or disaster, various audiences are distinct from one another.

4.3.3.1. Public Health Institutions

Communication plays a key role in public health. It happens in multiple directions. Public health experts must first communicate with individuals, vulnerable populations, population groups, and the entire population that is affected by the implementation of a particular public health initiative. The term "publicity" of healthcare organizations describes the openness, reach, and knowledge that the general public has regarding the operations, guidelines, offerings, and outcomes of these institutions. A democratic society is one in which the people have the right to information about issues on their health and the healthcare system. Public health institutions are important for many reasons.

Transparency in information is essential, to start. Healthcare facilities should guarantee transparency and easy access to information regarding their operations, expenses, outcomes of treatments, caliber of care, and plans and policies. This makes it possible for the public to get more information about how the healthcare system is run and how to get the services they require.

Second, citizens must participate in the decision-making process. The right to participate in the decision-making process regarding health institution policies that affect them is granted to citizens. This could entail taking part in advisory committees, offering recommendations and remarks on proposed modifications, and assessing the performance of healthcare facilities.

Third, it is crucial to inform and educate the general public. Public education on the value of disease prevention, leading a healthy lifestyle, access to services, and patient rights should be provided by healthcare facilities. Knowledgeable people are better able to make decisions about their own health and take an active role in maintaining their well-being.

Fourth, patients are entitled to information regarding their medical condition and course of care. Access to your medical records and thorough explanations of your diagnosis, course of treatment, potential risks, and available alternatives are included in this. The public should be heard, and the health system should analyze its surroundings. It's critical to comprehend the needs of patients and the general public, how they view the health system's current policies, pinpoint their complaints, identify the important healthcare facilities that require extra attention, and look into any potential trouble spots.

"Consultations with the interested public" refers to the section of the Ministry of Health of the Republic of Croatia's website where information about the interests, views, suggestions, and concerns of all parties involved in the adoption of laws and other regulations is gathered. Additionally, the section highlights the importance of identifying any previously unnoticed weaknesses and negative effects of the public policy that must be corrected as soon as possible. Establishing channels for complaints and feedback is crucial. The public has the right to voice concerns about the caliber of care received from healthcare organizations and to register complaints if they are dissatisfied with the treatment they received. These mechanisms facilitate ongoing assessment and enhancement of healthcare quality and foster a relationship of trust between patients and healthcare organizations.

4.3.4. Crisis Communication Plan

The management of institutions, corporations, and other organizations needs to be aware of potential systemic crises. They need to begin preparing for contingencies in this regard. This entails planning and reaching as many decisions as you can ahead of a crisis. Pre-crisis planning allows individuals ample time to weigh all available options, analyze situations, weigh the pros and cons of various options, and assess readiness for action. Performing these crucial duties effectively is simpler during regular times, but becomes exceedingly challenging and stressful during a crisis. Crisis communication specialists identify five processes that can assist in creating a successful plan: form a planning team in step one; evaluate the problem's scope in step two; create a plan in step three; test the plan in step four; and update the plan in step five. S. Black, a British scientist, highlights six phases in the crisis plan. He states that these are:

- **Examining Potential Crisis Causes:** It is imperative to evaluate potential challenges, whether internal or external. It is frequently impossible to foresee every potential crisis. On the other hand, after the causes are evaluated, a list and an official designation should be made for them.

- **Getting the Plan Ready**: Pre-crisis communication planning, crisis communication, and post-crisis communication should all be included in the plan.
- **Personnel Selection**: The corporate administration ought to compile a list of people who are available in case of emergency when drafting the plan. That team's primary responsibility is fielding phone and media inquiries. These team lists need to be monitored around the clock after they are created.
- **Communication Abilities:** From a technical standpoint, when developing the plan, the issue of the load on permanent communication lines needs to be carefully considered. Recall that there was a communication blockade across the entire city at the time of the World Trade Center buildings' demolition in New York. It is important to anticipate and give this problem a high priority. However, one needs to be aware of the members of the crisis communication group and their responsibilities.
- **Instruction**: To ensure that everyone involved in the crisis plan understands their responsibilities, education and training programs must be set up. This will guarantee that personnel are prepared to respond in an emergency.
- **A Crisis Scenario Simulation**: After the crisis plan is established, it is imperative to repeatedly and covertly mimic the crisis scenario at various intervals. How the staff responds to the crisis and the crisis plan will be revealed by the simulation. It is, of course, a chance to rectify any potential flaws.

4.3.4.1. Crisis Communication Team

Everyone in a crisis-affected organization can't decide, coordinate, and be as knowledgeable about everything as possible. This is the reason a crisis team made up of the organization's top executives is formed, i.e., it needs to involve everyone who can professionally contribute to the crisis resolution. The CEO, the head of the organization's PR department, the vice president, the general manager of the region where the crisis originated, the head of protection, the organization's attorney, and anybody else who could provide insight into the matter should all be on the team.

Making contact with the crisis team ought to be the first step towards resolving the ensuing crisis. The team's first assignment is to design a crisis management strategy and select a spokesperson. It is crucial to remember that, even though a company might have a crisis plan in place, every crisis is unique and calls for either a new plan to be created or an adaptation of an existing one to take into account the situation as it is expected or predicted. During a crisis, the company should appoint a single person to serve as its primary spokesperson, making official statements and responding to inquiries from the media.

Appointing a deputy spokesperson is also important, as it allows for his replacement in case of need. It is anticipated that other parties involved in the crisis, such as the police, firefighters, and health officials, will also have spokespersons in addition to replacements. It is critical to ascertain these individuals' identities as soon as possible to coordinate all remarks and interactions with the media. As per Coombs (1999), a crisis communication team is defined as "a cross-functional group of people within an organization." In times of crisis, prompt and decisive action is necessary. The crisis team bears the majority of the load. The crisis information center needs to be set up because the crisis team's current tasks will prevent it from fully satisfying the public's curiosity.

4.3.5. Three Stages of the Crisis

The life cycle and developmental stages of crises are approached from various angles. We are familiar with the three-, four-, five-, and even six-stage models of crisis development in this regard. We will examine crisis and crisis communication in three stages, per various theoretical perspectives. This is the most popular model and approach for organizing and implementing crises.

Stage I- Preparation for the Crisis

The definition of the crisis, along with its types and causes, occurs during the first phase of the crisis. This stage includes the segmentation of the public during a crisis, which is crucial. Establishing a crisis communication team and a crisis communication plan are essential to crisis management.

i. **Causes of the Crisis:** The question of what causes crises in organizations emerges if we consider the crisis to be an unplanned process. Though the reasons vary, they can be broadly classified as internal and external. As the name implies, external causes originate in the surroundings and occur outside of the organization. It is believed that the organization has little to no impact on these factors. Natural disasters and accidents, political and social upheavals, economic crises, recessions, shifts in the market, the security environment, etc., are examples of external causes of crises that occur nowadays. Problems inside an organization are common. These crises are frequently invisible. These include a lackluster corporate culture; poor working conditions; unattainable union goals; strained interpersonal relationships; corruption; unhealthy rivalry; incompetence and immorality of management; etc. When considering the social and natural phenomena that can lead to crises, the causes can be broadly categorized into three groups.

- Natural phenomena – can be divided into two subgroups: a) geophysical phenomena such as earthquakes, floods, weather disasters, etc., and b) biological phenomena such as large epidemics (COVID-19).
- Technical factors – they are related to the technical and technological development of human civilization (major traffic accidents, major fires and explosions, nuclear accidents).
- Social phenomena (wars, armed conflicts, economic crises, mass hunger, etc.).

ii. **Research – Types of Crises:** As demonstrated, there are a variety of reasons why crises can occur. We can identify certain types of crises when we attempt to categorize all these crises into groups:

- Types of crises according to the environment they come from (physical crises, public opinion crises, administrative error crises, and crises in the political and economic spheres).
- Types of crises in terms of warning time: covert crises, such as audits or internal factors, and crises, such as accidents and deaths.

- Types of crises in terms of how they are experienced (perceptual crises and unusual crises). Some scientists list the following as potential crisis causes: natural disasters and accidents; health and environmental emergencies; technological mishaps; forces of the market and economy; and uncontrollably acting employees.

Stage II- Crisis Communication

The second stage is marked by the course of the crisis, i.e., the behavior of key publics during the crisis, workers, and external publics. It is crucial to draw attention to the strained relationships with the media during this time.

i. **The Course of the Crisis:** American crisis management specialist P. McCue described how the crisis developed. "A special interest group (active public) that sends negative information to the public and thereby activates the alarm," was how he put it in the beginning. As the explanation of the crisis trajectory continues, it is claimed that the media regularly instills a sense of general danger and plays a crucial role in reporting on the incident. When faced with a crisis, a company makes a statement that is more grounded in facts than in emotions. Because of the bad media coverage, people are starting to steer clear of dubious products from companies impacted by the crisis. Under such circumstances, product sales decline. The public's negative campaign against the impacted organization is stepped up by the crisis instigators, a special interest group, and the media is more likely to cover anything the instigators say. For a while, everyone loses sight of the true issue causing the crisis as the impacted company makes every effort to combat it and boost sales. After a while, everything becomes apparent, the organization gains momentum for more work, and the media searches for a fresh participant impacted by the crisis.

ii. **Implementation of the Crisis:** Five presumptions that should be remembered in times of crisis are listed by General Electric Company CEO and Manager of the Century in the USA, Jack Welch, in his book Winning.

- Always approach a problem with the assumption that it is more challenging than it initially appears. Crises tend to escalate quickly and become bigger and more serious than anticipated. They also have a longer duration than expected, causing more discomfort over time. More people are affected than imagined, leading to increased legal involvement and negative publicity. It is crucial to be proactive and assume that the worst has occurred within your organization and that it is your responsibility to resolve the issue. Always approach a crisis with the mindset that it is a significant problem that needs to be addressed promptly.
- Presume that everything will eventually come to light and that there are no secrets in the real world. Your lawyers will advise you to say as little as possible during a crisis. This advice is generally sound. However, don't accept it as infallible. Get as much time as you can to speak with your lawyers. All you need to do is make

sure that everything you say is completely truthful and devoid of any ambiguity. People will trust you more, both inside and outside the company, the more candidly you discuss the issue, its causes, and potential solutions.

- Expect that the media will present you and your organization's handling of the crisis in the worst possible light. The size of the market share is a key indicator of success in certain industries; in others, it may be an increase in revenue, the number of concessions secured over a year, or metrics indicating higher levels of customer satisfaction. Success in journalism is determined by how many empires are overthrown and emperors exposed. Being publicly defamed is difficult. However, that is entirely unimportant, regardless of how innocent you feel or how certain you are that your company is managing its problems admirably. A journalist's job is to present opportunities as they see them, not to interpret your interpretation of the situation. Although you might want to give up sometimes, you can't. In addition to outlining every facet of the issue, concisely describe your perspective on the recently formed predicament and offer your suggestions for resolving it. If you don't, people will take your ambiguity as an admission of guilt. Not every crisis is indeed made public. The same guidelines apply in this instance: discuss the issue honestly, express your viewpoint, explain how the issue came about, and outline your plan of action.
- Anticipate that following the crisis, both personnel and process changes will occur. A financial or legal settlement marks the end of most crises. Next is cleaning, which necessitates adjustments. Procedures are typically the first to suffer, though there are times when individuals who disregard the rules may also be the source of the issue. Changes are necessary in crises. This explains why bloodshed is a common outcome of crises.
- Think that your company will not only get through this crisis but will come out of it stronger. No crisis is so great that you cannot learn something from it, even though you will always despise it. You will always feel pressure to move on and forget about a crisis period quickly after it ends. Resolve from crises and seize every chance to tell others about your experiences.

iii. **Information Gap:** It is crucial to respond to the public right away, as demonstrated by the examination of crisis relations initiatives with the media. To prevent an information gap, the spokesperson, general manager, or other person authorized to communicate with the media must answer questions from the press, even if not all information is gathered. The period between a crisis's emergence and media communication is known as the "information gap." If the public is not informed promptly, the media will have to rely on rumors or incomplete information to enlighten them. Professionals and experts agree that a prompt response—within 24 hours—is necessary. However, in the modern era of new media and digital technology, you no longer have to consider 24 hours. "Eternity" is the term. Some people will argue that you must act as quickly as possible, even instantaneously. It is crucial to remember that accuracy and data verification must not be sacrificed in the name of a prompt response. When we have something to say, we must act quickly. When a crisis might arise, communications professionals need to consider a lot of things. People in the developed world take modern electronic communication for granted. One such question is, "What if communication channels are destroyed in a crisis?" The answers to this question are as follows. In actuality, we rely a great deal on fax, e-mail, the Internet, phones, radio, and television for mutual communication. It's not until the power goes out, our internet service fails, or the company server fails that we realize how dependent we are on these things. Thankfully, these incidents typically end after a few minutes. Crisis managers need to know that large-scale natural or man-made disasters can hinder their ability to communicate with staff and the general public and disrupt electronic communications for days or weeks at a time.

iv. **Tools in Crisis Public Relations:** The communication team can use a variety of channels to communicate with the media, including briefings, interviews, press conferences, statements, and press releases. Public statements are important communication tools for information mediation. With them, the company's management conveys its regret and other emotions as well as the essential details of the incident. Public statements in crises frequently need to be updated as soon as new information becomes available. A press conference that enables the administration to provide information to all journalists at once is unquestionably a useful communication tool in crises. Companies can explain any misunderstandings and live-tell their story at conferences. Press conferences should not be constrained in a crisis as this could give the impression that something is being covered up. This is an important principle to remember.

- Briefing. The first, urgent briefing usually kicks off the analysis of the crisis and the initial encounter with the crisis phenomenon. The campaign plan uses the briefing as a communication tool. The individuals taking part in the briefing are identified by the plan. Here, the circumstances are examined and agreed-upon actions and crisis management strategies are established.
- Interviews with spokespersons or representatives of management make good communication tools. Interviews allow management of the company to clarify events and eliminate any potential ambiguities. It would be ideal to conduct a mock interview in which the candidate would be presented with possible questions and asked to prepare responses.
- In media relations, press releases are also frequently utilized. Press releases assist in communicating the management's stance to the

public and media, as well as any new information. Background data is another frequently used crisis PR tool. This is the most crucial information available to journalists as an addendum to the current story about the organization, including its history, the makeup of the board, its accomplishments, pictures, and any other pertinent information. Since journalists can't always get to the scene, special phone lines and communication tools are required. Members of the crisis communication team, who must be well-prepared with all relevant information and materials regarding the crisis situation, should field calls from the media. Every question posed should be able to be addressed by members of the crisis communication team.

Stage III – Post-Crisis Communication

A crisis presents a company with both a chance to improve its reputation and a pivotal moment in its history. As soon as the crisis is over, the organization needs to get back to its regular operations and focus on enhancing and repairing its reputation. Regretfully, the majority of organizations continue to operate in the same manner following a crisis, failing to learn from the mistakes that brought them to that point. Ignoring the crisis is the biggest mistake. Only when experiences are carefully examined can they be instructive. Following the crisis, management needs to assess what went well and what didn't. If the crisis plan was followed by the management, it should be ascertained which aspects were carried out effectively and which were not. Determining whether and how the crisis might have been avoided is essential. Enhancing the action plan—which is never final—in crises is the primary goal of the analysis. After the crisis has passed, but not for more than 30 days, analysis of the situation should begin as new tasks come up.

i. **Consequence Analysis:** The final phase of the crisis involves communication and analysis of the fallout. The company or organization will take into account every aspect of the crisis, make deductions learn from it, and work to get back to business as usual as soon as feasible. Forgetting about the crisis too soon can be one of the worst mistakes. Consequently, the adage that lightning can strike the same spot twice is not unfounded. Both internal and external publics should be included in the analysis, i.e., the number of sales, public opinion, media publications, the number of employees involved in the crisis, material damage, and potential compensation lawsuits. To help the administration handle similar crises in the future, it is desirable to keep records and notices of events during a crisis. The management can avert similar crises in the future if the analysis is successful in identifying the crisis's causes and the individuals in charge.

ii. **Solving the Crisis:** This crisis stands alone as a narrative. Some are solely tied to internal issues within the company, and they typically have a speedy resolution. However, some crises develop into massive media sensations with a wide range of legal ramifications. The unique nature of every crisis makes it challenging to develop universal guidelines for resolving them. As we've already discussed, when resolving a crisis in your company, you need to consider the following five assumptions:

- Always assume that the issue is more complex than it initially appears.
- Assume that everyone will eventually know everything and that there are no secrets in the real world.
- It is reasonable to assume that the media will present you and your organization's handling of the crisis in the worst possible light.
- Presume that there will be personnel and process changes following the crisis.
- Think that your company will not only get through this crisis but will come out of it stronger.

It is a common occurrence for companies to take drastic measures after overcoming a crisis. To be prepared to combat the enemy who has already succeeded in breaching their ranks once, they arm themselves with a variety of regulations and establish certain protocols (Welch, 2005).

4.3.6. Crisis Caused by the Pandemic Covid 19

The global COVID-19 pandemic posed a significant challenge. The Chinese city of Wuhan saw the first case of an unidentified viral illness at the close of 2019 and the start of 2020. Scientists identified the virus as SARS-CoV-2 very quickly, i.e., the coronavirus, the causative agent of COVID-19. This virus causes pneumonia in humans, along with a few other symptoms like fever, chills, dyspnea, and dry cough. The coronavirus is a zoonotic virus, meaning that it spreads from humans to animals (. The health system had to deal with an increase in patients, a shortage of resources, and the possibility of health workers contracting infections. To stop the virus from spreading, state governments have put in place measures including mask-wearing, physical distance, and movement restrictions. The economy and daily living were greatly impacted by these policies.

On March 11, 2020, the World Health Organization declared a pandemic threat due to the virus's extremely quick spread. On January 13, 2020, cases were discovered in Thailand, marking the first instances of cases that left China. After a year, the coronavirus had spread to 191 nations and all activities were prohibited. Although vaccination has been crucial in the fight against the pandemic, issues with vaccine distribution and accessibility have surfaced. The pandemic had major psychological and social effects as well, with unemployment, social isolation, and uncertainty hurting people's mental health. Meeting these challenges also required a strong sense of community unity. Everyone had to work together during this crisis to overcome the obstacles and facilitate the community's speedy recovery. On May 5, 2023, the World Health Organization (WHO) finally announced that the COVID-19 pandemic had ended, ending the long-awaited global emergency.

4.4. Challenges

Giving people health-related information presents several difficulties. The disparity in health literacy between the general public and medical professionals and institutions, as well as the shortcomings in the dissemination of health information by the media, are among the most important concerns.

Cultural values also have an impact on health communication, and in certain situations, these influences can be a barrier to effective health communication. Effective health communication decreases when the sender and recipient come from different socioeconomic backgrounds, are not of the same race, or are even very different ages. This is because people are more likely to trust and be receptive to ideas from someone who looks like them.

4.4.1. Literacy-Communication Gap

The disparity that exists between health literacy and the application of health communication is one issue that health communication aims to solve. Health communication should effectively result in health literacy, but obstacles to patient healthcare literacy have been created by things like the use of medical jargon that isn't explained, poorly written messages, and frequently a general educational gap. Studies on senior populations in America have been conducted in particular to highlight a common audience that is disadvantaged as a result of this problem. Compared to other age groups, older adults typically have the highest number of chronic health conditions; however, research has shown that this group also has trouble understanding written health materials, comprehending health care and policies, and generally not understanding medical jargon. Inadequate health communication can result in a rise in hospital admissions, impaired response and management of illnesses, and a general deterioration in health.

Health communication specialists have suggested initiatives to enhance doctor-patient communication as a solution to these issues. One suggestion is to enhance the education of medical students by incorporating seminars, workshops, and closely monitored patient interactions to teach interpersonal and communication skills as essential competencies. It is also advised that practicing physicians participate in specialized on-site training programs and webinars to enhance their communication skills. Physicians who are better at communicating with patients will be able to address the issue of patients not understanding healthcare and help patients follow medical advice more closely.

In certain demographics, health-related websites (e.g., WebMD) and virtual support communities (e.g., Association for Cancer Online Resources) have made health information more widely available. Language has an important part in communication, particularly when it comes to the language that patients prefer that doctors speak to them in. Limited English proficient (LEP) patients have better health outcomes when they receive care from doctors who are fluent in their preferred language, according to the findings of a 2019 systematic review. A review of research on what happens when health information is unclear, how to help people understand health information, and which demographic groups may require additional support in understanding health content has been published by the National Institute for Health and Care Research (NIHR) for use by health information providers. It includes studies on choosing the right focus, employing straightforward, balanced language, and using different formats (e.g., films, images), and internet data.

4.4.2. Mass Media

The goal of mass communication is to encourage positive behavioral changes within populations. A significant critique of the mass media's role in health communication is its regrettable capacity to disseminate inaccurate and misleading information rapidly, often before experts have a chance to refute it. As technology develops, this problem might cause unjustified fear in individuals who receive the messages. An illustration of this can be seen in the persistent mistrust that people have for vaccinations as a result of multiple messages that incorrectly associate the childhood measles, mumps, and rubella (MMR) vaccination with the emergence and development of autism. Thanks to the new social networking technologies, this message spread quickly, making many parents distrust vaccinations and choosing not to give their children the shot. Public health is at risk because many people refuse vaccinations. After all, they have lingering misgivings about them, even though this panic is based on misleading information. (Tacheva et al., 2013; Vimala et al., 2017).

A Closer Look

The Evolution of Communication in the Healthcare Sector

The IT infrastructure of organizations and businesses involved in the healthcare industry has been significantly impacted by the numerous drastic changes that have occurred in communication over the years. Digitization has brought about a rapid technological change that has profoundly reshaped the patient journey, from care delivery to health data management, and from research and development to general operations. It has also had an impact on the quality and quantity of services offered. We will examine the most significant innovations of today and quickly recapitulate the key phases of the evolution of healthcare communication to get a sense of the scope of this shift.

From the 1960s to the 1980s: The First Computerized Systems

The United States saw the emergence of basic health databases and the first computerized medical data management systems in the 1960s. During this time, the first attempts were also made to digitize the electronic health records (EHRs) of patients. EHRs were initially so costly that governments could only use them in conjunction with large healthcare organizations. Over the following ten years, larger hospitals mostly used EHRs for scheduling and billing.

The 1960s also saw the emergence of a new, "problem-oriented," paper-based method for maintaining medical records that involved adding details to improve each patient's clinical picture. The medical record has evolved into a useful tool for healthcare teams to communicate with one another and coordinate the administration of preventive care.

Even though most records are still currently paper-based and must be physically filed and moved, business technology advanced to the point where in the 1980s electronic filing became commonplace and records could even be faxed electronically (at least in an emergency, like contacting a patient's family physician, for example). From this point on, the advancement of electronic health records gained momentum.

The 1990s: the Spread of Electronic Health Records

Electronic technology was widely used in most U.S. medical offices, although their use remained restricted (with the primary purpose being the updating of records). Electronic medical records, which included data exchange for processing requests and image scanning for document capture, were still mostly viewed at hospital medical facilities and academic outpatient clinics. Prescription history transfer and electronic medical record sharing were once sporadic activities; only with the introduction of the Internet did they gradually spread to a large scale. One of the biggest changes to the healthcare sector in a long time is the centralization of patient data through electronic medical records, which allows healthcare facilities to share, search, and access data at any time. As a result, there were fewer paper records and an increasing rationalization of the information. Patient data is now more accurate thanks to electronic health records, which have also made it simpler to obtain, update, and share important medical data. By doing this, EHRs successfully imposed a new paradigm of healthcare communication while also improving coordination amongst diverse healthcare providers and the quality of care.

The 2000s: From Telemedicine to Cloud Computing

Telemedicine services have grown since the 2000s, especially in the area of remote patient monitoring. This has been especially true since the 2010s. The capacity to overcome geographical barriers is the main advantage provided by the increasing use of telemedicine.

Telemedicine makes healthcare much more accessible by enabling remote monitoring, diagnosis, and consultation. The introduction of telemedicine marks a revolution in the provision of healthcare. Providers can diagnose, treat, and consult with patients anywhere by utilizing digital communication. This is especially important for providing care to patients in underserved or remote areas as well as during international health emergencies, such as the COVID-19 pandemic.

One important technology that makes data sharing and storage easier is cloud computing, which has grown significantly since the mid-2010s. Healthcare companies are moving more and more of their data and apps to the cloud because cloud-based systems are efficient, scalable, and flexible, and enable operators to safely store and analyze massive amounts of data. Applications for blockchain, IoT devices, and artificial intelligence are proliferating as well. Data analytics is also receiving more attention as it can be used to enhance the prompt management of patient populations.

Additional specialization is possible with electronic health records: using data in predictive analytics projects can yield insights that enhance clinical decision-making. The objective is to enhance physician-patient relationships, boost productivity, and further streamline workflows.

The development of digital communication in the healthcare industry has undoubtedly had a revolutionary impact. The healthcare industry has seen significant transformation, from the adoption of electronic health records to the growth of telemedicine, from the incorporation of cloud-based solutions to the launch of artificial intelligence applications. In addition to streamlining administrative procedures, digital communication tools have completely revamped the patient experience. They have increased patient involvement, made care coordination easier, and opened the door for more precise diagnosis and treatment.

As technology develops, it promises increased connectivity, ease of use, and individualized treatment. The history of digital communication in healthcare is one of advancement and constant change, with a seemingly limitless potential for creativity. In actuality, organizations still have obstacles to overcome before they can fulfill their ultimate objective, which is to deliver better, more effective, and increasingly patient-centered care.

Summary

- Healthcare leaders understand that effective communication in healthcare organizations starts with recognizing the importance of listening to one another.
- Health care facilities can develop patient portals, which allow patients to sign up and have confidential access to their individual health care information. Educational health information can be placed on the patient's portal that is relevant to the patient's specific health needs.
- Tailoring a health message is one strategy for persuasive health communication. For messages of health communication to reach selected audiences accurately and quickly, health communication professionals must assemble a collection of superior and audience-appropriate information that targets population segments. Understanding the audience for the information is critical to effective delivery.
- Communication is a basic clinical skill that, when performed competently and efficiently, enables the establishment of a true therapeutic alliance, a relationship of trust between medical staff and patients and clients.
- Verbal communication consists of spoken and written language that people use to convey their ideas. The language used by patients and healthcare providers in their encounters with healthcare has a significant impact on how well they understand each other.
- Nonverbal communication is another important part of good health habits. Scientists describe nonverbal communication as an aspect of communication in which information is exchanged via purely nonverbal communication signals such as gestures, touches, facial expressions, eye contact, clothing, and hairstyles.
- Crisis management can be defined as a series of factors organized to deal with a crisis, the main goal of which is to reduce its negative effects, i.e., damage to the organization.
- Crisis communication can be defined as a dialogue between an organization and its public immediately before a negative event, during a negative event and after a negative event. This dialogue implies the creation of strategies and tactics intending to minimize damage to the image of the organization.
- An audience is a homogeneous group of people who influence the corporation through their actions and vice versa. Its success and long-term survival depend on how successfully and efficiently the corporation manages its relations with the public.
- Management of corporations, management of institutions and organizations must be aware of possible crises in their system. In this regard, they must start planning for emergencies. This includes organization and making as many decisions as possible before a crisis occurs.
- There are many challenges in communicating information about health to individuals. Some of the most essential issues have to do with the gap between individual health literacy and healthcare workers and institutions, as well as flaws in communicating health information through mass media.

References

1. Adolphs, R. (2009). The social brain: Neural basis of social knowledge. *Annual Review of Psychology, 60*(1), 693–716. https://doi.org/10.1146/annurev.psych.60.110707.163514.
2. Ainsworth, M. S. (1989). Attachments beyond infancy. *American Psychologist, 44*(4), 709–716. https://doi.org/10.1037/0003-066X.44.4.709.
3. Al-Qarni, A. A., Alsharqi, O. Z., Qalai, D. A., & Kadi, N. (2013). The impact of marketing mix strategy on hospital performance measured by patient satisfaction: An empirical investigation on Jeddah private sector hospital senior managers' perspective. *International Journal of Marketing Studies, 5*(6), 210–221. https://doi.org/10.5539/ijms.v5n6p210.
4. Ambady, N., LaPlante, D., Nguyen, T., Rosenthal, R., Chaumeton, N., & Levinson, W. (2002). Surgeons' tone of voice: A clue to malpractice history. *Surgery, 132*(1), 5–9. https://doi.org/10.1067/msy.2002.122314.
5. Athanasiu, A. (1998). *Tratat De Psihologie Medicală*. Oscar Print.
6. Balaban, R. B. (2000). A physician's guide to talking about end-of-life care. *Journal of General Internal Medicine, 15*(3), 195–200. https://doi.org/10.1046/j.1525-1497.2000.98041.x.
7. Blair, A., & Wasson, K. (2015). Professionalism and appropriate expression of empathy when breaking bad news. *AMA Journal of Ethics, 17*(2), 111–115. https://doi.org/10.1001/journalofethics.2015.17.2.e111.
8. Boudreaux, E. D., Mandry, C. V., & Wood, K. (2003). Patient satisfaction data as a quality indicator: A tale of two emergency departments. *Academic Emergency Medicine, 10*(3), 261–268. https://doi.org/10.1197/aemj.10.3.261.
9. Brock, D., Abu-Rish, E., Chiu, C. R., Hammer, D., Wilson, S., Vorvick, L., & Zierler, B. (2013). Republished: Interprofessional education in team communication: Working together to improve patient safety. *Postgraduate Medical Journal, 89*(1057), 642–651. https://doi.org/10.1136/postgradmedj-2012-131282.
10. Chichirez, C. M., & Purcărea, V. L. (2018). Interpersonal communication in healthcare. *Journal of Medicine and Life, 11*(2), 119–121. https://doi.org/10.25122/jml-2018-0023.
11. Cole, K. (1993). *Crystal Clear Communication: Skills for Understanding and Being Understood* (2nd ed.). Prentice Hall.
12. Coombs, T. (2012). *Ongoing Crisis Communications*. Sage Publications.
13. Crandall, W., Parnell, J., & Spillan, J. (2014). *Crisis Management in the New Strategy Landscape*. Sage Publications.
14. Denio, G. (2013). "It'll be OK": The effects of supportive talk on patient perceptions of physicians in racially discordant medical interactions. *Journal of Health Communication, 18*(5), 561–577. https://doi.org/10.1080/10810730.2012.710570.
15. Duffy, F. D., Gordon, G. H., Whelan, G., Cole-Kelly, K., & Frankel, R. (2004). Assessing competence in communication and interpersonal skills: The Kalamazoo II report. *Academic Medicine, 79*(6), 495–507. https://doi.org/10.1097/01.ACM.0000120653.26068.8f.
16. Gorawara-Bhat, R., Dethmers, D. L., & Cook, M. A. (2013). Physician eye contact and elder patient perceptions of understanding and adherence. *Patient Education and Counseling, 92*(3), 375–380. https://doi.org/10.1016/j.pec.2013.06.013.

17. Gordon, T., & Edwards, W. S. (1997). *Making the Patient Your Partner: Communication Skills for Doctors and Other Caregivers*. Auburn House.

18. Graham, S., & Brookey, J. (2008). Do patients understand? *The Permanente Journal, 12*(3), 67–71. https://doi.org/10.7812/tpp/07-153.

19. Hall, J. A., Stein, T. S., Roter, D. L., & Rieser, N. (1999). Inaccuracies in physicians' perceptions of their patients. *Medical Care, 37*(11), 1164–1168. https://doi.org/10.1097/00005650-199911000-00002.

20. Hirsch, E. M. (2007). The role of empathy in medicine: A medical student's perspective. *Virtual Mentor, 9*(6), 423–427. https://doi.org/10.1001/virtualmentor.2007.9.6.msoc1-0706.

21. Horton, J. A., Clance, P. R., Sterk-Elifson, C., & Emshoff, J. (1995). Touch in psychotherapy: A survey of patients' experiences. *Psychotherapy: Theory, Research, Practice, Training, 32*(3), 443–451. https://doi.org/10.1037/h0087815.

22. Hull, M. (2016). Medical language proficiency: A discussion of interprofessional language competencies and potential for patient risk. *International Journal of Nursing Studies, 54*, 158–172. https://doi.org/10.1016/j.ijnurstu.2015.12.003.

23. Joyce, A., Jain, B., Khoury, J., & Trodden, M. (2015). Beyond the cosmological standard model. *Physics Reports, 568*, 1–98. https://doi.org/10.1016/j.physrep.2014.12.002.

24. Khan, F. M., & Gibbons, J. P. (2014). *Khan's the Physics of Radiation Therapy* (5th ed.). Lippincott Williams & Wilkins.

25. Kupst, M. J., Schulman, J. L., & Dowding, J. (1979). Evaluation: Attitudes toward patient care and work satisfaction. *Hospital & Health Services Administration, 24*(1), 78–92.

26. Larson, E. B., & Yao, X. (2005). Clinical empathy as emotional labor in the patient-physician relationship. *JAMA, 293*(9), 1100–1106. https://doi.org/10.1001/jama.293.9.1100.

27. Mackenzie, E., Farah, C. S., & Savage, N. W. (2002). Effective communication for health care professionals. *Hygiene Today, 14*, 8–12.

28. Marcinowicz, L., Konstantynowicz, J., & Godlewski, C. (2010). Patients' perceptions of GP non-verbal communication: A qualitative study. *British Journal of General Practice, 60*(571), 83–87. https://doi.org/10.3399/bjgp10X483056.

29. Matusitz, J., & Spear, J. (2014). Effective doctor–patient communication: An updated examination. *Social Work in Public Health, 29*(3), 252–266. https://doi.org/10.1080/19371918.2011.642805.

30. McDonald, S. P., Marshall, M. R., Johnson, D. W., & Polkinghorne, K. R. (2009). Relationship between dialysis modality and mortality. *Journal of the American Society of Nephrology, 20*(1), 155–163. https://doi.org/10.1681/ASN.2008040370.

31. McGorry, S. Y. (1999). An investigation of expectations and perceptions of health-care services with a Latino population. *International Journal of Health Care Quality Assurance, 12*(2), 63–70. https://doi.org/10.1108/09526869910255628.

32. Oliver, R. L. (2014). *Satisfaction: A Behavioral Perspective on the Consumer*. Routledge.

33. Olson, D. P., & Roth, K. E. (2007). Diagnostic tools and the hands-on physical examination. *Virtual Mentor, 9*(2), 113–118. https://doi.org/10.1001/virtualmentor.2007.9.2.stas1-0702.

34. Roter, D. L., & Hall, J. A. (1989). Studies of doctor-patient interaction. *Annual Review of Public Health, 10*(1), 163–180. https://doi.org/10.1146/annurev.pu.10.050189.001115.

35. Roter, D., Stewart, M., Putnam, S. M., Lipkin, M., Stiles, W., & Inui, T. S. (1997). The patient–physician relationship: Communication patterns of primary care physicians. *Journal of the American Medical Association, 277*(4), 350–356. https://doi.org/10.1001/jama.277.4.350.

36. Silverman, J. L., Yang, M., Lord, C., & Crawley, J. N. (2010). Behavioral phenotyping assays for mouse models of autism. *Nature Reviews Neuroscience, 11*(7), 490–502. https://doi.org/10.1038/nrn2861.

37. Soo, K. C. H., David, M. K., Kia, L. S., & Pei, A. (2011). Openings and closings in front counter transactions of Malaysian government hospitals. *The Journal of the South East Asia Research Centre for Communication and Humanities, 3*(1), 13–30.

38. Sparks, L. (1998). *Health Care and Caregiving Research, Policy, and Practice: Multi-Disciplinary Coordinated Caregiving: Professional Contributions*. Springer.

39. Street, R. L. (1992). Communicative styles and adaptations in physician-parent consultations. *Social Science & Medicine, 34*(10), 1155–1163. https://doi.org/10.1016/0277-9536(92)90013-K.

40. Swinglehurst, D., Roberts, C., Li, S., Weber, O., & Singy, P. (2014). Beyond the "dyad": A qualitative reevaluation of the changing clinical consultation. *BMJ Open, 4*(9), e006017. https://doi.org/10.1136/bmjopen-2014-006017.

41. Tacheva, V. (2013). Communication–the master key to the patient's heart. *JAHR-European Journal of Bioethics, 4*(7), 601–620.

42. Tomić, Z., Vegar, V., & Radalj, M. (2024). Crisis communication in healthcare. *Medicina Academica Integrative, 1*(1), 11–25. https://doi.org/10.1016/j.medicina.2024.01.001.

43. Van Servellen, G. (2009). *Communication Skills for the Health Care Professional: Concepts, Practice, and Evidence*. Jones & Bartlett Publishers.

44. Vimala, G. (2017). Interpersonal communication skills used by cardiologists in doctor-patient communication at the National Heart Institute, Malaysia. *Proceedings of the International Conference on Business and Social Sciences*. http://psasir.upm.edu.my/id/eprint/67389/1/FBMK%202017%2061%20IR.pdf (accessed on 3 September 2024).

45. Women, P., Yawn, B., Yawn, R., & Uden, D. (1992). American Medical Association diagnostic and treatment guidelines on domestic violence. *Archives of Family Medicine, 1*(1), 39–48. https://doi.org/10.1001/archfami.1.1.39.

Chapter 5

HEALTH DISPARITIES

Contents

Introduction

The term "health disparities" describes the notable variations in health outcomes and healthcare service accessibility between different population groups. Disadvantages in the social, economic, and environmental spheres frequently impact these differences. They appear in a variety of contexts, such as those involving race, ethnicity, socioeconomic class, age, place of residence, gender, sexual orientation, and disability status. In addition to being a question of personal health, health disparities also represent larger structural problems in society that have an impact on equity and the well-being of communities. The difference in health outcomes between racial and ethnic groups is one of the most well-known instances of health disparities. Compared to their white counterparts, members of minority groups—especially African Americans, Hispanic Americans, Native Americans, and Pacific Islanders—frequently have greater incidence of chronic illnesses like diabetes, hypertension, and some types of cancer. African Americans, for example, have greater mortality rates from heart disease and stroke and are more likely to experience these conditions. These variations are mostly caused by social determinants of health, which include exposure to environmental hazards, lower socioeconomic status, limited access to high-quality healthcare, and educational disparities, rather than just genetic factors.

Another important factor that significantly contributes to health disparities is socioeconomic status (SES). People from lower socioeconomic backgrounds frequently encounter obstacles when trying to obtain healthcare, such as not having insurance, being unable to pay for treatment, and having few healthcare providers in their areas. This results in poorer chronic condition management, delayed disease diagnosis and treatment, and ultimately worse health outcomes. Inequalities in health are further exacerbated by the fact that those with lower SES are more likely to reside in places where environmental pollutants are more prevalent and have less access to safe recreational areas and wholesome food options. Health disparities are significantly influenced by geographic location as well. Longer travel times to medical facilities, a shortage of healthcare providers, and fewer public transportation options are just a few of the particular difficulties faced by rural communities. In comparison to urban populations, these obstacles lead to lower rates of preventive care, a higher incidence of untreated medical conditions, and generally worse health outcomes. Furthermore, access to advanced treatments and specialized medical services is frequently limited for residents living in rural areas, which can cause delays in receiving necessary care.

Age and gender differences exacerbate health disparities even more. For example, women may face different health risks during pregnancy and childbirth and have unequal access to reproductive health services. Conversely, age-related biases in the healthcare system may affect elderly people, underdiagnosing and undertreating conditions that have a substantial negative influence on their quality of life. A multifaceted strategy including systemic reforms targeted at enhancing social determinants of health, community engagement, and policy changes is needed to address health disparities. The main goals should be to improve health literacy, expand access to high-quality healthcare, and advance fair economic and educational opportunities. Interventions in public health must be customized to the unique requirements of marginalized communities to guarantee that everyone has the chance to reach optimal health. Society can advance toward greater health equity and enhance overall public health outcomes by addressing the underlying causes of health disparities.

Orientation and Directional Terms:

Term	Definition	Illustration
Ableism	Characterizes people as they are defined by their disabilities and it also classifies disabled people as people who are inferior to non-disabled people.	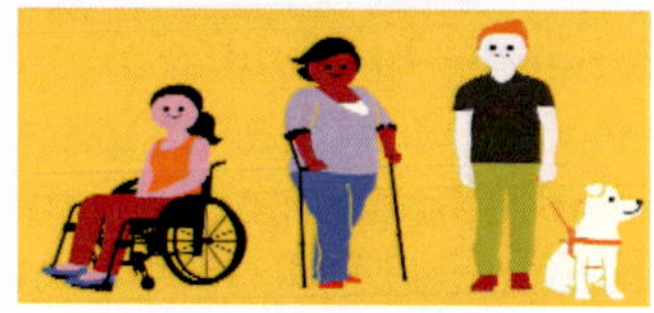
Homophobia	Encompasses a range of negative attitudes and feelings toward homosexuality or people who identify or are perceived as being lesbian, gay, or bisexual.	
Racial disparities	The imbalances and incongruities between the treatment of racial groups, including economic status, income, housing options, societal treatment, safety, and myriad other aspects of life and society.	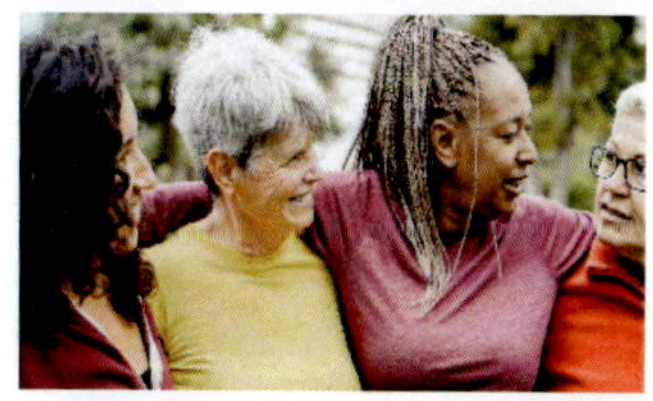
Hispanic patients	Hispanic patients are individuals receiving medical care who identify as Hispanic or Latino. This term refers to people with cultural ties to Spanish-speaking countries, primarily in Latin America and the Iberian Peninsula (Spain and Portugal).	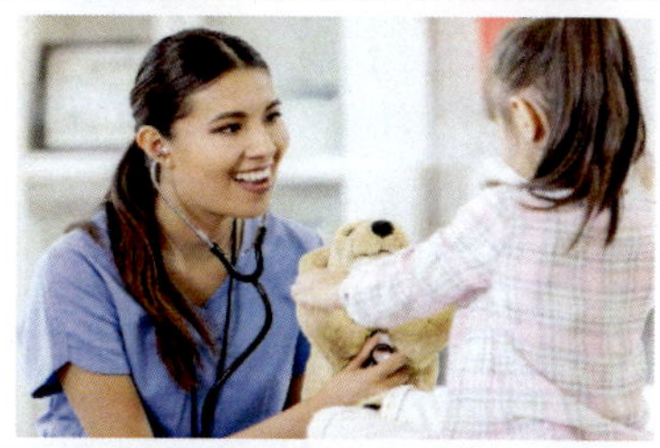
Social desirability	A type of response bias that is the tendency of survey respondents to answer questions in a manner that will be viewed favorably by others.	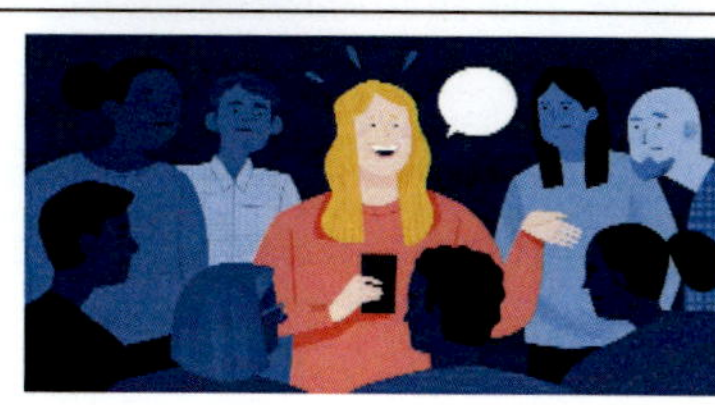

5.1. Basics of Health Disparities

When people and communities face greater rates of obesity, heart disease, breast cancer, and other illnesses due to particular factors like race and ethnicity, access to care, poverty, and environmental risk, it is known as a health disparity. The causes of these health disparities are numerous. For example, mistrust of the healthcare system can exacerbate Black people's difficulties in preventing HIV infection. Not only can transportation make it difficult for elderly people to keep appointments, but it can also be a problem for people who live in areas known as "food deserts," which are areas lacking supermarkets that sell wholesome foods. Complex factors are at the heart of health disparities. Since so many factors affect health, it can be challenging to identify the precise reason why differences in health can exist between individuals and groups.

Some examples include:

- **Infant Mortality:** Babies born to Black people in the United States die at more than double the rate of babies born to white people.
- **Dementia:** Access to care for Alzheimer's disease is more difficult for Black Americans, who report a 50% rate of discrimination in seeking health care, and other minorities facing dementia.
- **Cancer:** There are many examples. Black females are less likely than White females to live 5 years after being diagnosed with cervical cancer. Native people are more likely to face colorectal cancer, in part due to access issues with screening.
- **Obesity:** Childhood obesity is far more common in Black and Latinx kids (25% or more) than White kids (17%), as reported through 2020 data.
- **Smoking:** Low-income people use tobacco more often, have a higher risk of related illness, and may live and work in environments where secondhand smoke exposure is more common.
- **Binge Drinking:** Young people ages 18–34 are more likely than other groups to binge drink and it's more common in males.
- **Mental Health:** Racial and ethnic minorities may experience more stress in their lives, due to racism or its indirect consequences, like distrust in the healthcare system.

One example of a health disparity that affects generations is maternal health. A developing fetus's health is influenced by a variety of environmental and social factors, including chronic stress, access to high-quality prenatal care, and the ability to pay for vitamins and nutritious foods. Additionally, low-income individuals may be more susceptible to type 2 diabetes due to inadequate treatment for gestational diabetes.

5.1.1. Causes of Health Disparities

Although there are several significant injustices in the US that are known to contribute to health disparities between groups, disparities frequently have several underlying causes. For instance, there are typically fewer affordable neighborhoods for Black people in communities where housing options were historically restricted by redlining (banking and loan denials) and segregation. This may entail a greater chance of lead contamination in paint or water, restricted access to wholesome foods, or difficult access to parks and recreational areas. Lack of good jobs and health insurance can make mental health therapy inaccessible or prohibitively expensive. Transportation issues can also make it difficult to schedule. The broader community is also impacted by general challenges and new consequences resulting from these health disparities. For instance, parents who are too ill to work may lose their jobs. Those without jobs and those with low incomes are less likely to have health insurance. If they can't afford medical care, their pre-existing conditions may get worse if they don't receive treatment.

5.1.1.1. Income Inequality

With almost twice as much spent on healthcare as other high-income countries, the healthcare system is among the priciest in the world. Prescription medication, hospital stays, and clinic visits cost more to Americans. Health disparities are a result of a widening income divide between the rich and the poor, many of whom have limited access to healthcare.

5.1.1.2. Systemic Discrimination or Exclusion

Social drivers—like racism, sexism, ableism, classism, or homophobia—can perpetuate inequities by prioritizing one group over another through factors like housing policies that affect long-term health.

5.1.1.3. Health Inequities and Future Generations

Scientist Camara Phyllis Jones compares two flower boxes—one with lower productivity because of poor soil quality—using a gardening analogy. Because their early access to resources impacted subsequent generations, the seeds from the following generation will fall into the same soil year after year, with one flower box flourishing and the other struggling.

5.1.1.4. Environmental Factors

Exercise and diet are two examples of lifestyle decisions that can affect health outcomes. Some of those decisions are influenced by the surroundings. Older people may be prevented from walking healthily by unsafe neighborhoods and poorly maintained sidewalks if they are afraid of falling or becoming victims of crime. People's options can be influenced by the availability of parks, bike lanes, hygienic public transportation, supermarkets, social opportunities, and more (for people of all ages).

5.1.2. Strategies for Reducing Health Disparities

It's not simple to close the gap in health outcomes. The causes are frequently complex. Both the original context and the underlying cause of a particular disparity would need to be addressed in any solution. As for the Healthy People 2030 objectives, a list of targets outlined by the U.S. government's efforts to enhance American health—by addressing important variables referred to as social determinants of health—aims to lessen health disparities. These include factors that contribute to health disparities, such as education and economic stability. The initiative is in line with numerous others that aim to address health disparities and enhance access to healthcare, including those from the Office of Health Equity, medical groups and professionals, social and community activists, and many more. Numerous medical conditions and mental health diagnoses have their roots in health disparities, which disproportionately affect vulnerable populations due to factors such as race, income, and other variables. Health equity can be established by implementing deliberate policies and approaches that address these causes of health disparities. Widely varying initiatives and interventions range from straightforward methods to enhance access to healthful foods to intricate regulations to enhance access to reasonably priced healthcare and intricate procedures.

5.1.3. Gender Health Disparities

The term "gender health disparities" describes how people's access to healthcare services and health outcomes differ depending on their gender. These differences in health outcomes between men, women, and non-binary people are caused by a complex interaction of biological, social, economic, and cultural factors. To advance health equity and enhance general public health outcomes, it is imperative to recognize and address these disparities. Men and women are biologically predisposed to distinct health risks and conditions. Men are more likely to develop certain cancers, such as prostate and bladder cancer, whereas women are more likely to experience autoimmune diseases like lupus and multiple sclerosis. Furthermore, certain healthcare services are needed for women's reproductive health needs, such as pregnancy, childbirth, and menopause, but not for men. Despite these variations, social determinants of health have a substantial impact on gender disparities in health, which go well beyond biology. Differential access to healthcare services is one of the main causes of gender health disparities. Women frequently encounter obstacles to receiving care, especially those from lower socioeconomic backgrounds. These obstacles include a lack of insurance, financial limitations, and a dearth of services tailored to the needs of women. Gender norms and cultural expectations can prevent women from seeking prompt medical attention, even in situations where services are available. Women prioritize the health of their families over their own in many cultures, which causes delays in their medical conditions' diagnosis and treatment.

Gender health disparities are significantly influenced by economic disparities as well. Women are less likely than men to be wealthy and to live in poverty, which has a direct effect on their capacity to pay for healthcare. The gender pay gap makes these economic difficulties worse, as does the greater probability of women working in low-paying and unstable jobs. Furthermore, women frequently take on unpaid caregiving duties, which may restrict their access to employer-sponsored health insurance as well as their employment options. The way that healthcare systems handle mental health is another area where gender health disparities are visible. Women are more likely than men to experience depression and anxiety disorders, in part because of social stressors like discrimination, gender-based violence, and the strain of juggling work and family obligations. However, because of the stigma associated with mental illness and cultural expectations of masculinity, men are less likely to seek treatment for mental health problems. This may result in underdiagnosis and undertreatment of mental health issues in men, which raises the suicide rate in men relative to women.

Furthermore, stigma, discrimination, and a shortage of medical professionals who are culturally competent present particular health disparities for non-binary and transgender people. The aforementioned individuals may face considerable obstacles in obtaining essential medical services, such as care that is gender-affirming, and consequently may suffer from inferior health outcomes. Furthering health disparities, the healthcare system frequently lacks the necessary resources and training to address the unique needs of transgender and non-binary people. Gender health disparities must be addressed through a multimodal strategy that includes targeted public health interventions, enhanced healthcare access, and policy changes. Ensuring equitable access to healthcare for all genders, promoting gender-sensitive health services, and lowering financial barriers to healthcare should be the main objectives of policy. To provide care that is culturally competent and addresses gender-specific health issues, healthcare providers need to undergo training. Campaigns for public health should support gender equity in health and increase public awareness of the disparities in health between genders. We can work toward a more equitable healthcare system that better meets the needs of all people, regardless of gender, by addressing the underlying causes of gender health disparities and putting comprehensive strategies to address them into practice.

5.1.4. Disability and Health Disparities

Disability and health disparities describe how people with disabilities experience different health outcomes and have less access to healthcare services than people without disabilities. Numerous variables, such as obstacles connected to the healthcare system and the social, economic, and environmental spheres, have an impact on these disparities. These complex barriers frequently make it difficult for people with disabilities to achieve optimal health. First, one of the main causes of the exacerbation of health disparities is the presence of physical barriers to healthcare facilities and services. People with mobility impairments may find it difficult to access certain healthcare environments, which can impede their ability to receive timely and appropriate care. Accessible medical equipment, like diagnostic machines and examination tables, makes it more difficult to provide basic healthcare services. Furthermore, people with sensory impairments—such as the deaf or hard of hearing—often face communication obstacles that make it difficult for them to communicate with healthcare professionals efficiently. This may result in misinterpretations, incorrect diagnoses, and insufficient care.

Significantly, health disparities among individuals with disabilities are also influenced by economic factors. People with disabilities are more likely to be poor and unemployed, which makes it harder for them to pay for essential medications and medical care. Access to health services may be further hampered by the high costs of specialized care, assistive technology, and other disability-related expenses. In addition, a large number of individuals with disabilities depend on government healthcare programs like Medicaid, which may have restrictions on the services that are available and the coverage that is provided. The health outcomes of people with disabilities are also influenced by social determinants of health, such as social support, housing, and education. People with disabilities who have less education may be less health literate, which can make it difficult for them to properly manage chronic conditions and navigate the healthcare system. Poor living circumstances and housing can aggravate existing medical conditions and raise the possibility of developing new ones. Social isolation can result in mental health issues and limit opportunities for engaging in behaviors that promote health. It is more prevalent among people with disabilities.

Lack of provider education and awareness of health issues unique to people with disabilities is one of the factors affecting the healthcare system. Inadequate training prevents many medical personnel from meeting the special needs of patients with disabilities, which leads to poor treatment and unfavorable health consequences. Because people with disabilities might not receive the same quality of care as those without disabilities, implicit biases and discrimination within the healthcare system can also contribute to disparities. A comprehensive strategy that includes improved training for healthcare professionals, policy changes, and increased funding for accessible healthcare infrastructure is needed to address health disparities and disabilities. Encouraging inclusive healthcare practices, increasing coverage of disability-related healthcare costs, and enhancing accessibility to healthcare facilities should be the main objectives of policy. Public health campaigns should also promote the inclusion of people with disabilities in all facets of health planning and service delivery, as well as increase awareness of the special health needs of this population.

5.2. Racial Disparities and Health

It is important to consider racial injustices in societal institutions when analyzing racial differences in health care. Unconscious bias based on unfavorable stereotypes and institutional policies frequently serves as the foundation for systematic discrimination, which is not the aberrant behavior of a select few. To effectively address disparities in the quality of care, new initiatives to recruit more providers from underrepresented minority backgrounds and appropriately train medical professionals are needed, as well as enhanced regulatory vigilance and data systems. It should be a national priority to identify and put into practice efficient methods to end racial disparities in health and medical care.

According to national data, there has been a positive improvement in the health of Black and White Americans over the last 50 years, as indicated by rising life expectancies and falling infant and adult mortality rates. Nonetheless, for the majority of physical health indicators, Black people continue to experience greater rates of morbidity and mortality than White people. American Indians and Hispanics also have higher rates of illness and mortality for a variety of ailments. Medical care can have a significant impact on health, even though its significance as a determinant of health is somewhat limited (Bunker, Frazier, & Mosteller, 1995). This is especially true of preventive care, early intervention, and the proper management of chronic disease. Racial disparities in health status are therefore probably caused in part by differences in the quantity and quality of care received by different racial and ethnic groups. Due to their higher unemployment rates and underrepresentation in well-paying jobs where health insurance is provided as part of the benefits package, Black people and other minorities in the United States have less access to medical care than White people (Blendon et al., 1989; Trevino et al., 1991).

Even after accounting for insurance status and disease severity, a significant and increasing number of studies reveal racial disparities in the use of major therapeutic procedures for a wide range of conditions. These findings are startling and unsettling to many. The racial disparities in environments like the Veterans Health Administration System, where variations in insurance coverage and economic status are minimized, are particularly startling to many people (Whittle et al., 1993) as well as the Medicare scheme. According to additional research, Hispanic patients are significantly less likely than non-Hispanic White patients to receive appropriate analgesia, even though doctors' abilities to assess the degree of pain do not differ for either group. According to recent research, members of minority groups experience negative health outcomes as a result of these disparities in the therapeutic procedures they receive. How do we reconcile these discrepancies and develop a research and policy agenda that will effectively end these disparities?

5.2.1. Race, Racism, and Discrimination

These results have surprised and confused many observers. But only if we approach the data with an ahistorical and decontextualized perspective will we be able to regard these findings as surprising. Following the United States Constitution's Article 1, Section 2, and Paragraph 3, the first Census, which took place in 1790, listed three racial categories: whites, blacks, who made up three-fifths of the population, and only "civilized Indians"—those who filed taxes (Anderson, 1988). It became necessary to track newly marginalized immigrant groups, so in the late 19th century and beyond, new racial categories were added (Chinese in 1870, Japanese in 1890, and Mexican in 1930) (Anderson & Feinberg, 1995). Race was and still is a social construct that describes unequal access to resources and positions of power in society (Williams, 1997). Non-dominant racial groups have historically been treated less favorably in important societal institutions, either by statute or custom. Healthcare is not an exception.

Thus, an understanding of the ways that racism has operated and still operates in society is necessary to comprehend racial disparities in medical care. The word "racism" describes a systemic approach, based on an inferiority complex that assigns social resources to human population groups based on their classification, ranking, and disparate distribution (Bonilla-Silva, 1996). Prejudice on an individual basis may or may not accompany it. By taking into account access to housing and employment, we will demonstrate the nuanced nature of race, racism, and discrimination in society. First, as Table 5.1 shows, there have been significant improvements in white people's racial attitudes toward black people in recent decades, and there is currently widespread support for the idea of housing and employment equality (Schuman et al., 1997). When it came to the statement, "White people have a right to keep Black people out of their neighborhoods if they want to, and Black people should respect that right," in 1963, 60% of white people agreed. Merely 13% of Caucasian individuals concurred with that assertion in 1996, indicating a significant improvement in the demographic's attitude. Comparably, in 1944, most white people (55%) said that white people should get the first shot at any kind of job, but by 1972, only 3% of white people still held that opinion, with 97% saying that black people should have an equal opportunity to get any kind of job.

Table 5.1. *Racial Attitudes of White Persons in the United States: Selected Years, 1944–1996*

Question	**Year of Survey**								
	1944	**1963**	**1964**	**1972**	**1973**	**1980**	**1983**	**1990**	**1996**
	Percent in Agreement								
Access to Housing Principle Item									
White persons have a right to keep black persons out of the neighborhood.	—	60	—	41	—	34	—	24	13
Implementation Item									
They would support a law to let homeowners discriminate if they want to.	—	—	—	—	67	60	54	47	33

Access to Employment Principle Item									
White persons should have the first chance at any job.	55	15	—	3	—	—	—	—	—
Implementation Item									
Government should ensure no discrimination in jobs.	—	—	38	40	—	—	—	—	28
No interest in the issue.	—	—	13	18	—	—	—	—	36

*Source: Schuman, Steeh, Bobo, & Krysan (1997).*https://www.ncbi.nlm.nih.gov/pmc/articles/PMC4194634/.

Second, legal authority was granted to these affirmative feelings. Refusing to sell or rent a home to someone based on their race became unlawful in 1968 when the Fair Housing Act (Title VIII) came into effect. Before this, employers were not allowed to fire employees, reject applications for employment or promotions, or restrict their pay or working conditions in any other way due to their race under the Civil Rights Act of 1964 (Title VII). Third, Table 5.1 also shows that policies that would genuinely achieve equal access to housing and employment are met with much less support (Schuman et al., 1997). A 1973 national survey of white people found that 67% of them would back legislation that guaranteed a homeowner the freedom to choose who to sell their home to, even if they didn't want to sell to black people. A third of white people in 1996 would still grant that right to a homeowner. Likewise, there is scant support for laws that outlaw discrimination in the workplace. 13% of white people said they were too uninterested in the issue to support either side in 1964, while 38% of white people said the government in Washington should ensure that black people receive fair treatment in employment. In 1996, the proportion of white individuals who supported government intervention to guarantee equitable treatment in employment fell to 28%, while the proportion who showed no interest in the matter rose to 36%. Fourth, statistics on national stereotypes show that white people still have a bad opinion of black people, which presumably makes them unwelcome as neighbors and coworkers. For instance, according to Davis & Smith (1990), 56% of white people think that black people would rather live on welfare, 51% think that black people are violent, 29% think that black people are stupid, and 44% think that black people are lazy. In contrast, white people believe that only 4% of white people would rather live on welfare, that 16% are violent, that 6% are stupid, and that 5% are lazy. Hispanics and Asians were viewed more negatively by white people than by themselves, but black people were viewed more negatively than any other group, and Asians were viewed twice as negatively as Hispanics. This information is instructive. Social desirability concerns have probably understated the reported levels of negative stereotypes of minority groups.

The high degree of acceptance of derogatory stereotypes about minority groups portends widespread discrimination in society. Numerous psychological studies show that discrimination against minority groups results from the acceptance of unfavorable racial stereotypes. Furthermore, well-learned stereotypes are resistant to disconfirmation (Stangnor & McMillan, 1992), and the process of activating them is automatic; people become aware of pertinent stereotypes on their initiative after meeting someone who fits the mold. Racial stereotypes have a real-world impact on minority groups' access to housing and jobs in the United States. The majority of white people express a strong preference for living in racially segregated neighborhoods due to negative stereotypes of black people, and black people looking for housing are still consistently directed toward neighborhoods with higher minority populations, lower home values, and lower median incomes. "On any given encounter between a black home-seeker and a realtor, the odds are at least 60% that something will happen to limit that black renter or buyer's access to housing units that are available to white persons," according to a review of the data on the persistence of housing discrimination in the United States.

Research on white employers shows that black job applicants are frequently denied opportunities due to racial stereotypes. Furthermore, both U.S.-based and international businesses specifically consider the racial makeup of labor market regions when choosing locations for new plants. It should come as no surprise that a Wall Street Journal review of more than 35,000 U.S. Businesses discovered that during the 1990–1991 recession, black people lost 59,000 jobs net, while white people gained 71,100, Asian people gained 55,100, and people of Latin descent gained 60,000 jobs (Sharpe, 1993). The migration of employment facilities to areas with a lower concentration of Black people was reflected in these job losses. Racial disparities are also observed in audit studies of employment discrimination in terms of eligibility for application submission, interview opportunities, and job offers. According to these studies, discrimination favored white job applicants over black applicants in one out of every five audits where trained individuals with identical qualifications applied for jobs. The fact remains that racial discrimination in housing and employment has not been eradicated by policies. When Congress passed the Fair Housing Act in 1968, there was almost the same level of residential racial segregation as there was in 1990. In a similar vein, from 1950 until the present, the unemployment rate for Black people has continuously been roughly twice that of White people. Therefore, the introduction of civil rights laws and modifications to white people's racial attitudes have not been enough to end discrimination. On a number of racial inequality-related dimensions, there has been notable stability over time despite these changes. For instance, in 1996, the median income of Black people was the same as it was in 1978: 59 cents for every dollar earned by White people.

The body of research on societal discrimination indicates that racism still exists in modern America, even though it has evolved from overt "Jim Crow racism" to covert "laissez-faire racism" (Bobo, Kluegel, & Smith, 1997). Even though it may hurt to admit it, we have to start by realizing that discrimination is normal and commonplace in society and probably also occurs in the medical field. The literature on racial disparities in medical care, with rare exceptions, is reluctant to acknowledge and address provider racial bias as a significant contributing factor. On the other hand, there is ample and convincing evidence that racial discrimination is a pervasive social issue rather than the aberrant behavior of a small number of "bad apples." It is improbable that inequalities in health care are the result of personal prejudice on the part of providers. The causes of racial differences are multifaceted and multifaceted in any area of societal evaluation; discrimination is merely one of them. Furthermore, discrimination in institutions is frequently at least as significant as discrimination in individuals. Other possible explanations for racial disparities in medical care include the unequal distribution of medical resources across geographic regions, racial variations in patient preferences, pathophysiology, economic status, insurance coverage, and levels of trust, knowledge, and comfort with medical procedures. The alternative explanation that would seem to be most in line with all of the available data would be the patient's preferences. Nonetheless, discrimination is still a major plausible explanation for these disparities, according to recent research that shows patient preferences cannot account for these differences.

Most importantly, a lot of discrimination nowadays takes place through actions that the perpetrator does not personally perceive as deliberate. Nowadays, a lot of discriminatory behavior is unintentional, thoughtless, and unconscious. As was previously mentioned, prejudices stemming from racial stereotypes happen instinctively and unconsciously, even in people who do not support racism. According to recent psychological research, when other negative traits are present, people who do not consider themselves to be prejudiced will make decisions about the distribution of health care that negatively impact Black people. For instance, when it came to patients who were presented as black and unemployed versus White and unemployed, respondents showed more resentment, scored health care lower on the priority scale, and were less willing to pay for their care. Stereotypes can automatically activate during real-life medical encounters, providing the negative characterization that sets off unconscious bias. Because they concentrate on deliberate or purposeful discrimination, the majority of anti-discrimination laws, programs, and policies have proven to be ineffectual. Furthermore, our review indicates that it is not sufficient to guarantee that discrimination does not occur in healthcare settings based solely on the presence of laws against it or on the declared racial attitudes of White people.

5.2.2. Policy and Research Directions

5.2.2.1. Improving Equity in Access to Medical Care

Equal access to care must be the first step in any comprehensive strategy to address inequities, even though the focus of this article is on racial disparities in the quality of care. Comprehensive efforts by various societal sectors to address larger inequities in significant societal institutions will be necessary to effectively address health care disparities. To improve the socioeconomic status (SES) of underprivileged minority populations and thereby give them greater access to medical care, there is an evident need for coordinated efforts across society to confront and eradicate discrimination in housing, employment, education, criminal justice, and other areas of society. As a fundamental civic duty, the United States must also commit politically and morally to ensuring that everyone has access to healthcare. The removal of financial obstacles alone, however, is not enough to guarantee equitable access to healthcare. Patient alienation and avoiding contact with the health care system until necessary can result from a wide range of system barriers, including lengthy wait times, convoluted bureaucratic processes, and the failure to treat patients with dignity and respect. Long-standing research has shown that low-income patients receive subpar care from medical professionals and are not seen as desirable patients. Low SES individuals experience more communication problems between themselves and their healthcare providers; conversely, higher SES patients receive more positive communication and superior technical and interpersonal care.

To prevent two factors that might make racial disparities in access to care worse, efforts must be made to ensure equitable access to care. First, an increasing number of healthcare facilities are closing, with hospitals in minority and low-income communities closing more frequently than those in other areas. Second, and perhaps more importantly, minorities and other vulnerable populations' access to medical care is likely to suffer as a result of the transition from a fee-for-service (FFS) to a managed care system. Critics contend that managed care will probably worsen the racial disparities in access to healthcare that already exist in several ways. Due to increased competition in the financing and delivery of healthcare, treating patients with private insurance may result in lower profits, which could force providers to reduce the amount of uncompensated care they offer (Schlesinger, 1987). Managed care plans also frequently restrict access for physicians of color and other medical professionals who treat underprivileged patients. Managed care plans seek out cost-effective doctors who write few prescriptions, order few procedures, and refer few patients. On the other hand, patients from minority and low-income populations tend to require more intensive management of chronic illness due to higher rates of morbidity, comorbidity, and greater severity of disease at the time of diagnosis. This can result in higher costs associated with medical services. As a result, managed care plans may restrict the doctors that their enrollees, who may include low-income patients and residents of low-income communities, can consult, and they may also regard doctors who practice in minority communities as undesirable. As a result, many doctors who practice in minority communities might see a decrease in patient volume, and some might not even be able to continue running a profitable practice.

It's unclear, though, if these worries have come true. In a 1994 national conference survey, 92% of black physicians responded that they were more likely than white doctors to have their contracts terminated by managed care plans (Lavizzo-Mourey et al., 1996). In actuality, 71% of them had lost patients to a managed care organization (MCO) they were not affiliated with, and 88% had experienced an MCO rejecting their request for a contract. In addition, 75% of respondents said their practice had expanded or stayed the same the year prior, and 71% reported having at least one managed care contract. Moreover, some observers point out that under managed care plans, minority populations' access to healthcare need not always deteriorate. Enhanced competition may offer a financial incentive to certain healthcare providers to treat populations they may have previously considered undesirable (Schlesinger, 1987).

5.2.2.2. Improved Data Systems and Monitoring the Quality of Medical Care

Systematic and regular data on the occurrence of racial bias in the medical field is necessary for any concerted effort to address it. As previously mentioned, significant changes are occurring in the administration and delivery of healthcare services in the United States, and it is crucial to keep an eye on how these changes will affect vulnerable populations' access to and quality of care. At the moment, significant efforts are being made to determine which data elements belong in nationally uniform, standardized data sets. Racial and ethnic status must be consistently and thoroughly evaluated in these minimum core data sets. According to Williams (1996), a comprehensive assessment necessitates the inclusion of identifiers for significant ethnic subgroups inside the conventional racial/ethnic categories in data systems. For instance, it's important to distinguish between the three largest Hispanic populations: Mexicans, Puerto Ricans living on the mainland, and Cubans. Indicators of SES should be included in any uniform data set due to the importance of SES in health and the strong correlation between SES and race/ethnicity.

Given how common discrimination is, racial information ought to be accessible for each medical encounter. The evaluation of race/ethnicity and SES in an enrollment database that could subsequently be connected to information on medical encounters has been demanded by the National Committee of Vital and Health Statistics, a public advisory body to the Department of Health and Human Services. The most useful and practical SES indicator in this situation was proposed to be the number of years of formal education. If these identifiers were included in an enrollment database, there would be no need for the resource-intensive hassle of trying to get racial data at each medical visit. To guarantee the consistent collection of racial/ethnic and SES data, healthcare personnel would need to receive the required training in addition to strict measures to protect patient privacy and confidentiality. The examination of racial disparities in the HCFA data files shows how useful administrative databases can be in generating information about the scope and character of the issue. But because "black, white, and other" were the only racial identifiers identified, these analyzes have only examined differences between black and white people. The Social Security Administration (SSA) and HCFA made significant efforts to enhance racial/ethnic identifiers in the SSA and Medicare data systems in the early 1990s. Routine data reporting and analysis for all racial/ethnic groups is now required. Regular data reporting would show which healthcare facilities, if any, provide medical care in a racially equitable way. Probably, racial disparities vary significantly between different contexts. By establishing benchmarks—levels of excellence attained by industry leaders—this type of data can help us better understand these best practices and make replication easier (Weissman et al., 1999). Additionally, research is required to determine the best-targeted approaches that healthcare facilities can use, if not continuously, then at least occasionally, to identify and address patterns of discrimination in medical treatment. It has been proposed that hospitals create a system for anonymous reporting to help identify instances of systematic bias in medical decision-making patterns. However, as part of a constructive problem-solving approach, it will be imperative to establish a reporting-friendly environment (Leape, 1997). In general, direct observation, chart review, computer screening, focus groups, and voluntary reporting are the five methods for identifying inappropriate medical treatment, ranked by yield and intensity of effort. Data on disparities in medical care between races would also help with at least some civil rights enforcement initiatives. The fact that many modern antidiscrimination laws depend on demonstrating subjective discriminatory intent is one of their drawbacks. It is frequently challenging to establish discriminatory intent because the great majority of white Americans support non-discrimination in theory. Disparate impact claims in the legal system need statistical evidence to support the different ways that policies affect different racial groups. It is not a common tactic employed by people pursuing relief under civil rights statutes since proving a discriminatory effect typically necessitates the collection and examination of substantial amounts of data. On the other hand, regular racial data collection would make it easier to evaluate racial group disadvantage in the medical field.

According to Smith (1998), the managed care environment's emphasis on tracking clinical and financial data opens up new possibilities for improved civil rights monitoring of the provision of healthcare. He suggests that the development of report cards that could be used to track disparities in health plans, healthcare facilities, and communities would be made easier by the addition of racial identifiers to already-existing data systems. The widely recognized measures of health and health care delivery (such as mortality rates and the use of particular screening tests) that are suggested by different standards organizations for the comparative assessment of medical care would be included in these report cards. Similar reporting requirements in the banking sector, according to Smith (1998), have resulted in a sharp rise in the number of loans approved for racial minorities. Report cards, however, need to be a part of a bigger system to function.

5.2.2.3. Renewed Regulatory Vigilance

Enhanced regulatory vigilance is another policy approach to address the issue of discrimination in medicine. The history of overt discrimination in healthcare suggests that until institutional commitment and the ability to enforce laws and regulations were established, they were ineffective. Some legal experts contend that certain laws already in place aren't being followed right now. For instance, Title VI of the Civil Rights Act of 1964 offers a potential legal pathway to address discrimination in the provision of healthcare. Title VI forbids any organization receiving federal funding from engaging in racial discrimination when offering goods or services to the program's beneficiaries. Since Medicare and Medicaid funds are included in federal financial assistance, almost all hospitals, nursing homes, and other healthcare facilities in the US are covered by this anti-discrimination law. The documentation of adverse impact would offer a potent tactic for addressing and resolving discrimination in care, as courts have ruled that Title VI forbids both deliberate discrimination and disproportionate adverse impact.

Noah (1998) adds that if the disparate impact was documented, many neutral policies that might have a disproportionate effect on racial and ethnic minorities receiving medical care could also be addressed. Certain hospitals impose restrictions on Medicaid patients' admission, such as requiring large deposits before inpatient care, delivering babies only to mothers who have received a certain level of prenatal care, and only admitting patients whose doctors have staff privileges at the facility. Even though the policies do not expressly address race, minority patients are more likely to suffer from them. Therefore, one way to effectively challenge these policies could be to apply a disparate impact analysis. Noah (1998) cautions that while Title VI covers institutional policies that have a disproportionate impact, it does not cover the actions of individual doctors who discriminate, either intentionally or unintentionally, as long as the healthcare organization can demonstrate that this is not its institutional policy.

Regarding racial disparities in health care, another regulatory body that might be more involved is the Joint Commission on Accreditation of Health Care Organizations (JCAHO). For instance, one of the conditions for maintaining accreditation could be that health care organizations set up protocols for the observation and rectification of unexplained discrepancies in the provision of services. In the past, the JCAHO has been a major force behind progressive change in the medical field. The initiatives to encourage hospitals to create and implement policies to address communication issues with patients who do not speak English are one recent example. To determine whether more effective ways can be created to recognize and address observed patterns of racial disparities in the provision of services to Medicare and Medicaid beneficiaries, HCFA may also evaluate its current utilization review procedures.

5.2.2.4. Monitoring Managed Care

Since that managed care fosters an environment that is favorable to discrimination and some have suggested that discrimination will become more pervasive under managed care, increased regulatory efforts must also specifically target managed care plans. In managed care, there are frequently pressures to restrict the quantity and cost of services provided to members of the prepaid health plan, in contrast to the FFS system where a physician's income increases as the number of services provided increases. A lot of managed healthcare plans reward providers financially for reducing the number of specialist referrals they make. A financial reserve is frequently set aside for diagnostic testing and specialists, with the provider receiving a portion of the fund that is not used. In certain managed care programs, doctors are held financially responsible for exceedingly high hospitalization rates for their patients, regardless of whether the expenses were medically necessary. It has been demonstrated that these monetary incentives influence providers' decisions.

The current body of research is insufficient to conclusively state whether managed care plans or the FFS system provides better overall medical care. According to certain data, people enrolled in managed care plans have a higher likelihood of getting cancer screening tests than those enrolled in FFS plans. The use of inpatient care, emergency rooms, and surgeries did not differ between health maintenance organizations (HMOs) and other types of insurance, according to recent national data collected from 35,000 non-elderly people. Simultaneously, HMO patients reported higher levels of unmet medical needs, lower levels of satisfaction, and less trust in doctors. According to this study, HMOs had higher administrative barriers to care and offered fewer specialized services than they did primary and preventive care. According to additional data, managed care plans worsen the quality of health care for vulnerable groups, including the elderly and the chronically ill.

The possible threat that managed care organizations pose to the health of minorities has been addressed in several ways (Harvard Law Review, 1995). First, the government, consumer advocacy groups, and professional medical associations need to conduct more systematic audits of the managed care providers' services. The federal government currently has minimal control over and monitoring of the relatively quick changes in health care delivery. Additionally, new laws or rules must be created in order to guarantee that doctors who work in minority communities are appropriately included in managed care programs. For instance, managed care plans that hire from underrepresented communities might be compelled to employ a specific percentage of physicians with prior experience working in those communities. Legislation could also be implemented to prevent the categorical exclusion of service providers from underprivileged communities. For instance, they might forbid the exclusion of healthcare providers from managed care plans on the grounds of their patients' SES, race, or general health. Lastly, MCOs and other healthcare organizations may be prevented from practicing discrimination by using sanctions. If there is consistent proof of discrimination, there may be severe penalties or even the possibility of losing one's license to practice.

Wallace et al., (1998) stress that the quality of medical care provided to minority populations could be enhanced by managed care. There is a chance for better care coordination in MCOs because of the increased bureaucratic oversight, which could guarantee that patients receive the right medical attention. That is to say, managed care plans could help buck the trend of minorities receiving less aggressive treatment and fewer medical procedures for a wide range of illnesses if the right incentives were included in them. Similarly, the more than 60 standards that currently serve as the foundation for evaluating health plans could be expanded to include racial disparities in care by organizations like the National Committee for Quality Assurance (NCQA), which voluntarily accredits nearly half of the HMOs in the US. The primary performance evaluation for managed care, the Health Plans Employer Data and Information Set (HEDIS), was developed under the direction of NCQA. It compares health plans using a set of uniform metrics. At the moment, HEDIS assesses how well a health plan performs in critical areas of care like member satisfaction and immunization rates. One more performance metric that needs to be included is the degree of racial/ethnic disparities.

5.2.2.5. Education and Training

Comprehensive and organized education campaigns regarding the issue of racial disparities in health care are also necessary. It is necessary to increase public and professional community awareness, particularly in the medical field. It will take research to determine the best ways to increase sensitivity to and awareness of racial issues in medical practice. While awareness of education's limitations is important, it's also helpful to know that awareness campaigns can achieve a lot. For instance, over the last century, there has been a decline in tobacco consumption per capita in the United States anytime there has been a significant media campaign on the harmful effects of cigarette smoking (Warner, 1985). Changes to the medical school curriculum are required to guarantee that racial concerns and sensitivity to them are sufficiently addressed. Geiger (1996) states that "every physician's training should include awareness of the dilemmas associated with race and health care." The way that cultural sensitivity is currently stressed and approached may not be sufficient to solve the structural issue of discrimination. Unconscious prejudice remains unaddressed, even in the case of model cultural sensitivity programs for medical students and residents. Programs that promote cultural sensitivity may strengthen and accentuate unfavorable stereotypes. Certain cultural sensitivity training seems to concentrate mainly on the "strange" behavior of patients and ignores the unique behavioral patterns of population subgroups. Further studies on the attitudes and actions of healthcare providers are also required, particularly to determine the best ways to recognize and lessen unconscious prejudice in the medical community.

Increasing the proportion of minority professionals should be a key objective of medical education. Research unequivocally shows that doctors of color, specifically black and Hispanic doctors, are far more likely than other doctors to treat Medicaid recipients and uninsured patients, as well as to work in underserved urban and rural areas where a high proportion of the population belongs to their racial or ethnic group. According to a recent study, the United States must triple the number of Native American residents and double the number of Black and Hispanic first-year residents to achieve racial and ethnic population parity. Asian first-year residents would need to be lowered by two-thirds, and White first-year residents by two-fifths. These objectives are not likely to be accomplished based on current trends. Over the past 30 years, there hasn't been much of an increase in the percentage of doctors from underrepresented minority backgrounds. Black physicians, for instance, now make up 20.5% of all U.S. doctors before 1968 to 21.9% at the moment. Beginning in the late 1960s, there was an increase in the proportion of underrepresented minorities in medical schools, including American Indians, Black Americans, Mexican Americans, and mainland Puerto Ricans. After reverse discrimination lawsuits, minority enrollment fell after reaching a peak in 1974 at 10% of total enrollment. The Association of American Medical Colleges started a new initiative to have 3000 minority first-year medical students by the year 2000 to buck the trend. The initial success of this project was demonstrated by the high enrollment of underrepresented minorities (12% of all new entrants) in 1994. Over half of all U.S. medical schools received fewer applications from underrepresented minorities in 1996. S. minority enrolment in medical schools is declining. The four states (California, Texas, Louisiana, and Mississippi) where affirmative action policies have been outlawed and public medical schools experiencing the biggest decline were these states.

To determine the best practices for attracting and keeping doctors from underprivileged backgrounds, more research is required. But we also ought to take advantage of the data that is currently available regarding successful tactics. Federal initiatives known as affirmative action programs, which permit employers and educational institutions to consider an applicant's race, sex, national origin, or disability, have proven to be effective. According to estimates, affirmative action accounts for 40% of all U.S.-trained medical professionals from marginalized minority backgrounds. While underrepresented minority students typically score lower on exams than other medical students, there is no difference in their clinical performance, indicating that other non-cognitive factors play a crucial role in the selection of qualified doctors. Furthermore, affirmative action policies are justified for many reasons, including the need for society to provide for the healthcare needs of all racial and ethnic groups, even though they are currently unpopular. Furthermore, current research shows that the primary source of opposition to affirmative action is racial prejudice, particularly subtle prejudice that exists in the modern world. These findings highlight how important it is to address and eradicate societal racism to create workable plans for overcoming the terrible history of exclusion and discrimination in America.

McClellan (1999) points out that it is insufficient to just match the client's race with the physician's race. He presents a sobering yet illuminating example from the Tuskegee Syphilis Study. The Macon County Medical Society approved the Tuskegee Syphilis Study's continuation in 1969. Nearly every member of the Society at that time was black. According to McClellan (1999), the behavior of those black physicians can be explained by their social class. That is, middle-class physicians, their families, and friends were not threatened by the Tuskegee study because the majority of the patients were poor and illiterate. He contends that healthcare workers may become less emotionally attached to and self-interested in their original groups as a result of professional and educational socialization. The endorsement of negative societal stereotypes about patients by medical professionals, regardless of their race, is likely to result in unconscious discrimination. To determine how much these processes function and what might be the best ways to combat them, more research is required. Efforts to lessen racial/ethnic disparities in the quality of medical care should aim to change the systems that govern the delivery of care rather than concentrating solely on individual traits. Leape (1997) emphasizes that in medicine, as in other occupations, work conditions can be managed, tasks and processes can be designed, and workers can be trained in ways that minimize undesirable outcomes. A definitive answer to this question awaits the necessary research. Can systems for the delivery of medical care be designed and implemented in a way that can ensure appropriate behavior regardless of effect and unconscious stereotypes?(Schulman et al., 1999; Chen et al., 2001).

5.3. Health Disparities: Gaps in Access, Quality, and Affordability of Medical Care

Physicians and health policy experts are paying more and more attention to health disparities, also known as health inequities, and federal health agencies are refocusing on the issue. Numerous studies have validated the complex and multifaceted construct of differential access to medical care, treatment modalities, and disparate outcomes among different racial and ethnic groups. Preventive health services, primary care physicians, and the cost and accessibility of the healthcare system are some of the "drivers" that precede these disparities.

5.3.1. The Significance of Racial and Ethnic Disparities

There are several reasons why racial and ethnic disparities in healthcare are significant. They present the US healthcare system with serious moral and ethical challenges. As a country, we are the proud owners of an abundance of world-class healthcare facilities, state-of-the-art technologies, pharmaceuticals, and other resources that are inaccessible to large portions of the populace for a variety of reasons. Furthermore, the quality of life for our patients, our communities, and the country as a whole is closely linked to the concepts of social justice, opportunity, and healthcare as a resource. The health of our population as a whole and particular population groups is directly and indirectly correlated with the nation's economic health, which is a closely related concern. Therefore, insufficient, unaffordable, and/or subpar medical care exacerbates rising healthcare costs, which have significant effects on the general standard of care received by all Americans.

The evidence gathered in the last three to four decades is strong. Different population groups are not equally affected by health and disease conditions. A few examples serve as illustrations: the infant mortality rate for Black babies is still nearly 2.5 times higher than that of White babies; Black men and women have a life expectancy that is nearly ten years shorter than that of White people; the rates of diabetes are more than 30% higher in Native Americans and Latinos than in White people; the rates of heart disease, stroke, and breast and prostate cancer are still significantly higher in Black populations; and minorities are still disproportionately underrepresented in the health professions compared to their percentages in the population.

5.3.2. Health Disparities Defined

Disparities in healthcare quality between racial, ethnic, and socioeconomic groups are known as health disparities. It can also be understood as variations in disease prevalence, health outcomes, or healthcare access among different populations. The Institute of Medicine has offered another helpful definition, stating that health disparities are racial or ethnic variations in healthcare quality that are not brought on by variables relating to access, clinical requirements, patient preferences, or the suitability of an intervention. Even though these definitions are helpful, it's crucial to realize that racial, ethnic, and cultural differences within a population are not the only factors contributing to health disparities. Inclusions should also include lifestyle decisions, age, sexual orientation, accessibility issues, and environmental, socioeconomic, and personal traits.

5.3.3. The Landmark Malone-Heckler Report

The "Heckler Report" raised awareness of the

poor health status, poor results, and restricted access to medical care for over 300 years—issues that were anecdotally well-known by many African Americans and, in certain cases, by a small cohort of academicians and public health officials. The report presented an unbiased account of the significant differences in the disproportionate number of deaths and illnesses that African Americans and other minority Americans endured when compared to the overall population of the country. Furthermore, it asserted that these differences had existed for the duration that official federal health statistics were gathered. The report also stressed that nearly 45% of deaths in the black population up to the age of 70 (58,000 of 138,000) would have been preventable if better evaluation, detection, and treatment had been available. These six medical conditions were found to account for 86% of the excess black mortality. The six conditions were: cirrhosis (4.9%), infant mortality (26.9%), diabetes (1.0%), heart disease and stroke (14.4%), cancer (3.8%), and homicide and accidents (35.1%).

5.3.4. Unequal Treatment: Confronting Racial and Ethnic Disparities in Healthcare

The Heckler-Malone Report was well received initially, but was not followed up on until 2003 when the Institute of Medicine released the groundbreaking report "Unequal Treatment: Confronting Racial and Ethnic Disparities in Healthcare." This analysis rigorously reviewed over 600 articles from the medical literature over the previous 3 decades, focusing specifically on the top 100 studies covering various health conditions. The findings revealed significant differences in care, indicating biases and discrimination even among populations with equal access to healthcare. The report highlighted the complexities of the healthcare system and its impact on disparate treatment decisions and outcomes. Ultimately, the IOM report contributed to a better understanding of health disparities by offering an integrated model that considers the multifactorial factors influencing unequal care (Figure 5.1).

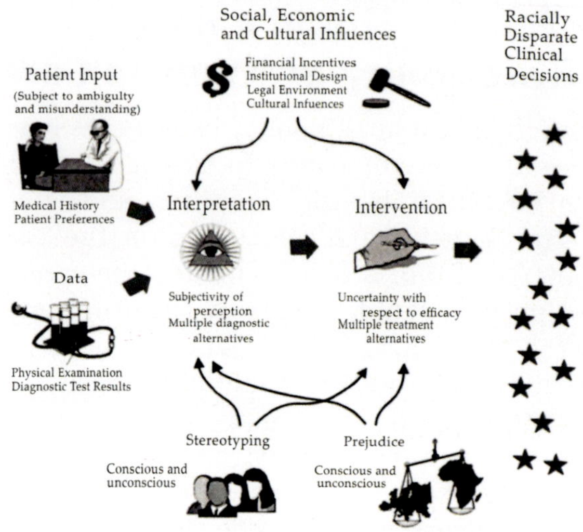

Figure 5.1. *Integrated model of health disparities from the institute of medicine (IOM).*

Source: *https://www.ncbi.nlm.nih.gov/pmc/articles/PMC3540621/bin/zsd0011228280001.jpg.*

5.3.5. Disparities in Cardiovascular Care

Many in the House of Medicine had reasonable doubts after the publication of "Unequal Treatment," believing that treatment decisions made differently based on racial, ethnic, or cultural differences might be partially to blame for the health disparities. The American Heart Association and the Henry J. Together, the Kaiser Family Foundation analyzed the cardiology services. Following a thorough analysis of 81 out of 158 studies, they concluded that, even in cases where patient characteristics were similar, there was reasonable evidence that African Americans were less likely than Whites to undergo thrombolytic therapy, diagnostic procedures, and revascularization. Whittle et al., study was one of the important ones that was included. Absent financial barriers, Whittle et al. discovered a glaring disparity in the rates of cardiac catheterization, angioplasty, and coronary artery colon bypass grafting among Black and White veterans in a retrospective study of cardiovascular procedures: Blacks were less likely to have invasive cardiac procedures performed in the Veterans Healthcare System. Similar disparities in the application of cardiac catheterization following acute myocardial infarction were also observed by Chen et al., and Schulman et al., in another study that also discovered racial and sexual differences in cardiac catheterization recommendations.

5.3.6. Disparities in Cost and Affordability

Numerous data point to one of the main causes of health disparities in America: the expense and accessibility of the necessary medical care for many citizens. There are glaring differences in the percentages of Latino and Black population groups that have health insurance. Significant negative effects of not having insurance include using fewer preventive services, having worse health outcomes, having higher rates of death and disability, having lower yearly earnings due to illness and disease, and having an advanced stage of illness (i.e., many become "sicker" upon diagnosis). As a result, the uninsured are disproportionately young, from racial or ethnic minorities, and impoverished. The Joint Center for Political and Economic Studies and Johns Hopkins University analyzed the financial impact of health disparities in the US and found that it is substantial. Over three years, the elimination of health disparities for minorities would have resulted in a $1.05 trillion reduction in overall costs.

5.3.7. The Challenges Ahead

In the 27 years since the release of the Heckler Report, significant strides have been made in addressing health disparities. The report served as a catalyst for the coordination of federal and state responses to address disparities and the establishment of the Office of Minority Health within the US Department of Health and Human Services. However, despite such progress, it is clear that much work remains to be done to fully address health inequities. As documented by Benz et al., overall awareness of ethnic and health disparities remains somewhat disappointing, particularly in racial and ethnic groups, about certain disease conditions such as HIV/AIDS. In addition, although medical education has made perceptible progress in what is commonly referred to as cultural competency training for students, trainees, and physicians in general, recent evidence emphasized by Haider et al., reveals worrisome implicit preferences for whites and upper-class patients in implicit association testing instruments. Furthermore, in the emerging era of health reform, cost-conscious care, and pay-for-performance reimbursement schemes for hospitals and physicians, recent evidence by Jha et al., emphasizes the challenge in even more stark terms: Lower-performing hospitals, as manifested by quality performance data and metrics, tend to treat higher percentages of minority patients and have higher overall costs. Failure to address these disparities will only serve to worsen pre-existing disparities in access, quality, and costs of medical care for most our most vulnerable populations. Indeed, much work remains.

5.4. Disparities in Health and Health Care

Health equity has become more important as a result of the COVID-19 pandemic and the national racial justice movement, which have both raised awareness of health disparities and their underlying causes in recent years. These differences are not recent; rather, they are the result of persistent structural and systemic injustices that have their roots in racism and prejudice. Even though efforts to address disparities have increased recently, there is a chance that progress will be undone and disparities will widen if certain COVID-19 pandemic-related policies—like Medicaid continuous enrollment and the Children's Health Insurance Program (CHIP)—are ended. In addition to being crucial for equity, addressing health disparities will also enhance the general health and economic well-being of the country. In this brief, the definition of health and health care disparities, the significance of addressing disparities, their current state, recent federal initiatives to address disparities, and significant issues about addressing disparities in the future are all covered. Disparities in health and healthcare received by different groups resulting from wider injustices are referred to as health and healthcare disparities. Health disparities are defined in a variety of ways. A health disparity is "a particular type of health difference that is linked with social, economic, and/or environmental disadvantage," according to Healthy People 2030, and it is harmful to groups of people who have consistently faced more health-related barriers. Health disparities are "preventable differences in the burden, disease, injury, violence, or in opportunities to achieve optimal health experienced by socially disadvantaged racial, ethnic, and other population groups and communities," according to the Centers for Disease Control and Prevention (CDC). Disparities in health insurance coverage, affordability, access to and utilization of care, and quality of care are commonly referred to as health care disparities. Inequities and health inequality are other terms that are occasionally used to characterize unfair disparities. The CDC defines racism as the systems, laws, customs, and behaviors that determine a person's worth and opportunities based on their appearance or skin color. Racism leads to unfair advantages for some and disadvantages for others, increasing the risk of negative health outcomes for people of color.

When disparities in health and healthcare are eliminated, people can attain their optimal level of health. This is commonly referred to as health equity. According to Healthy People 2030, achieving health equity means valuing each individual equally and focusing and continuing social efforts to address historical and current injustices, preventable inequalities, and disparities in health and health care. When everyone has the chance to be as healthy as possible, that is what the CDC refers to as health equity. Disparities in health and health care are caused by a wide range of factors both inside and outside the health care system (Figure 5.1). Research indicates that a variety of factors, including underlying genetics, health behaviors, social and environmental factors, and access to healthcare, influence health outcomes, even though access to care is crucial for good health. Research indicates that social and economic factors—often referred to as social determinants of health—as well as health behaviors are the main drivers of health outcomes and that social and economic factors influence people's health behaviors, even though there is currently disagreement in the literature regarding the relative contributions of each of these factors to health. Furthermore, racism creates disparities across the social determinants of health, which has a direct detrimental impact on mental and physical health (Figure 5.2).

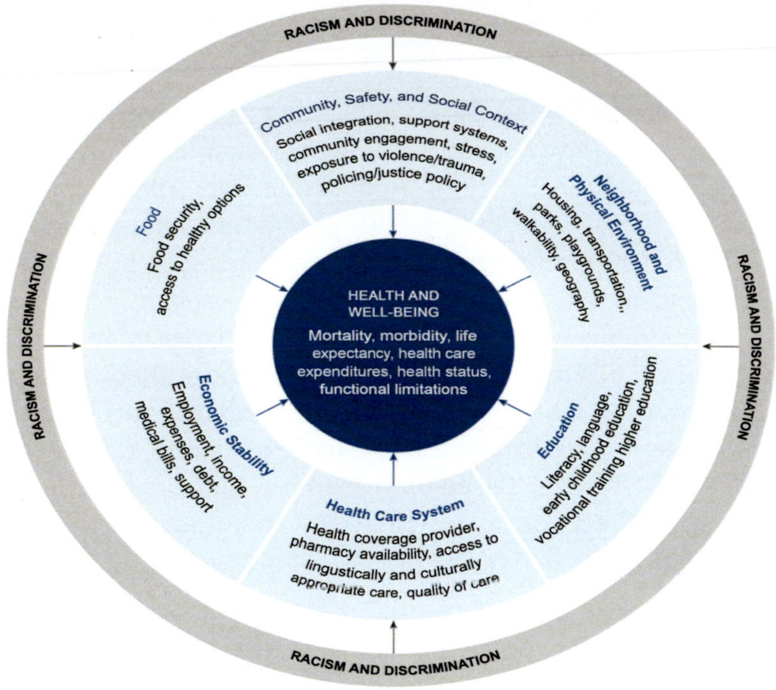

Figure 5.2. *Health disparities driven by social and economic inequalities.*

Source: https://www.kff.org/wp-content/uploads/2023/04/8396–06-Figure-1.png?resize=1024,1024.

Although they occur across a wide range of dimensions, health, and healthcare disparities are frequently seen through the prism of race and ethnicity. Disparities exist, for instance, in relation to socioeconomic status, age, location, language, gender, citizenship status, disability status, and sexual identity and orientation. Additionally, research indicates that differences exist among older adults as well as throughout the life course, from birth to midlife. "Members of underserved communities: Black, Latino, and Indigenous and Native American persons, Asian Americans and Pacific Islanders and other persons of color; members of religious minorities; lesbian, gay, bisexual, transgender, and queer (LGBT+) persons; persons with disabilities; persons who live in rural areas; and persons otherwise adversely affected by persistent poverty or inequality" are among the designated priority populations that are the focus of federal efforts to reduce disparities. These groups frequently cross in significant ways and are not mutually exclusive. Within population subgroups, disparities also exist. For instance, based on immigration status, length of stay in the nation, and primary language, there are variations in the health and medical care received by Hispanics. Additionally, data frequently conceal underlying differences between Asian population subgroups.

5.4.1. Important to Address Disparities

In addition to being crucial for equity, addressing health and healthcare disparities will also enhance the general health and economic well-being of the country. The general health of the country is hampered by the higher rates of illness and death among people of color and other marginalized groups for a variety of medical conditions. Additional research reveals that health disparities are expensive, leading to annual increases in medical care expenses, lost productivity, and additional financial losses from preventable deaths.

Addressing health disparities is becoming more and more crucial as the population grows more diverse and income inequality keeps rising. People of color are expected to make up more than half (52%) of the population by 2050, with Asian and Hispanic individuals expected to experience the greatest growth (Figure 5.3). The population has grown more racially diverse over time as a result of changing immigration trends, an increase in the number of people who identify as multiracial, and modifications to the methods used by the Federal Census Bureau to measure racial and ethnic diversity. With time, income disparity in the U.S. has expanded as well. In 2021, the wealthiest 20% of households made up more than half of all households with an income of $149,132 or more, while the lowest 20% of households earned less than 3% of all households with an income of $28,007 or less. At least $286,305 was earned by the top 5% of households in the income distribution. Based on research, it appears that the COVID-19 pandemic's disproportionately negative effects on lower-paid jobs could have long-term repercussions that exacerbate income inequality.

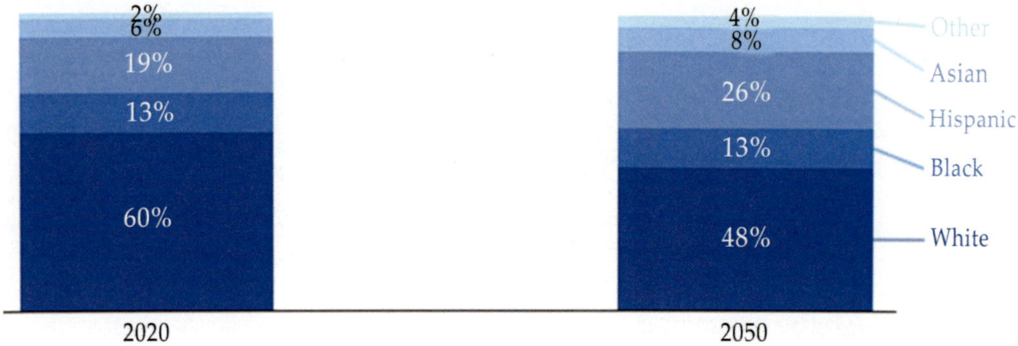

Figure 5.3. *People of color are projected to make up over half of the U.S. Population as of 2050.*

Source: *https://www.kff.org/racial-equity-and-health-policy/issue-brief/disparities-in-health-and-health-care-5-key-question-and-answers/.*

5.4.2. Status of Disparities Today

Health and healthcare disparities are enduring and pervasive. With the publication of the Report of the Secretary's Task Force on Black and Minority Health (Heckler Report) in 1985, which compiled strategies to promote health equity and detailed enduring health disparities that contributed to 60,000 excess deaths annually, the issue of health disparities was first widely acknowledged more than thirty years ago. The Heckler Report prompted the establishment of the U.S. Influenced by the Office of Minority Health at the Department of Health and Human Services, numerous facets of health equity have received federal recognition and funding. Systemic racism was identified as a primary cause of health disparities in the United States in the 2003 report Unequal Treatment: Confronting Racial and Ethnic Disparities in Health Care, which was published by the Institute of Medicine's Committee on Understanding and Eliminating Racial and Ethnic Disparities in Health Care. Many disparities have continued and, in some cases, widened over time, although they have been recognized and documented for decades and that population health has generally improved over time.

People of color and other marginalized and underserved groups continue to have higher rates of uninsured individuals despite significant increases in coverage since the Patient Protection and Affordable Care Act (ACA) went into effect in 2014. As of 2021, there were still racial differences in coverage, with nonelderly American Indian or Alaska Native (AIAN), Black, Hispanic, and Native Hawaiian or Pacific Islander (NHOPI) individuals having greater rates of uninsured status than White individuals (Figure 5.4). Uninsured status persisted for other groups as well, such as immigrants and members of lower-class households. Many uninsured individuals can obtain coverage through Medicaid, CHIP, or the ACA Marketplaces; however, there are obstacles to enrollment, such as unclear eligibility rules, challenging enrollment procedures, and issues with language and literacy. Even though they are eligible, some immigrant families are afraid to enroll themselves or their children in Medicaid or CHIP due to immigration-related concerns. Others continue to be ineligible. After all, they have access to an affordable Marketplace plan or an offer of employer coverage, because their state did not expand Medicaid, or because of their immigration status.

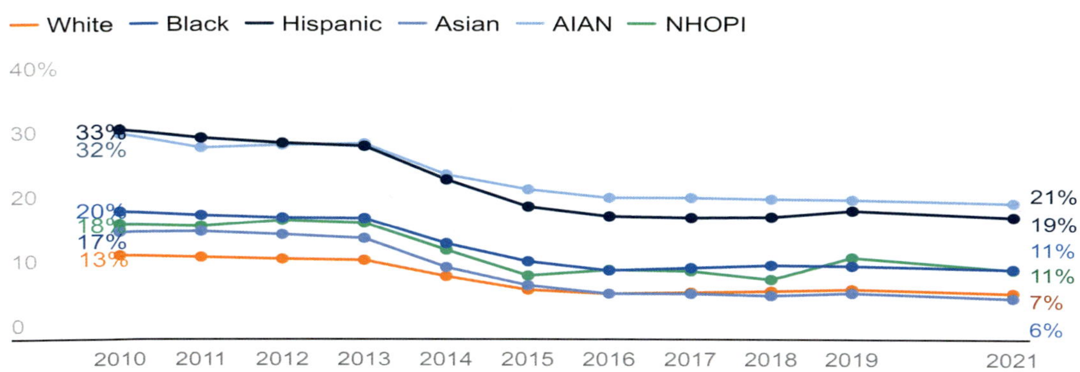

Figure 5.4. *Uninsured rates for nonelderly population by race/ethnicity, 2010–2021.*

Source: https://www.kff.org/racial-equity-and-health-policy/issue-brief/disparities-in-health-and-health-care-5-key-question-and-answers/.

Beyond coverage, there are still significant differences in the ways that people of color and other marginalized and underprivileged groups can obtain and receive healthcare. For instance, the low provider density, longer travel times to care, and more restricted access to health coverage present challenges for those living in rural areas when trying to get healthcare. Additionally, there are disparities in how different groups experience getting medical care. For instance, according to the KFF/The Undefeated 2020 Survey on Race and Health, one in five Black adults and one in five Hispanic adults say they have received unfair treatment when seeking medical care for themselves or a family member in the previous year because of their race or ethnicity. In a 2021 KFF survey, nearly one in three (34%) potentially undocumented Hispanic adults and nearly one-quarter (24%) of Hispanic adults said it was very or somewhat difficult to find a doctor who explains this in an easy-to-understand way. According to additional KFF survey data from 2022, 9% of adult women who are not elderly and visited a healthcare provider in the previous two years reported that they were subjected to discrimination during their visit due to their age, gender, race, sexual orientation, religion, or any other personal characteristic. Additionally, according to KFF data, LGBT+ individuals were more likely than their non-LGBT+ counterparts to report specific negative experiences related to receiving medical care, such as a doctor who mistrusted them, implied that they were personally at fault for a health issue, made assumptions about them without seeking clarification, or discounted their concerns. Compared to cisgender adults, trans adults were more likely to report difficulty finding affordable health care or a provider who treated them with dignity and respect, according to the 2023 KFF/The Washington Post Trans Survey.

Health disparities continue to exist for people of color and other marginalized communities. For instance, as of 2021, Black, Hispanic, and AIAN individuals all had lower birth weights than White people, and between 2019 and 2021, these groups' life expectancies declined more than White people, indicating the effects of COVID-19 (Figure 5.5). As of 2021, infant mortality rates were more than twice as high for Black babies and nearly twice as high for Asian babies compared to White babies. Among all groups, Black and Asian women exhibited the highest rates of pregnancy-related mortality. Racial and ethnic differences exist in the rates of cancer and chronic illnesses. Black people were more likely to die from cancer in 2019 even though they did not have higher cancer incidence rates than White people overall or for the majority of cancer types. There are also notable differences in health according to income. Studies indicate that individuals residing in regions with elevated rates of poverty are more susceptible to experiencing unfavorable health consequences throughout their lifespan. Despite being a younger population than non-LGBT+ people, KFF analysis also revealed that LGBT+ people were more likely to report being in fair or poor health and having a continuous medical condition that necessitates ongoing monitoring, care, or medication.

People of color and other marginalized groups have suffered disproportionately from the COVID-19 pandemic in terms of health and well-being. Age-adjusted cumulative data indicated that individuals who identify as AIAN or Hispanic have a higher risk of contracting COVID-19 and that individuals who identify as Black, Hispanic, or AIAN have a higher risk of hospitalization and death from COVID-19. In addition to these immediate health effects, the pandemic has had a detrimental effect on people of color and other marginalized groups, such as LGBT+ individuals, in terms of their mental health, general well-being, and access to social and economic resources. Therefore, in the future, the pandemic might exacerbate health disparities.

Since the pandemic's start, worries about substance abuse and mental health have grown, especially among certain populations. A 2022 KFF/CNN survey found that 90% of people believe there is a mental health crisis in the U.S. Many adults reported experiencing symptoms of anxiety and depression during the pandemic. In addition, there has been a noticeable rise in drug overdose deaths, mostly attributable to fentanyl, and following a brief dip, suicide deaths are once again on the rise. Certain populations, especially communities of color and young people have been disproportionately impacted by these detrimental effects on mental health and substance use. AIAN and Black people had the highest rates of drug overdose deaths in 2021. Throughout the pandemic, the number of alcohol-related deaths rose significantly; individuals of color and those residing in rural areas saw the fastest increases in rates. Compared to White people, many people of color saw a higher increase in suicide death rates between 2019 and 2021. Furthermore, adolescent females' self-harm and suicide ideation have increased more quickly than that of their male peers. According to a Washington Post survey, transgender adults reported experiencing significant mental health problems at a rate that was six times higher than that of cisgender adults. They were also six times more likely to have self-harmed in the previous year (17% vs. 3%). Additionally, there are significant differences in the mental health of LGBT+ youth compared to their non-LGBT+ peers, including suicidality.

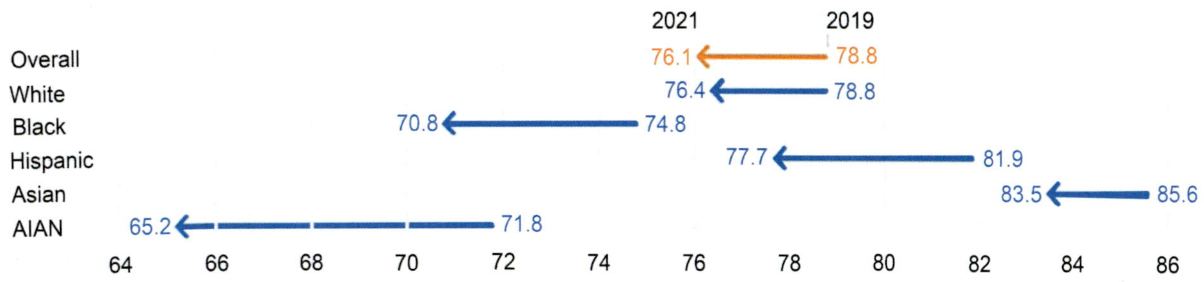

Figure 5.5. *Life expectancy in years by race/ethnicity, 2019–2021.*

Source: https://www.kff.org/racial-equity-and-health-policy/issue-brief/disparities-in-health-and-health-care-5-key-question-and-answers/.

5.4.3. Federal Actions to Address Disparities

Addressing health disparities has received more attention and awareness since the COVID-19 pandemic. Racial disparities in health and their underlying causes, including racism, have come to light as a result of the disparate effects of COVID-19 and the concurrent racial reckoning that followed the police killing of George Floyd. President Biden prioritized health equity early in his presidency, issuing several executive orders outlining the government's general priorities and including equity in the response to and recovery from pandemics. Federal agencies were tasked with creating Equity Action Plans that detailed specific tactics and pledges to remove systemic obstacles throughout the federal government. The Department of Health and Human Services (HHS) outlined many new strategies in its Health Equity Plan, including addressing the higher rates of pregnancy and postpartum morbidity and mortality among Black and Asian women; addressing the difficulties faced by people who do not speak English well to obtain information, services, and benefits from HHS programs; utilizing grants to incorporate equity consideration into funding opportunities; putting equity assessments into practice across all of its major policies and programs; financing civil rights advancements; and increasing contracting opportunities for small, underprivileged businesses. To address structural racism and racial inequities in biomedical research, the plan expands on past initiatives that established the National Institutes of Health UNITE Initiative, increased stakeholder engagement, and established the Office of Climate Change and Health Equity. HHS has taken steps to strengthen patient protections, including nondiscrimination protections, and to ensure that telehealth services are accessible to individuals with disabilities and limited English proficiency since releasing its Equity Action Plan. It has also issued regulations to strengthen postpartum coverage through Medicaid and CHIP.

To promote health equity, increase access to care, and enhance health outcomes for those enrolled in Medicare, Medicaid, CHIP, and the Health Insurance Marketplaces, the Centers for Medicare and Medicaid Services (CMS) has updated its framework. The framework outlined five priorities: increasing the amount of standardized data on social determinants of health and demographics that are collected, reported, and analyzed; identifying policy and operational inequalities and assessing the reasons behind program disparities within CMS; enhancing language access, health literacy, and the provision of culturally appropriate services; and boosting accessibility in all forms for health services and coverage. Additionally, the Administration has emphasized the importance of addressing social determinants of health and promoting health equity within Medicaid. States have been urged to submit Section 1115 Medicaid waiver proposals that increase coverage, lessen health disparities, and/or promote "whole-person care." States are asking for and/or getting approved for waivers more frequently to advance equity. Furthermore, an increasing number of states have authorized or are in the process of approving waivers that contain clauses addressing social needs related to health, like food and housing, and are frequently targeted at high-risk or needy populations.

A variety of steps have been taken by the Administration and Congress to stabilize the situation and broaden access to health care amid the pandemic. Congress enacted the Families First Coronavirus Response Act (FFCRA) early in the pandemic, which included an interim mandate that Medicaid programs maintain continuous enrollment for the duration of the COVID-19 Public Health Emergency in exchange for increased federal funding. Medicaid enrollment has increased significantly since the beginning of the pandemic, largely because of the continuous enrollment provision. Additionally, the percentage of people without insurance has decreased, with the gaps between those of people of color and White people becoming less pronounced. Gains in coverage also probably resulted from increased outreach and enrollment efforts, a Special Enrollment Period for the Marketplaces offered in response to the pandemic, low Marketplace attrition, and enhanced ACA Marketplace subsidies made available by the American Rescue Plan Act (ARPA) of 2021 and renewed for an additional three years in the Inflation Reduction Act of 2022. Furthermore, the Trump Administration's modifications to public charge immigration policies were undone by the Biden Administration in 2019, which made some immigrant families more reluctant to sign up for public services, such as health coverage. To support the stability of children's coverage, the Consolidated Appropriations Act of 2023 most recently mandated that all states implement a 12-month continuous coverage requirement for children. However, it also established March 31, 2023, as the termination date for the more comprehensive Medicaid continuous enrollment provision. This could result in millions of people losing their coverage, undoing recent gains in coverage.

The federal government is making more of an effort to address maternal health disparities. The Administration has started a number of programs aimed at resolving disparities in maternal health during the last few years. President Biden proclaimed in April 2021 recognizing the need to address the high rates of morbidity and mortality among Black women who give birth. The first-ever White House Maternal Health Day of Action was held at the end of 2021. During the event, the Administration unveiled plans to address the maternal health crisis and highlighted areas of concern in maternal health outcomes. The

Biden Administration unveiled its Blueprint for Resolving the Maternal Health Crisis in June 2022. The Blueprint delineates the priorities and measures that federal agencies will undertake to augment and refine data collection and research, broaden and diversify the perinatal workforce, fortify social and economic support, and augment training and incentives to facilitate women's active involvement in their prenatal, perinatal, and postpartum care. To aid in the execution of the Biden-Harris Administration's Blueprint for Addressing the Maternal Health Crisis, CMS released a Maternity Care Action Plan in July 2022. The action plan improves health outcomes and lessens disparities for individuals during pregnancy, childbirth, and the postpartum period by using a comprehensive and coordinated approach across CMS. The Consolidated Appropriations Act made permanent the ARPA option that permitted states to increase the duration of Medicaid postpartum coverage from 60 days to 12 months. Most states have taken action to extend postpartum coverage as of April 2023. Additionally, the Rural Maternal and Obstetrics Management Strategies Program (RMOMS), which aims to create models and put strategies into practice to enhance maternal health in rural communities, was awarded $12 million by the Human Resources and Services Administration.

In addition, the Administration has taken action to address discrimination against LGBT+ individuals as well as health disparities. An Executive Order on "Preventing and Combating Discrimination based on Gender Identity or Sexual Orientation" was signed by President Biden on his first day of office. Subsequently, the Administration has implemented various measures to specifically tackle discrimination in the healthcare industry. In May 2021, the Biden Administration reversed the course taken by the Trump Administration and declared that the HHS Office for Civil Rights (OCR) would take gender identity and sexual orientation into account when interpreting and enforcing the ACA's Section 1557 prohibition against sex discrimination. The Administration has also opposed state initiatives that limit transgender and gender nonconforming people's access to care that affirms their gender identity, especially those that target young people. The Federal Evidence Agenda on LGBTQI+ Equity, which the Administration views as essential to comprehending the inequalities and discrimination this community faces, was published in January 2023. It serves as a "roadmap for federal agencies as they work to create their own data-driven and measurable SOGI Data."

5.4.4. Issues Related to Health Disparities

Insurance losses and a rise in disparities could result from the Medicaid continuous enrollment provision's termination. State Medicaid redeterminations began on March 31, 2023, the day the Medicaid continuous enrollment provision expired. KFF projects that 5–14 million people, many of whom obtained coverage for the first time during the pandemic, may lose their Medicaid coverage. The expiration of the continuous enrollment provision is likely to disproportionately affect Black and Hispanic people, according to other research. Furthermore, completing the Medicaid renewal process can be more difficult for some people, such as those with disabilities and limited English proficiency, increasing their risk of losing coverage even if they are still eligible for it. To prevent coverage lapses during the termination of the continuous enrollment provision, OCR has reminded states of their legal responsibilities under federal civil rights laws to take reasonable measures to furnish meaningful language access for people with limited English proficiency and to guarantee effective communication with people with disabilities. To lower the number of people who lose coverage while still qualifying, CMS released guidance that gives states a road map for streamlining procedures and putting strategies into place. Losses of coverage and possible effects on coverage disparities will be determined by how much states streamline the processes for renewing or switching to other types of coverage and reach out to and help those who are more likely to have trouble with the renewal process.

The COVID-19 Public Health Emergency (PHE) is coming to an end, and some people—especially those without insurance—may have less access to COVID-19 vaccines, treatments, and tests as a result of the possible exhaustion of the federally purchased supply. The federal government used emergency funds worth billions of dollars to buy COVID-19 vaccinations, treatments, and tests to give the public at no cost. This was done in response to the COVID-19 pandemic. Additionally, the Administration released guidelines and regulations to safeguard patient access and advance equitable distribution, and Congress passed legislation that included unique requirements for their coverage by both public and private insurers. Though these effects may vary by product and type of health coverage an individual has, the impending expiration of the PHE on May 11, 2023, as well as the possible depletion of federally purchased supplies in the absence of any additional funding, could result in new or higher cost-sharing and/or reduced access to these products. Uninsured or underinsured individuals are most vulnerable to access issues, such as restricted availability of free vaccines and lack of coverage for diagnostics or treatments. People of color and those with lower incomes are more likely to be uninsured, so once the PHE ends and the federal supply runs out, they may be disproportionately at risk of encountering obstacles in getting access to COVID-19 tests, treatments, and vaccines. The decision to overturn Roe v. Wade might make the significant racial differences in maternal and newborn health that already exist worse. There is now more variance in state laws protecting or restricting abortion as a result of the decision to overturn the long-standing constitutional right to an abortion and to remove federal standards on abortion access. Due to their higher abortion rates, less access to healthcare, and structural injustices that make it more difficult for them to travel out of state for an abortion than for their White counterparts, women of color may be disproportionately affected by these changes. Limiting access to abortions could exacerbate the glaring racial differences in mother and child health that already exist, since certain racial groups are more likely than White people to die during pregnancy, during infancy, or from birth complications. It might also have detrimental effects on employment and educational opportunities, not to mention the direct costs of raising children. Furthermore, in a post-Roe world, women from marginalized communities might be more vulnerable to criminalization because, even before the decision, many low-income or women of color had been criminalized for miscarriages, stillbirths, or infant deaths.

In addition to other legal actions that jeopardize LGBT+ people's access to care, numerous states have enacted policies prohibiting or restricting access to gender-affirming healthcare, particularly for young people. Restrictions on access to care that is gender-affirming may have serious negative effects on the health of transgender and nonconforming individuals, especially in the youth. These effects may include worsening mental health and a higher risk of suicide. Furthermore, the treatment of Pre-Exposure Prophylaxis (PrEP) among LGBT+ individuals is directly impacted by the recent Braidwood case regarding access to preventive care. The plaintiff's allegation that the drug "facilitate[s] and encourage[s] homosexual behavior, prostitution, sexual promiscuity, and intravenous drug use" is the basis for some of the arguments made in favor of religious protections. HIV incidence may rise as a result of the Braidwood ruling, disproportionately affecting people of color and LGBT+ individuals if PrEP use falls. The Braidwood ruling and efforts to restrict access to gender-affirming healthcare are incompatible with the Administration's professed commitment to LGBT+ health equity. The courts will have a major say in how such policies turn out in the long run.

The health and happiness of immigrant families may be impacted by changing immigration laws. Title 42 restrictions that prohibited people from entering the U.S. after May 11, 2023, will expire. s. boundaries to safeguard public health amid the COVID-19 crisis are anticipated to close. It is expected that there will be a surge in immigration activity at the U.S. border once the authority expires. s. boundary. The Biden Administration has made plans to strengthen border enforcement and security in order to decrease unauthorized crossings; to extend "legal pathways for orderly migration"; to allocate more funds to the border region; and to collaborate with Mexico in carrying out the aforementioned initiatives. It is unclear, nevertheless, how changing policies will affect border trends, local health, and medical services. Deferred Action for Childhood Arrivals (DACA) program implementation is currently limited by court orders, and its future is still unclear. People would lose their DACA status and, consequently, their work authorizations, if the DACA program is determined to be illegal in future court decisions. People who lose their work authorization and status may also lose their employer-sponsored health insurance, which would leave them without insurance and unable to apply for Medicaid, CHIP, or the Marketplace. Furthermore, many families still have reservations about enrolling in government assistance programs like Medicaid and CHIP, which contributes to continuous gaps in coverage for immigrants and their children. This is despite the Biden Administration overturning public charge regulations that the Trump Administration had put in place in an attempt to allay immigration-related fears that had limited immigrant families' participation in these programs.

Health disparities may be exacerbated by persistent racism, discrimination, and violence, as well as growing concerns about mental health and drug abuse. As was previously mentioned, since the pandemic's start, concerns about mental health and drug use have grown, with some groups being disproportionately impacted. These patterns could result in growing inequalities. For instance, the death rate from drug overdoses has increased more for people of color than for White people. As a result, by 2020, the death rate for Black people will have surpassed that of White people for the first time. In addition, Black and Asian individuals have reported detrimental effects on their mental health as a result of an increase in anti-Black and anti-Asian racism and violence in recent years. Studies have shown that exposure to violence, including that which occurs between police and people, has detrimental effects on one's health, including mental health and general well-being. Compared to their White counterparts, research indicates that Latino men and women, as well as African American and Asian men and women, are more likely to be killed by police. Data from the 2023 KFF survey also show that adults who identify as Black or Hispanic are more likely than White adults to be concerned about gun violence. Additional KFF analysis reveals that during the pandemic, firearm-related deaths among Black and Hispanic youth rose significantly, mainly as a result of gun assaults and suicides. Additional research reveals that prolonged and frequent exposure to racism and discrimination is linked to detrimental effects on one's physical and mental well-being, including early aging and the health risks that go along with it—a process known as "weathering"—as well as a higher death rate.

People of color still face disproportionate obstacles to receiving mental health care, despite the growing concern about mental health. Research indicates that structural injustices resulting from larger disparities in social and economic factors may be a factor in the disparities in the use of mental health care. These injustices include a lack of health insurance coverage and logistical and financial barriers to accessing care. People of color may receive less mental health treatment than other populations due to a variety of factors, including a lack of culturally sensitive treatment options, a lack of a diverse workforce in the mental health field, and prejudice and stereotypes connected to poor mental health. Many states expanded access to behavioral health care during the pandemic by implementing telehealth behavioral health services, and the majority of these states plan to maintain these services. States are also implementing plans to deal with the lack of workers in the behavioral health field. As states work to increase access to mental health services, it will be crucial to make sure that the linguistic and cultural needs of various populations are taken into account. Furthermore, the suicide and crisis lifeline number, which offers a single three-digit number (988) to access a network of more than 200 locally and state-funded crisis centers, was mandated by the federal government in 2022. It's anticipated that the 988 number will enhance the provision of crisis mental health care, but it's unclear how well it will meet the needs of people of color and other marginalized groups. (Schulmanet al., 1999; Chen et al., 2001).

A Closer Look

Role of Community Health Initiatives in Reducing Disparities

Community health initiatives play a pivotal role in reducing health disparities by addressing the social determinants of health and improving access to healthcare for underserved populations. These initiatives are designed to meet the specific needs of communities, particularly those experiencing significant health inequities due to socioeconomic status, race, ethnicity, geographic location, and education. Community health initiatives can bridge the gap between healthcare services and marginalized groups by focusing on prevention, early intervention, and providing culturally competent care.

One of the primary ways community health initiatives reduce disparities is by enhancing access to healthcare services. Many underserved communities face barriers such as lack of transportation, financial constraints, and limited availability of healthcare providers. Community health programs often establish local clinics, mobile health units, and health fairs that bring essential services directly to these areas. These efforts ensure that residents can receive preventive care, screenings, and treatment without the burden of traveling long distances or incurring high costs. Additionally, community health workers, who often come from the communities they serve, play a crucial role in building trust, providing education, and connecting individuals to necessary resources.

Community health initiatives also address the root causes of health disparities by tackling social determinants of health such as housing, nutrition, education, and employment. Programs that provide affordable housing, food assistance, job training, and educational opportunities can significantly impact the overall health and well-being of community members. For example, initiatives that promote access to healthy foods and physical activity can help reduce rates of obesity, diabetes, and cardiovascular diseases, which are disproportionately high in low-income and minority communities. By creating environments that support healthy lifestyles, these initiatives contribute to long-term improvements in public health.

Culturally competent care is another critical component of effective community health initiatives. These programs often employ a diverse workforce that reflects the demographics of the community, ensuring that language barriers and cultural differences do not hinder access to care. Health education materials are tailored to be culturally relevant and linguistically appropriate, which enhances understanding and compliance with medical advice. Additionally, community health initiatives frequently involve collaboration with local leaders and organizations to ensure that programs are culturally sensitive and resonate with the community's values and beliefs.

Prevention and early intervention are central strategies in community health initiatives aimed at reducing disparities. Programs that focus on vaccination drives, chronic disease management, maternal and child health, and mental health services can prevent the onset of diseases and manage existing conditions more effectively. Early detection and treatment of health issues reduce the risk of complications and lower healthcare costs, ultimately leading to better health outcomes for individuals in underserved communities.

Moreover, community health initiatives often advocate for policy changes at the local, state, and national levels. By raising awareness about the health needs of disadvantaged populations and lobbying for supportive policies, these initiatives work to create systemic changes that promote health equity. This can include advocating for expanded healthcare coverage, improved funding for community health programs, and the implementation of policies that address social determinants of health.

Summary

- Socioeconomic status (SES) is another critical factor contributing to health disparities. Individuals from lower socioeconomic backgrounds often face barriers to accessing healthcare, including lack of insurance, inability to afford medical care, and limited availability of healthcare providers in their communities.
- Health disparities occur when people and communities experience higher rates of breast cancer, obesity, heart disease, and other challenges for specific reasons that include race and ethnicity, access to care, poverty, and environmental risk.
- Disparities often have multiple root causes, but there are a few major inequities in the United States that are known to contribute to health gaps between groups.
- Closing the gap in health outcomes is no easy task. Causes are often multi-layered. Solutions would need to address not only the root cause of a given disparity but also the original context.
- Gender health disparities refer to the differences in health outcomes and access to healthcare services between individuals based on their gender. These disparities are rooted in a complex interplay of biological, social, economic, and cultural factors that differentially impact the health of men, women, and non-binary individuals.
- Economic disparities also play a crucial role in gender health inequalities. Women are more likely to experience poverty and have lower incomes compared to men, which directly impacts their ability to afford healthcare.
- Disability and health disparities refer to the unequal health outcomes and access to healthcare services experienced by individuals with disabilities compared to those without disabilities.
- Addressing disability and health disparities requires a comprehensive approach that includes policy changes, increased funding for accessible healthcare infrastructure, and enhanced training for healthcare providers.
- Racial disparities in medical care should be understood within the context of racial inequities in societal institutions. Systematic discrimination is not the aberrant behavior of a few but is often supported by institutional policies and unconscious bias based on negative stereotypes.

References

1. Schulman KA, Berlin JA, Harless W, et al. The effect of race and sex on physicians' recommendations for cardiac catheterization. *N Engl J Med.* 1999;340:618–26.
2. Chen J, Rathore SS, Radford MJ, Wang Y, Krumholz HM. Racial differences in the use of cardiac catheterization after acute myocardial infarction. *N Engl J Med.* 2001;344:1443–9.
3. Benz J, Espinosa O, Welsh V, Fontes A. Awareness of racial and ethnic health disparities has improved only modestly over a decade. *Health Affairs.* 2011;30:10.
4. Haider A, Sexton J, Sriram N, Cooper LA, et al. Association of unconscious race and social class bias with vignette-based clinical assessments by medical students. *JAMA.* 2011;306:9.

5. Jha AK, Orav EJ, Epstein AM. Low quality, high-cost hospitals, mainly in south, care for sharply higher shares of elderly black, Hispanic, and medicaid patients. *Health Affairs.* 2011;30:10.
6. Allen J. A Remedy for Unthinking Discrimination. *Brooklyn Law Review.* 1995 Winter;61:1299–1345.
7. Anderson MJ. *The American Census: A Social History.* New Haven, CT.: Yale University Press; 1988.
8. Anderson M, Feinberg SE. Black, White, and Shades of Gray (and Brown and Yellow) *Chance.* 1995;8(1):15–18.
9. Blendon R, Aiken L, Freeman H, Corey C. Access to Medical Care for Black and White Americans. *Journal of the American Medical Association.* 1989;261(2):278–281.
10. Bobo L, Kluegel JR, Smith RA. Laissez Faire Racism: The Crystallization of a "Kinder, Gentler" Anti-Black Ideology. In: Tuch SA, Martin JK, editors. *Racial Attitudes in the 1990s: Continuity and Change.* Westport, CT.: Praeger; 1997.
11. Bobo L, Zubrinsky CL. Attitudes on Residential Integration: Perceived Status Differences, Mere In-Group Preference, or Racial Prejudice? *Social Forces.* 1996;74(3):883–909.
12. Bonilla-Silva E. Rethinking Racism: Toward a Structural Interpretation. *American Sociological Review.* 1996;62(3):465–480.
13. Bunker JP, Frazier HF, Mosteller F. The Role of Medical Care in Determining Health: Creating an Inventory of Benefits. In: Amick BCI, Levine S, Tarlov AR, Walsh DC, editors. *Society and Health.* New York: Oxford University Press; 1995.
14. Carlisle DM, Gardner JE, Liu H. The Entry of Underrepresented Minority Students Into U.S. Medical Schools: An Evaluation of Recent Trends. *American Journal of Public Health.* 1998;88(9):1314–1318.
15. Cleeland CS, Gonin R, Baez L, et al. Pain and Treatment of Pain in Minority Patients with Cancer: The Eastern Cooperative Oncology Group Minority Outpatient Pain Study. *Annals of Internal Medicine.* 1997;127(9):813–816.
16. Cole RE, Deskins DR., Jr Racial Factors in Site Location and Employment Patterns of Japanese Auto Firms in America. *California Management Review.* 1988;31(1):9–22.
17. Council on Ethical and Judicial Affairs. Black-White Disparities in Health Care. *Journal of the American Medical Association.* 1990;263(17):2344–2346.
18. Davis JA, Smith TW. *General Social Surveys, 1972-1990.* Chicago: National Opinion Research Center; 1990.
19. Devine PG. Prejudice and Out-Group Perception. In: Tesser A, editor. *Advanced Social Psychology.* New York: McGraw-Hill; 1995.
20. Devine PG. Stereotypes and Prejudice: Their Automatic and Controlled Components. *Journal of Personality and Social Psychology.* 1989;56:5–18.
21. Duff R, Hollingshead A. *Sickness and Society.* New York: Harper and Row; 1968.
22. *Economic Report of the President.* Washington, DC.: U. S. Government Printing Office; 1998.
23. Editorial. Affirmative Action. *Lancet.* 1999;353(9146):1.
24. Fix M, Struyk RJ. *Clear and Convincing Evidence: Measurement of Discrimination in America.* Washington, DC.: Urban Institute Press; 1993.

25. Geiger HJ. Race and Health Care - An American Dilemma? *New England Journal of Medicine.* 1996;335(11):815–816.

26. Hall JA, Roter DL, Katz NR. Meta-Analysis of Correlates of Provider Behavior in Medical Encounters. *Medical Care.* 1988;26(7):212–229.

27. Hannan EL, van Ryn M, Burke J, et al. Access to Coronary Artery Bypass Surgery by Race/ Ethnicity and Gender Among Patients Who Are Appropriate for Surgery. *Medical Care.* 1999;37(1):68–77.

28. Harris DR, Andrews R, Elixhauser A. Racial and Gender Differences in Use of Procedures for Black and White Hospitalized Adults. *Ethnicity and Disease.* 1997;7(2):91–105.

29. Harvard Law Review. The Impact of Managed Care on Doctors Who Serve Poor and Minority Patients. 1995 May;108:1625–1642.

30. Hillman A. Financial Incentives for Physicians in HMOs. Is There a Conflict of Interest? *New England Journal of Medicine.* 1987;317(27):1743–1748.

31. Hilton JL, von Hippel W. Stereotypes. *Annual Review of Psychology.* 1996;47(250):237–271.

32. Horner RD, Oddone EZ, Matchar DB. Theories Explaining Racial Differences in the Utilization of Diagnostic and Therapeutic Procedures for Cerebrovascular Disease. *Milbank Quarterly.* 1995;73(3):443–462.

33. Johnson SL. Unconscious Racism and the Criminal Law. *Cornell Law Review.* 1988 Jul;73:1016–1037.

34. King G. Institutional Racism and the Medical/Health Complex: A Conceptual Analysis. *Ethnicity and Disease.* 1996;6(1,2):30–46.

35. Kirschenman J, Neckerman KM. "We'd Love to Hire Them, But...": the Meaning of Race for Employers. In: Jencks C, Peterson PE, editors. *The Urban Underclass.* Washington, DC.: The Brookings Institution; 1991. pp. 203–232.

36. Komaromy M, Grumbach K, Drake M, et al. The Role Of Black And Hispanic Physicians In Providing Health Care For Underserved Populations. *Black and Hispanic Physicians and Underserved Populations.* 1996;334(20):1305–1310.

37. Krieger N. Embodying Inequality: A Review of Concepts, Measures, and Methods for Studying Health Consequences of Discrimination. *International Journal of Health Services.* 1999;29(2):295–352.

38. Krieger N, Williams DR, Moss N. Measuring Social Class in U.S. Public Health Research: Concepts, Methodologies, and Guidelines. *Annual Review of Public Health.* 1997;18:341–378.

39. Lavizzo-Mourey R, Clayton LA, Byrd M, et al. The Perceptions of African-American Physicians Concerning Their Treatment By Managed Care Organizations. *Journal of the National Medical Association.* 1996;88(4):210–214.

40. Lawrence CRI. The Id, the Ego, and Equal Protection: Reckoning with Unconscious Racism. *Stanford Law Review.* 1987 Jan;39:317–38.

41. Leape LL. A Systems Analysis Approach to Medical Error. *Journal of Evaluation in Clinical Practice.* 1997;3(3):213–222.

42. Libby DL, Zhou Z, Kindig DA. Will Minority Physician Supply Meet U. S. Needs? *Health Affairs (Millwood)* 1997;16(4):205–214.

43. Massey DA, Gross AB, Shibuya K. Migration, Segregation, and the Geographic Concentration of Poverty. *American Sociological Review.* 1994;59(3):425–445.

44. Massey DS. The Age of Extremes: Concentrated Affluence and Poverty in the Twenty-First Century. *Demography.* 1996;33(4):395–428.

45. McBean AM, Gornick M. Differences by Race in the Rates of Procedures Performed in Hospitals for Medicare Beneficiaries. *Health Care Financing Review.* 1994;15(4):77–90.

46. McClellan FM. Is Managed Care Good for What Ails You? Ruminations on Race, Age and Class. *Villanova Law Review.* 1999;44:227–255.

47. McLafferty S. Neighborhood Characteristics and Hospital Closures: A Comparison of the Public, Private, and Voluntary Hospital Systems. *Social Science Medicine.* 1982;16(19):1667–1674.

48. Murphy-Berman VA, Berman JJ, Campbell E. Factors Affecting Health-Care Allocation Decisions: A Case of Aversive Racism? *Journal of Applied Social Psychology.* 1998;28(24):2239–2253.

49. National Center for Health Statistics. *Health, United States and, Socioeconomic Status and Health Chartbook Hyattsville, MD.* U.S. Department of Health and Human Services; Washington, DC.: 1998.

50. National Committee on Vital and Health Statistics. *1. Diversity and Health Care Data Base: A Preamble for Policymakers.* 1993. pp. 3–19. DHHS Publication PHS 93-1205.

51. Neckerman KM, Kirschenman J. Hiring Strategies, Racial Bias, and Inner-City Workers. *Social Problems.* 1991;38(4):433–447.

52. Nickens HW, Cohen JJ. On Affirmative Action [Policy Perspectives] *Journal of the American Medical Association.* 1996;275(7):572–574.

53. Noah BA. Racial Disparities in the Delivery of Health Care. *San Diego Law Review.* 1998 Winter;35:135–178.

54. Oppenheimer DB. *Negligent Discrimination.* Vol. 141. University of Pennsylvania Law Review; Jan, 1993. pp. 899–972.

55. Pauly MV, Hillman AL, Kerstein J. Managing Physician Incentives in Managed Care: The Role of For-Profit Ownership. *Medical Care.* 1990;28(11):1013–1024.

56. Peterson ED, Shaw LK, DeLong ER, et al. Racial Variation in the Use of Coronary-Revascularization Procedures--Are the Differences Real? Do They Matter? *New England Journal of Medicine.* 1997;336(7):480–486.

57. Potosky AL, Breen N, Graubard BI, Parsons PE. The Association Between Health Care Coverage and the Use of Cancer Screening Tests. Results from the 1992 National Health Interview Survey. *Medical Care.* 1998;36(3):257–70.

58. Randall VR. Impact of Managed Care Organizations on Ethnic Americans and Under Served Populations. *Journal of Health Care for the Poor Underserved.* 1994;5(3):224–226.

59. Reschovsky JD, Kemper P, Tu HT, et al. Do HMOs Make a Difference?: Comparing Access, Service Use and Satisfaction Between Consumers in HMOs and Non-HMOs. *Issue Brief: Findings From Health System Change.* 2000 Mar;28:1–8.

60. Robins LS, Fantone JC, Hermann J, et al. Culture, Communication, and the Informal Curriculum: Improving Cultural Awareness and Sensitivity Training in Medical School. *Academic Medicine.* 1998;73(10):S31–S34.

61. Schlesinger M. Paying the Price: Medical Care, Minorities, and the Newly Competitive Health Care System. *Milbank Quarterly.* 1987;65(2):270–296.

62. Schuman H, Steeh C, Bobo L, Krysan M. *Racial Attitudes in America: Trends and Interpretations.* Rev. Edition. Cambridge, MA.: Harvard University Press; 1997.

63. Sharpe R. In Latest Recession, Only Blacks Suffered Net Employment Loss. *Wall Street Journal.* 1993 Sep 14;:A-1.

64. Smith DB. Addressing Racial Inequities in Health Care: Civil Rights Monitoring and Report Cards. *Health Politics, Policy, and Law.* 1998;23(1):75–105.

65. Stangnor C, McMillan D. Memory for Expectancy-Congruent and Expectancy-Incongruent Information: A Review of the Social and Social Development Literatures. *Psychological Bulletin.* 1992;111(1):42–61.

66. Tekian A. A Thematic Review of the Literature on Under Represented Minorities and Medical Training, 1981-1995: Securing the Foundations of the Bridge to Diversity. *Academic Medicine.* 1997;72(10):S140–S146.

67. Todd KH, Lee T, Hoffman JR. The Effect of Ethnicity on Physician Estimates of Pain Severity in Patients With Isolated Extremity Trauma. *Journal of the American Medical Association.* 1994;271(12):925–928.

68. Todd KH, Samaroo N, Hoffman JR. Ethnicity as a Risk Factor for Inadequate Emergency Department Analgesia. *Journal of the American Medical Association.* 1993;269(12):1537–9.

69. Trevino FM, Moyer ME, Valdez RB, Stroup-Benham CA. Health Insurance Coverage and Utilization of Health Services by Mexican Americans, Mainland Puerto Ricans, and Cuban Americans. *Journal of the American Medical Association.* 1991;265(2):233–237.

70. van Ryn M, Burke J. The Effect of Patient Race and Socio-Economic Status on Physicians' Perceptions of Patients. *Social Science & Medicine.* 2000;50(6):813–828.

71. Wallace SP, Enriquez-Haass V, Markides K. The Consequences of Color-Blind Health Policy for Older Racial and Ethnic Minorities. *Stanford Law and Policy Review.* 1998;9(2):329–346.

72. Warner K. Cigarette Advertising and Media Coverage of Smoking and Health. *New England Journal of Medicine.* 1985;312(6):384–388.

73. Weissman NW, Allison JJ, Kiefe CI, et al. Achievable Benchmarks of Care: the ABC's of Benchmarking. *Journal of Evaluation in Clinical Practice.* 1999;5(3):269–281.

74. Wenneker MB, Epstein AM. Racial Inequalities in the Use of Procedures for Patients with Ischemic Heart Disease in Massachusetts. *Journal of the American Medical Association.* 1989;261:253–257.

75. Whiteis DG. Hospital and Community Characteristics in Closures of Urban Hospitals, 1980-87. *Public Health Reports.* 1992;107(4):409–416.

76. Whittle J, Conigliaro J, Good CB, Lofgren RP. Racial Differences in the Use of Invasive Cardiovasular Procedures in the Department of Veterans Affairs. *New England Journal of Medicine.* 1993;329(9):621–626.

77. Williams DR. Race and Health: Basic Questions, Emerging Directions. *Annals of Epidemiology.* 1997;7(5):322–333.

78. Williams DR. Race/Ethnicity and Socioeconomic Status: Measurement and Methodological Issues. *International Journal of Health Services.* 1996;26(3):483–505.

79. Williams DR. *Race, SES, and Health: The Added Effects of Racism and Discrimination.* Vol. 896. Annals of New York Academy of Sciences; 1999. pp. 173–188.

80. Williams DR, Jackson JS, Brown TN, et al. Traditional and Contemporary Prejudice and Urban Whites' Support for Affirmative Action and Government Help. *Social Problems.* 1999;46(4):503–527.

81. Zweifler J, Gonzalez AM. Teaching Residents to Care for Culturally Diverse Populations. *Academic Medicine.* 1998;73(10):1056–1061.

Chapter

6

TOBACCO CONTROL AND PREVENTION

Contents

Introduction

Efforts to control and prevent tobacco use are crucial to public health initiatives worldwide. These efforts aim to reduce the prevalence of tobacco use and its health consequences through a variety of strategies, policies, and interventions. One important aspect of tobacco control is the implementation of comprehensive policies at the national, regional, and local levels. These policies often include measures such as tobacco taxation, smoke-free laws, advertising and promotion restrictions, and packaging regulations. Research consistently shows that these policies are effective in reducing tobacco use and preventing initiation, especially among youth and vulnerable populations. Educational campaigns and public awareness initiatives also play a key role in tobacco prevention by informing the public about the health risks of tobacco use and the benefits of quitting. These campaigns use various media channels to reach diverse audiences and convey compelling messages, ultimately contributing to changing attitudes and behaviors related to smoking.

Programs for quitting tobacco use offer vital resources and support to people who want to stop using tobacco products or smoking. To address the needs of various populations, these programs frequently combine behavioral counselling, medication, and support services. Pharmacotherapy options include prescription medications, alternative therapies, and nicotine replacement therapy; behavioral interventions include counselling, phone helplines, online programs, and individual or group counselling. Tobacco users need to receive evidence-based, easily accessible services to effectively quit and maintain their smoke-free lifestyle.

To reach tobacco users and give them the support they need to quit, tobacco control and prevention initiatives must be integrated into healthcare systems. Physicians, nurses, pharmacists, and other allied health professionals are among the healthcare professionals who are essential in identifying tobacco users, providing brief interventions, and directing patients to cessation services. Healthcare systems can effectively address tobacco use as a chronic disease and improve patient outcomes by integrating tobacco screening, counselling, and cessation support into routine clinical practice.

Moreover, equitable tobacco control outcomes require addressing the social determinants of tobacco use. Patterns of tobacco use and cessation behavior are influenced by several factors, including socioeconomic status, education, employment, and access to healthcare services. Targeted interventions, laws, and initiatives that remove structural obstacles and advance health equity are necessary to address these underlying social determinants in the context of efforts to lessen tobacco-related health disparities. To lower tobacco use, encourage quitting, and address the larger social determinants of health, tobacco control, and prevention initiatives take a multimodal approach. Public health stakeholders can significantly reduce the global burden of tobacco-related diseases and improve the health and well-being of individuals and communities by putting evidence-based strategies, policies, and interventions into practice at the individual, community, and population levels.

Orientation and Directional Terms:

Terms	Definition	Illustration
Tobacco	Tobacco is the common name of several plants in the genus Nicotiana of the family Solanaceae, and the general term for any product prepared from the cured leaves of these plants.	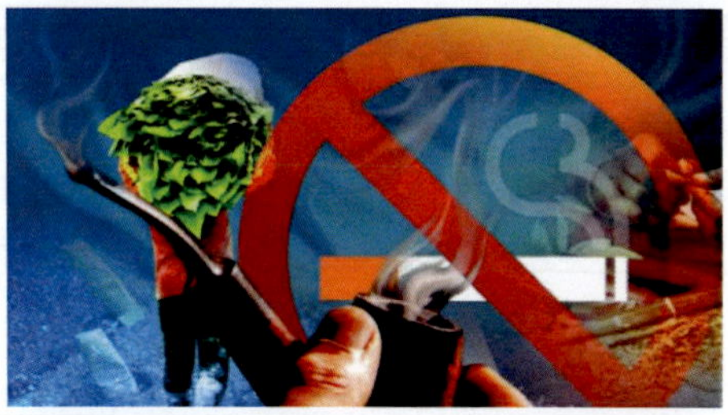
Disease	A disease is a particular abnormal condition that adversely affects the structure or function of all or part of an organism and is not immediately due to any external injury.	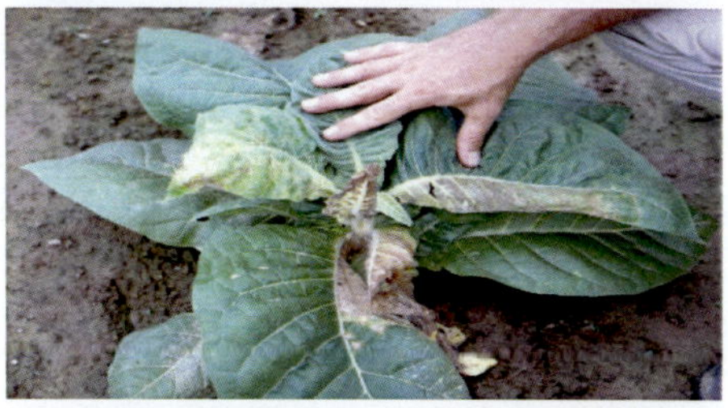
Cardiology	Cardiology is the study of the heart. Cardiology is a branch of medicine that deals with disorders of the heart and the cardiovascular system.	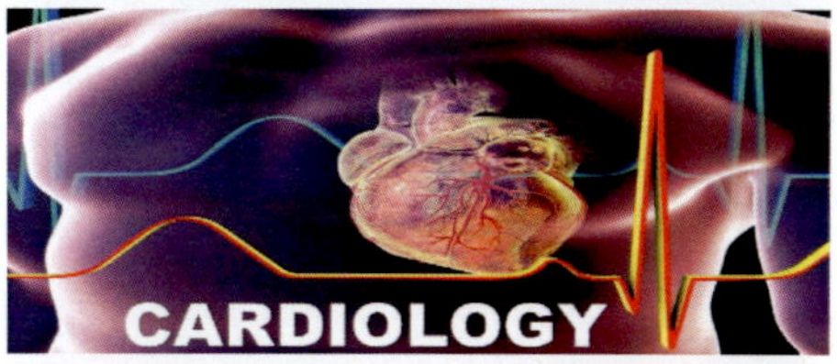
Low-density lipoprotein	Low-density lipoprotein is one of the five major groups of lipoprotein that transport all fat molecules around the body in extracellular water.	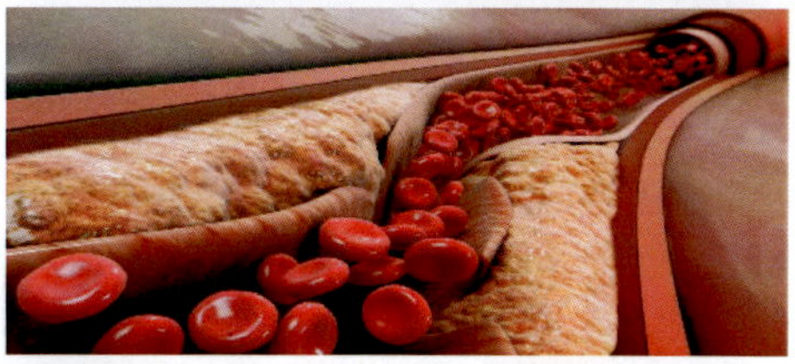
	Diagnosis is the endpoint of a complex process centered on a patient, collaborating with both the patient and other sources of clinical information to reason backward as to the potential health issue causing the patient's current condition.	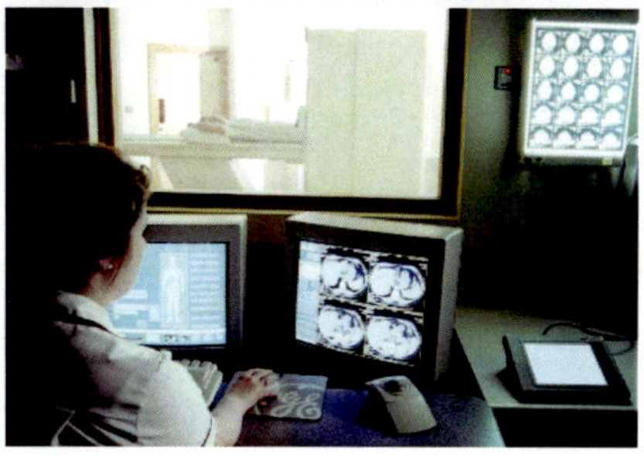

6.1. Overview of Tobacco Control

The goal of tobacco control in international public health science, policy, and practice is to address tobacco use and minimize the associated morbidity and mortality. Tobacco control also affects cigars, hookahs, and cigarettes since most of them contain or use tobacco. Nicotine is frequently present in e-cigarettes but tobacco is not. Through the Framework Convention on Tobacco Control, the World Health Organization (WHO) has made tobacco control a top priority. Depending on the commentator, references to a tobacco control movement can have a positive or negative connotation. The goal of tobacco control is to lower the prevalence of tobacco use, and the age-standardized prevalence of current tobacco use among people 15 years of age and older is used to measure this.

6.1.1. Connotations

The field of tobacco control encompasses the efforts of various health, policy, and legal research organizations as well as reform advocacy groups worldwide. The first article in the first edition of the Tobacco Control journal suggested that developing as a diffusely organized movement was necessary to bring about effective action to address the health effects of tobacco use. It took some time for these to come together into a sufficiently organized coalition to advance measures such as the World Health Organization Framework Convention on Tobacco Control. Reluctant supporters of the tobacco control movement have also referred to it as an anti-smoking movement, as internal tobacco industry memos attest to.

6.1.2. Early History of Tobacco Control

Shortly after tobacco was introduced to Europe, efforts to address the health risks associated with tobacco use began. During his thirteen-day pontificate, Pope Urban VII instituted the first tobacco use ban in history in 1590, threatening to excommunicate anyone found using tobacco in a church porchway or within its walls, whether through chewing, pipe smoking, or sniffing powdered tobacco through the nose. Tobacco was condemned to excommunication under this restriction, not so much. It was unhealthy as it was because its use inside the churches was unbearable. After all, it degraded the general ambiance. Therefore, these penalties would be for the inappropriate use of tobacco in locations regarded as holy and public, rather than against tobacco use in general (whose personal use was not punished as long as it was moderate). Even in modern Catholic doctrine, improper use is still condemned. The first smoking bans in European cities were implemented in the late 17th century in Bavaria, Kreisachsen, and some regions of Austria.

In Britain, the still-new habit of smoking met royal opposition in 1604, when King James I wrote *A Counterblaste to Tobacco*, describing smoking as: "A custom loathsome to the eye, hateful to the nose, harmful to the brain, dangerous to the lungs, and in the black stinking fume thereof, nearest resembling the horrible Stygian smoke of the pit that is bottomless." His commentary was accompanied by a doctor of the same period, writing under the pseudonym "Philaretes," who as well as explaining tobacco's harmful effects under the system of the four humors ascribed an infernal motive to its introduction, explaining his dislike of tobacco as grounded upon eight 'principal reasons and arguments' (in their original spelling):

1. First, that in their use and custom, no method or order is observed. Diversity and distinction of persons, times, and seasons considered.
2. Secondly, for it is in quality and complexion hotter and dry then may be conveniently used daily of any man:

much less of the hot and choleric constitution.

3. Thirdly, for it is experimented on and tried to be a strong and violent purge.
4. Fourthly, for that it withereth and drieth up natural moisture in our bodies, thereby causing sterility and barrenness: In which respect it seemeth an enemy to the continuance and propagation of mankind.
5. Fifthly, for that it decayed and dissipate natural heat, that kindly warmth in us, and thereby is cause of crudities and resumes, occasions of infinite maladies.
6. Sixthly, for that, this herb is rather weed, seems not void of venom and poison, and thereby seemeth an enemy to the life of man.
7. Seventhly, for that the first author and finder hereof were the Devil, and the first practisers of the same were the Divells Preiests, and therefore not to be used of us Christians.
8. Last of all, because it is a great augmenter of all sorts of melancholy in our bodies, a humor fit to prepare our bodies to receive the prestigious and hellish illusions and impressions of the Divell himself: in so much that many Physicians and learned to mean doe hold this humor to be the very seate of the Divell in bodies possessed.

Later in the seventeenth century, Sir Francis Bacon identified the addictive consequences of tobacco use, observing that it "is growing greatly and conquers men with a certain secret pleasure, so that those who have once become accustomed thereto can later hardly be restrained therefrom." Smoking was forbidden in Berlin in 1723, in Königsberg in 1742, and in Stettin in 1744. These restrictions were repealed in the revolutions of 1848. In 1930s Germany, scientific research for the first time revealed a connection between lung cancer and smoking, so the use of cigarettes and smoking was strongly discouraged by a heavy government-sponsored anti-smoking campaign.

6.1.3. Origins of Modern Tobacco Control

The development of contemporary tobacco control programs dates back to the middle of the 20th century when medical studies started to show how seriously smoking cigarettes could affect one's health. An important turning point was the groundbreaking 1964 Surgeon General's Report on Smoking and Health, which showed how smoking causes lung cancer and other illnesses. This report sparked a change in societal perceptions about tobacco use and increased public awareness.

Comprehensive tobacco control initiatives and policies emerged in the following decades to reduce tobacco use. Among these initiatives were the introduction of warning labels on tobacco products, the adoption of smoke-free laws in public areas, and the passing of legislation prohibiting tobacco advertising. International cooperation, like the Framework Convention on Tobacco Control (FCTC) established by the World Health Organization in 2003, further sparked a global push to reduce tobacco use through coordinated action and policy development. Furthermore, public health campaigns, grassroots advocacy groups, and the mobilization of civil society organizations have all contributed significantly to the global advancement of tobacco control agendas. Modern tobacco control initiatives are constantly evolving in an attempt to safeguard public health, lessen tobacco-related inequalities, and establish smoke-free environments for coming generations. These efforts combine scientific evidence, policy advocacy, and community engagement.

German research was essentially suppressed following World War II because of its alleged ties to Nazism. But Richard Doll's research in the UK, which proved smoking and lung cancer were causally related in 1952, raised awareness of this issue once more. Eventually, most of the developed world saw the implementation of partial controls and regulatory measures, such as minimum age of sale requirements, partial advertising bans, and basic health warnings on tobacco packaging. However, in the first three decades after Richard Doll's discovery, the prevalence of smoking and the illnesses it causes continued to rise in the developed world. Governments were occasionally reluctant to restrict a habit that was seen as popular as a result, and the tobacco industry and its proxies increasingly coordinated disinformation campaigns. Gradually, it became clear that the health effects of smoking and tobacco use could only be addressed by a multifaceted policy response that included effective marketing restrictions, medical assistance to stop tobacco use, and positive health messages. This was first suggested in a 1962 overview by the British Royal College of Physicians and the 1964 report of the U. S. General Surgeon. An objective synthesis of the evidence regarding the health effects of smoking based on causal criteria was included in the groundbreaking 1964 report of the Advisory Committee to the Surgeon General, which was issued in the United States.

6.1.4. Comprehensive Tobacco Control

6.1.4.1. At the Global Level

The idea of multifaceted, and thus "all-encompassing," tobacco control emerged from scholarly developments (e.g., the special Tobacco Control journal), government policy initiatives, and nonprofit advocacy organizations like Action on Smoking and Health. Progress was first noticeable at the state or federal level, especially with the introduction of the groundbreaking smoke-free public places laws in New York City in 2002 and the Republic of Ireland in 2004. There were also efforts made in the UK to deliver on the coordinated approach outlined in the white paper "Smoking Kills" by encapsulating the essential components of tobacco control activity in the 2004 "six-strand approach" and its local equivalent, the "seven hexagons of tobacco control." To negotiate and support the first international public health treaty, the World Health Organization Framework Convention on Tobacco Control, or FCTC for short, this loosely organized group of health research and policy development bodies formed the Framework Convention Alliance.

WHO subsequently produced an internationally applicable and now widely recognized summary of the essential elements of tobacco control strategy, publicized as the mnemonic MPOWER tobacco control strategy.

The six components are:

- **M**onitor tobacco use and prevention policies;
- **P**rotect people from tobacco smoke;
- **O**ffer help to quit tobacco use;
- **W**arn about the dangers of tobacco;
- **E**nforce bans on tobacco advertising, promotion and sponsorship; and
- **R**aise taxes on tobacco.

Enhancing the implementation of the WHO Framework Convention on Tobacco Control in all nations, as appropriate, is one of the goals of the United Nations Sustainable Development Goal 3, which is to be accomplished by 2030.

The age-standardized prevalence of current tobacco use among people aged 15 and older serves as a progress indicator. The Tobacco Products and Cigarettes (Prohibition of Advertisement and Regulation of Trade and Commerce, Production, Supply, and Distribution) Act, 2003 was enacted in India in 2003. It prohibited smoking in public areas, limited the advertising of tobacco products, and imposed additional regulations on the trade of tobacco products. The Hindi-language anti-smoking short film Swing was released in 2010, and Bhutan passed the Tobacco Control Act of Bhutan 2010 to regulate tobacco and tobacco products, outlawing their cultivation, harvesting, production, and sale within the country.

6.1.4.2. Tobacco Control Policies

1. **Age Restriction:** Policies about tobacco that prohibit smoking in public areas and limit the sale of cigarettes to minors are crucial tools in the fight against youth access to and consumption of cigarettes. Youth in the United States, for instance, were more likely to smoke every day among young adolescents living in states with no or minimal restrictions than among students in states with strict regulations. This was especially true for high school students. Despite other tobacco control measures, these effects were lessened when logistic regressions were adjusted for sociodemographic variables and cigarette prices. This suggests that higher cigarette prices may deter youth from accessing and consuming cigarettes.

   In December 2022, New Zealand became the first country to pass a bill that effectively raises the minimum age for cigarette consumption annually, to prohibit their sale to future generations. The bill specifically prohibits the sale of cigarettes to anyone born on or after 1 January 2009.

2. **Graphic Warning Labels:** Some smokers do not know all the dangers associated with smoking. Graphic, larger, and more thorough tobacco package warning messages are more effective at conveying smoking-related health risks and information. Smokers who were aware of the warnings were much more likely to support heart disease and lung cancer as health risks. Smokers who lived in nations where government-mandated warnings on labels were mandatory reported knowing more about health in every case where labeling policies varied between nations. The majority of teenagers are aware of the graphic warning labels on cigarette packs, which also enhance the messages' cognitive processing and may reduce the desire of teenagers to smoke. The use of graphic warning labels has significantly decreased among teenagers who smoke.
3. **Smoke-Free Public Places:** Smoking in indoor workplaces was first prohibited nationwide by the Republic of Ireland in 2003, with most other leading economies following suit with similar ordinances in subsequent years.

6.2. Prevention and Treatment of Tobacco Use: JACC Health Promotion Series

Because tobacco use carries substantial health risks, prevention and treatment of tobacco use remain vital public health priorities. Many approaches are described in the Journal of the American College of Cardiology (JACC) Health Promotion Series to deal with this widespread problem. First, prevention initiatives concentrate on decreasing tobacco initiation, particularly in young people and other vulnerable groups. Entire tobacco control laws, such as those about taxes, restrictions on advertising, and smoke-free settings, are essential in halting the initiation of tobacco use. Another crucial element of prevention efforts is the promotion of resources for quitting smoking and educational campaigns that highlight the negative health effects of smoking.

For those who are already using tobacco products, comprehensive programs for quitting are essential. These programs frequently combine pharmacotherapy—such as nicotine replacement therapy or prescription drugs like varenicline or bupropion—with behavioral interventions, like counselling and support groups. Success rates for cessation interventions are higher when they are customized to each person's needs and preferences. Reaching a wide audience requires integrating tobacco cessation interventions into a variety of healthcare settings, such as primary care, cardiology clinics, and mental health facilities. To identify tobacco users, offer brief interventions, and refer people to specialized cessation services when necessary, healthcare providers are essential. It is crucial to address the larger social determinants of tobacco use in addition to individual-level interventions. This entails tackling environmental factors like tobacco industry marketing strategies and smoking-related social norms, as well as socioeconomic factors like education and poverty.

To successfully implement tobacco prevention and treatment strategies, community organizations, healthcare professionals, legislators, and the general public must work together. Considerable progress can be made in lowering the burden of tobacco-related diseases and enhancing public health outcomes by implementing a multifaceted strategy that incorporates prevention, cessation, and addressing underlying social determinants.

Tobacco use is the leading preventable cause of death worldwide, accounting for over 6 million deaths annually. In the US, secondhand tobacco smoke exposure and cigarette smoking cause over 480,000 deaths annually, and smokers typically have a life expectancy that is at least 10 years lower than that of nonsmokers. > 150,000 U.S. About 20% of deaths in this age group from cardiovascular diseases (CVD) are attributable to smoking in adults 35 years of age and older. Clinicians who treat patients with cardiovascular disease (CVD) should prioritize managing tobacco use just as much as other cardiovascular risk factors, such as hypertension or hyperlipidemia, due to the significant risk associated with tobacco use.

Over a billion people use tobacco products worldwide, although the prevalence varies greatly by gender and location. According to estimates from the 2015 Global Burden of Disease Study, which covered 195 countries and territories, 54% of women and 25% of men smoked every day worldwide. While tobacco use was once more prevalent in high-income nations, an estimated 80% of smokers today reside in low- and middle-income countries, where the burden of tobacco use has now shifted. Within the U. S. Since the 1960s, when the health risks of tobacco use were first made public and various tobacco control initiatives were implemented by federal, state, and local governments, adult cigarette consumption has been declining (Figure 6.1). In the United States, combustible cigarettes are the most widely used tobacco product. S. grownups. In 2016, 15.5% of adults said they were current smokers, with 76% reporting daily smoking and 24% reporting less frequent smoking. Adults with co-occurring psychiatric and other substance use disorders, lower incomes, and lower levels of education are disproportionately more likely to smoke. With 8.0% of high school students and 2.2% of middle school students in 2016 reporting that they had smoked in the previous 30 days, the definition of current smoking among adolescents, and cigarette smoking rates among teenagers are at their lowest point in decades.

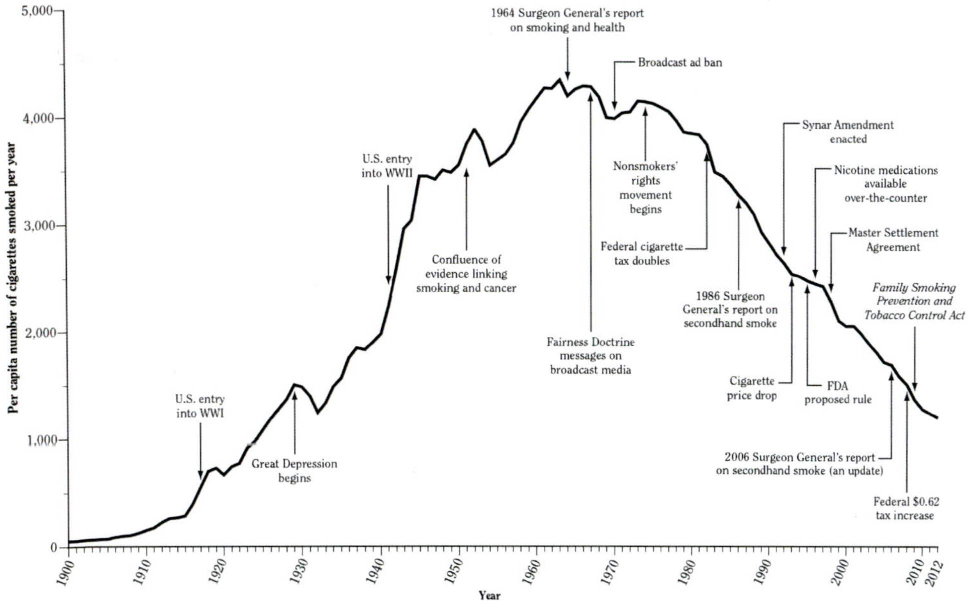

Figure 6.1. *Per capita cigarette consumption per year among U.S. adults from 1900 to 2012. Cigarette consumption has been declining since the 1960s, during which time tobacco control policies have been adopted at local and national levels. From: US Department of Health and Human Services.*

Source: https://www.ncbi.nlm.nih.gov/pmc/articles/PMC6261256/bin/nihms-1506688-f0002.jpg.

A growing number of people who smoke cigarettes also use other tobacco products. In the Population Assessment of Tobacco and Health survey conducted in 2013–2014, 40% of U.S. Adult and teenage tobacco users reported utilizing several different products. These consist of smokeless tobacco, pipes, waterpipes (also known as hookah or shisha), cigars, and cigarillos. But the most widely used non-cigarette tobacco product among adults and youth in the U.S. is the e-cigarette or electronic cigarette. This product is an aerosol that the user inhales after a liquid—typically containing nicotine—is heated by a battery-operated device. It is the first in a new line of substitute tobacco products designed to lessen the harmful effects of smoking by burning tobacco instead of producing smoke. In 2015, roughly 35% of U.S. Adults reported using e-cigarettes within the last 30 days, compared to 11.3% of high school students and 4.3% of middle school students.

6.2.1. Pathophysiological Effects of Tobacco Smoking on the Cardiovascular System

6.2.1.1. Epidemiologic Risks of Tobacco Use for Cardiovascular Disease

One of the main risk factors for a variety of cardiovascular diseases is cigarette smoking. Present smokers have a two- to three-fold increased risk of dying from ischemic heart disease compared to non-smokers, as well as significantly higher odds of myocardial infarction (MI) (OR 2.87, 95% CI 2.58–3.19). In addition, compared to never smokers, smokers with known coronary artery disease have a higher risk of sudden cardiac death (hazard ratio 2.47, 95% CI 1.46–4.19). For those who smoke now, the risk of dying from a stroke is about twice as high as for those who have never smoked.

Due to the non-linear nature of the relationship between smoking and CVD, the risk of cardiovascular disease is disproportionately increased by even a few cigarettes per day. A heightened risk of stroke is also linked to even one daily cigarette smoker. According to these findings, there is no such thing as a safe level of cigarette use, and total quitting should be the aim of treatment. Although smoking causes a temporary increase in blood pressure, epidemiological research has not consistently demonstrated a link between smoking and hypertension. Smoking has been linked to a higher risk of hypertension-related complications, including a higher chance of dying from hypertensive heart disease and a decline in renal function.

Compared to nonsmokers, current smokers have two to three times the risk of developing peripheral artery disease (PAD), and over five to six years, their arterial stiffness will worsen. According to one study, hospitalizations for acute MI and coronary heart disease (CHD) were more common among smokers with PAD than among nonsmokers over one year. Additionally, smokers are more likely to develop an abdominal aortic aneurysm (AAA). Higher odds of AAA have been linked to both the number of years spent smoking and the distinction between current and past smokers. A 2012 meta-analysis found that current smokers had a faster aneurysm growth rate than those who had smoked in the past or never smoked.

Compared to never smokers, the incidence of atrial fibrillation is roughly 1.5 and 2 times higher in former and current smokers, respectively. Smokers have a higher risk of developing ventricular arrhythmias. Compared to never-smokers, smokers have a higher risk of heart failure and worse outcomes. The Healthy Aging and Body Composition Study included adults aged 70–79. Those who currently smoked had a higher risk of heart failure than those who had never smoked. The Studies of Left Ventricular Dysfunction study discovered that current smokers had a higher relative risk of all-cause mortality and congestive heart failure (CHF)-related mortality than current non-smokers. The study included patients with a left ventricular ejection fraction below 35%. Additionally, compared to non-smokers, that study indicated that current smokers had a higher risk of MI and a higher risk of hospitalization for CHF.

After a cardiovascular event or revascularization, people who smoke still have worse outcomes, which emphasizes how important it is to offer tobacco use treatment in these situations. Smokers who continue to smoke after a MI are more likely to experience subsequent coronary events than those who give up (RR 1.51, 95% CI 1.10–2.07). Compared to quitting, smoking after a stroke or transient ischemic attack increases the risk of another stroke, MI, or death within five years. Negative consequences also result from continuing to smoke following a coronary artery disease intervention. Smokers who continued to smoke had a higher risk of all-cause mortality (RR 1.68, 95% CI 1.33–2.13) and cardiac death (1.75, 1.30–2.37) than those who stopped smoking among 985 coronary artery bypass graft surgery (CABG) patients followed for a median of 20 years. Additionally, smokers who persisted had a higher likelihood of needing a second procedure (e.g., angioplasty, or CABG). Persistent smoking was linked, compared to never smoking, to an increased risk of all-cause mortality (RR 1.76, 95% CI 1.37–2.26) and Q-wave MI (2.08, 1.16–3.72) among 5450 smokers followed for up to 16 years following successful percutaneous revascularization.

6.2.1.2. Secondhand Tobacco Smoke Exposure

Secondhand tobacco smoke exposure (TSE) by nonsmokers is associated with an increased risk of both CHD and stroke. In a meta-analysis, the relative risk for CHD among nonsmokers with TSE compared to nonsmokers without TSE was 1.31 (95% CI 1.21–1.41). In another meta-analysis, TSE by nonsmokers was associated with an increased risk of stroke (RR 1.25, 95% CI 1.12–1.38).

6.2.1.3. Smokeless Tobacco

Smokeless tobacco has the benefit of not exposing users to combustion byproducts, but it also exposes them to different concentrations of nicotine and metals and nitrosamines that are specific to tobacco that cause cancer. The majority of epidemiologic data regarding the risk of CVD from smokeless tobacco originates from Sweden, where a significant segment of the male population uses snus, a product that contains fewer nitrosamines and other contaminants than most other smokeless tobacco products. The majority of research has not revealed that users of smokeless tobacco have a higher risk of non-fatal CVD. On the other hand, a 2009 meta-analysis utilizing information from Sweden and the U.S. discovered that using smokeless tobacco increased the risk of fatal MI (RR 1.13, 95% confidence interval 1.06–1.21) and stroke (1.40, 1.28–1.54). Those who continue using snus after MI have a significantly higher two-year mortality rate than those who stop. Chewing tobacco use was linked to higher odds of acute MI compared to never using tobacco in the 52-country INTERHEART case-control study. Those who used both chewing tobacco and cigarettes had higher odds of acute MI than those who used either product alone.

6.2.2. Pathophysiologic Mechanisms of Increased Risk

More than seven thousand harmful substances, including many linked to cardiovascular disease and 69 recognized carcinogens, are found in cigarette smoke. Tobacco smoke's constituents affect hemodynamics negatively, endothelial dysfunction, thrombosis, inflammation, lipid abnormalities, and arrhythmogenesis, among other mechanisms that lead to CVD (Figure 6.2, Table 6.1). While nicotine is the main component of cigarette smoke that leads to addiction and produces the hemodynamic effects of smoking, other components of cigarette smoke are mostly responsible for the excess cardiovascular risk associated with smoking. Through the oxidation of low density lipoprotein (LDL), free radicals and reactive oxygen species from cigarette smoke induce endothelial dysfunction, platelet activation, and atherosclerosis. Particulate matter also affects the autonomic nervous system and induces oxidative stress, endothelial dysfunction, and platelet activation. It is possible to notice these effects even after being around secondhand smoke. Additional compounds found in cigarette smoke that could be linked to CVD include metals, carbon monoxide, carbonyls (like acrolein), and polycyclic aromatic hydrocarbons.

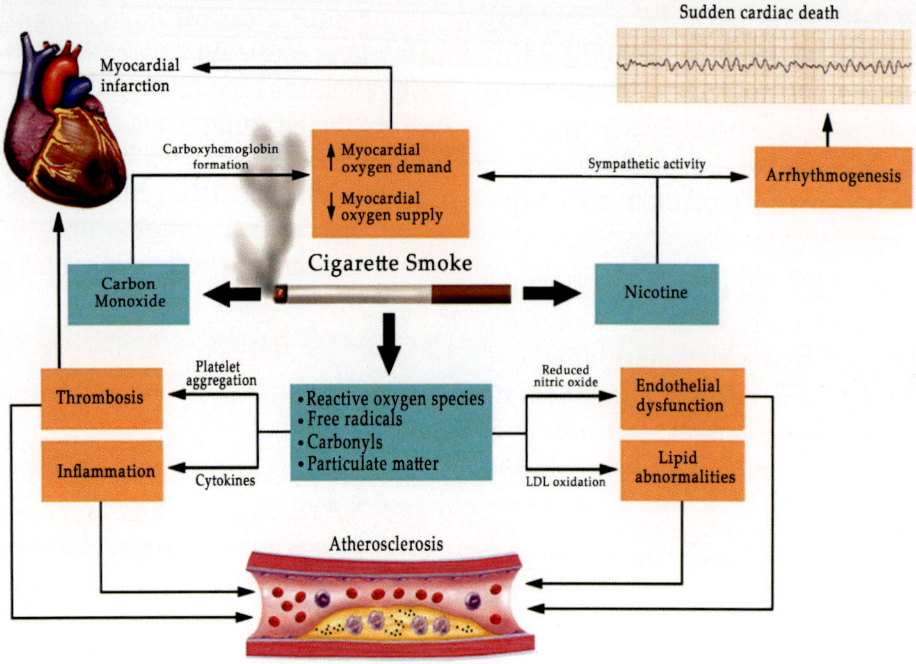

Figure 6.2. *Mechanisms by which smoking causes cardiovascular disease. The major components of cigarette smoke that contribute to cardiovascular disease include nicotine, carbon monoxide, reactive oxygen species, free radicals, carbonyls (such as acrolein), and particulate matter.*

Source: https://www.ncbi.nlm.nih.gov/pmc/articles/PMC6261256/bin/nihms-1506688-f0003.jpg.

Table 6.1. Mechanisms of Increased Cardiovascular Risk Associated with Cigarette Smoking

Cardiovascular Effect	Pathophysiological Mechanism
Hemodynamic changes • ↑ heart rate • ↑ contractility • ↑ blood pressure • ↑ Myocardial oxygen demand • ↓ myocardial oxygen supply • Altered coronary blood flow	• Nicotine activates the sympathetic nervous system • In general, nicotine ↑ coronary blood flow in response to increased myocardial work • Smoking leads to vasoconstriction in individuals with coronary artery disease • Reduced oxygen delivery by red blood cells containing carboxyhemoglobin (from carbon monoxide in cigarette smoke)

Endothelial dysfunction and damage	• Occurs as a consequence of oxidative injury and chronic inflammation • ↓ availability of nitric oxide, which normally acts as an endothelial cell vasodilator, reduces leukocyte adhesion, and prevents platelet aggregation
Hypercoagulability and thrombosis	• ↑ platelet activation • ↓ availability of nitric oxide • ↑ blood viscosity due to polycythemia from chronic carbon monoxide exposure and relative hypoxia • ↑ plasminogen activator inhibitor type 1 • ↓ tissue plasminogen activator (tPA) release from the coronary vasculature • ↑ expression of tissue factor in atherosclerotic plaques
Chronic inflammation	• Enhanced leukocyte adhesion to vascular endothelium • ↑ levels of inflammatory cytokines such as interleukin-6, interleukin-1b, and tumor necrosis factor-alpha • Smokers have higher levels of the inflammatory markers high-sensitivity C-reactive protein and fibrinogen
Lipid abnormalities	• ↓ high-density lipoprotein • ↑ low-density lipoprotein and triglycerides • ↑ levels of oxidized low-density lipoprotein
Arrhythmogenesis	• Nicotine may promote myocardial remodeling and fibrosis, likely related to beta-adrenergic stimulation • Nicotine-medicated catecholamine release may contribute to ventricular arrhythmia and sudden cardiac death
Other	• ↑risk of developing type 2 diabetes likely due to greater insulin resistance among smokers than nonsmokers, and believed to be mediated by the sympathomimetic effects of nicotine and nicotine-mediated activation of AMP-activated protein kinase • ↑ risk of coronary spasm

When combined, the effects of cigarette smoke create an environment that raises the risk of cardiovascular events by promoting the development of plaque and thrombosis, creating an imbalance between the supply and demand of blood in the heart, and raising the possibility of arrhythmogenesis. Furthermore, there seems to be an interaction between genetic factors that underlie CVD risk and cigarette smoking. For instance, compared to never smokers, the cardio-protective benefits of a variation in a gene locus close to the ADAMTS7 gene were lessened in smokers. Additional research on hereditary and environmental variables may help to clarify risk mechanisms and pinpoint those who are more vulnerable to smoking-related cardiovascular disease (CVD).

6.2.3. Factors Associated with Smoking Initiation and Cessation

6.2.3.1. Natural History of Tobacco Use

Because nearly all cigarette smokers report that they smoked their first cigarette during adolescence and have continued to use tobacco for decades after that, tobacco use can be described as a chronic disease that starts in childhood. Greater than 80% of U.S. adults who say they have ever tried cigarettes did so by the time they were 18 and 98% by the time they were 26. Furthermore, 96% of adults who have ever smoked cigarettes every day say they began doing so by the time they were 26 years old. Teenagers start out experimenting with smoking cigarettes once in a while, and some of them eventually become regular smokers over different periods. Quitting smoking is necessary to lower the risk of tobacco-related disease once it has become ingrained in one's behavior. The main responsibility of clinicians providing care for adults is to encourage cessation.

Periods of regular smoking, reduced smoking, and no smoking are characteristics of the dynamic process of quitting smoking. The majority of smokers try quitting multiple times before they are successful. Only 7% of adult smokers who participated in the 2015 National Health Interview Survey said they had successfully quit smoking, even though 68% of them said they wanted to stop and 55% had tried to quit in the previous year. Nonetheless, the majority of smokers keep trying to stop, and eventually, a large number of them are successful because 59% of all living adults in the U. S. who had ever smoked have stopped as of 2016. The majority of smokers (69%) do not use evidence-based treatments that are effective in helping them quit, which contributes to the low success rate.

6.2.3.2. Nicotine Dependence

Because it is a deeply ingrained learned behavior as well as a physical nicotine dependence, tobacco use is tenacious. When nicotine binds to nicotinic acetylcholine receptors in the brain, rewarding and reinforcing neurotransmitters are released.

Tolerance, physical dependence, and the upregulation of nicotine receptors are the results of repeated use. Adolescents who have smoked a few cigarettes for a brief period may experience the onset of symptoms of nicotine dependence quickly, even before they make the switch from occasional experimenting to regular daily smoking. There appears to be a reciprocal relationship between nicotine dependence and cigarette consumption as symptoms of nicotine dependence are linked to increases in cigarette consumption in the future. When a smoker quits, they may experience cravings, irritability, anxiety, restlessness, dysphoria, difficulty concentrating, and hunger as withdrawal symptoms from nicotine. Smokers experience different withdrawal symptoms and times; some people experience symptoms that go away in two weeks, while others continue to have cravings even after quitting for six months.

Smoking is a learned behavior that arises from its correlation with particular triggers that elicit a desire to smoke and lead to recurrent usage. Triggers can include seeing other smokers, drinking coffee or alcohol, smoking in social or private settings, and even just looking at things like cigarette packs or ads. Many smokers claim that stress or other unpleasant emotional states are the reason they smoke, and these smokers find it especially difficult to stop. This behavior is probably caused by the benefits of nicotine as well as the fact that smoking helps addicted smokers overcome the dysphoria and cognitive decline brought on by nicotine withdrawal.

6.2.3.3. Smoking Initiation

Various factors play a role in starting and continuing to use tobacco. The socio-ecological model breaks down these factors into different levels of influence: individual, interpersonal, community/organizational, and societal/policy levels, arranged in order of increasing impact (see Central Illustration).

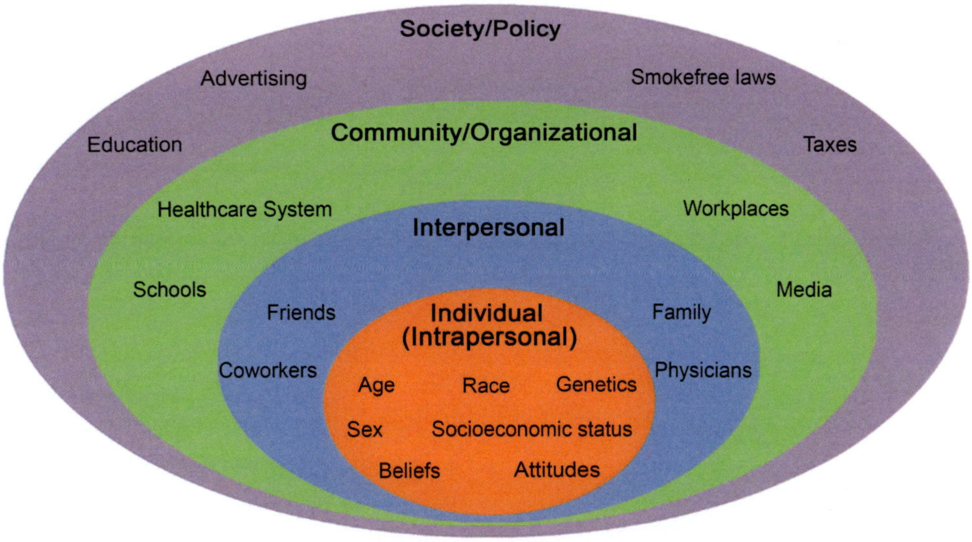

Central Illustration. Socio-ecological model of factors associated with smoking initiation and continued smoking. Various individual, interpersonal, community/organizations, and societal/policy factors play a role in why individuals start smoking and continue to smoke. Interventions targeting each of these factors can help to reduce smoking prevalence.

Source: https://www.ncbi.nlm.nih.gov/pmc/articles/PMC6261256/bin/nihms-1506688-f0001.jpg.

Individually, non-Hispanic white adolescents are more likely to smoke than black or Hispanic adolescents, as well as adolescents from lower socioeconomic backgrounds as indicated by their educational aspirations or parental educational attainment. Teenagers and young adults who start smoking do so for psychological reasons, such as increased risk-taking and impulsivity, stress, depressive symptoms, and anxiety. Both the beginning of smoking and the development of nicotine dependence are influenced by genetic factors, with the latter appearing to be more significant.

Peer pressure has the biggest impact on youth smoking at the interpersonal level. Teens who do not smoke but have friends who do are more likely to start smoking, and adolescents who smoke frequently hang out with other smokers. Adolescents' subsequent smoking has also been linked to their perception of their peers' smoking prevalence. Eighth-graders were the subjects of a study that revealed that nonsmokers who believed that a larger proportion of eighth-graders at their school were smokers were more likely to start smoking after a year. There is conflicting evidence regarding the impact of families on teenage smoking: although some studies have found that parental smoking predicts teenage smoking, other studies have not found this relationship. The initiation of smoking is also influenced by broader community and policy factors. A substantial amount of research indicates that tobacco product marketing and price have a significant impact on the decision to start smoking. Reduced prevalence of cigarette smoking has been directly linked to higher prices. This covers the impact of cigarettes on adult use as well as youth and young adult use. By increasing the tobacco excise tax rate, the federal, state, or local governments can raise the cost of cigarettes. One of the most effective legislative instruments for discouraging the start of smoking is this one.

Teenage smoking initiation and persistence are closely linked to tobacco marketing, which encompasses both commercials and promotional activities like sponsoring events that appeal to teenagers. Teens who are exposed to media portrayals of tobacco and tobacco advertisements have more positive attitudes toward tobacco use and are more likely to start smoking. Adolescents who were not predisposed to smoking were found to be more likely to start smoking cigarettes if they had tobacco promotional items or indicated they would use them.

Reduced rates of youth and young adult smoking are also linked to smoke-free laws and policies. Adolescents and young adults who live in an area where workplace smoke laws are completely smoke-free are less likely to start smoking (OR 0.66, 95% confidence interval [CI] 0.44–0.99). Additionally, there is a lower likelihood of current smoking among adolescents and young adults residing in areas with 100% smoke-free bars (OR 0.80, 95% CI 0.71–0.90). Adoption of voluntary smoke-free policies in homes and cars has also been linked to lower rates of adolescent smoking, and this is linked to smoke-free laws. Illegal sales can be decreased by limiting the supply of cigarettes, for example by upholding laws that forbid selling tobacco to minors. However, the fact that young people report obtaining cigarettes from a variety of sources other than just buying tobacco products may lessen the impact of such interventions on policies regarding smoking behavior. To decrease teen tobacco use, increasing the legal age of tobacco purchase from 18 to 21 has recently gained support. The National Academy of Science supported current advocacy efforts to raise the legal smoking age from 18 to 21 years old, concluding that "increasing the minimum age of legal access to tobacco products will likely prevent or delay initiation of tobacco use by adolescents and young adults."

6.2.3.4. Smoking Cessation

To quit smoking, a person must overcome their dependence on nicotine and give up a deeply rewarding behavior. The socio-ecological model can be used to conceptualize obstacles to quitting (Central Illustration). Nicotine dependence is a major contributing factor to smoking cessation difficulties at the intra-individual level. Some smokers—those with low socioeconomic status, mental illness, and other substance use disorders, for example—are more dependent than others. Whether receiving treatment or not, these people frequently experience less success when trying to stop smoking.

The spouse's and other household members' smoking status has an impact on interpersonal relationships. It has been shown that living with other smokers reduces the likelihood of quitting, but forbidding smoking inside the home increases the likelihood of quitting. According to one study, if a spouse or friend gave up smoking, a smoker's likelihood of starting again decreased by 67%

and 36%, respectively. According to a different study, smokers who had fewer smoking friends were more likely to give up than those who had no changes in their smoking circle. A smoker's perception of strong social support from friends and family to stop smoking is also linked to a higher likelihood of successfully quitting.

Interventions at the community and policy levels can also encourage quitting smoking. Compared to smokers without smoke-free workplaces, those with smoke-free policies have a higher chance of cutting back on their cigarette consumption and quitting. Prices for cigarettes have an inverse relationship with smoking behavior, so raising tobacco excise taxes can lower the percentage of adults who smoke. Adult cessation can be effectively encouraged by comprehensive tobacco control programs that include mass media campaigns educating smokers about resources for quitting.

6.2.4. The Role of Preventive Action

6.2.4.1. Health Benefits of Smoking Cessation

Adult smokers who stop smoking have a lower risk of dying from smoking overall, and there are health benefits even for those who stop smoking after turning 65 or after developing a tobacco-related illness. Smokers who give up by the age of forty have the largest mortality benefit, as they lower their risk of dying from smoking-related disease by 90%. However, smokers who are older than seventy-five can also benefit from the mortality benefit. Quitting smoking has benefits for mortality as well as lowering the risk of tobacco-related diseases like cancer, lung disease, and heart disease. Thus, quitting should be their top priority for smokers of all ages.

Quitting smoking has immediate health benefits, such as lowering heart rate and carbon monoxide levels in the blood. Platelet activation decreases within days, reducing the risk of tobacco-related diseases at different rates. The risk of coronary heart disease significantly decreases within one year of quitting and reaches the same level as nonsmokers within 15 years. The risk of stroke is nearly eliminated within 5 to 15 years of cessation. However, the reduction in excess lung cancer risk occurs more slowly and may still be elevated in long-time former smokers compared to those who never smoked.

Treating tobacco use is a priority for secondary CVD prevention because quitting smoking rapidly lowers the risk of CVD, even in smokers with pre-existing conditions. One systematic review found that among smokers with CHD, stopping was linked to a 36% lower cardiovascular death rate over two years when compared to continuing to smoke. After a MI, quitting smoking reduces subsequent mortality by 15 to 61%, improves the quality of life for health-related reasons, and reduces angina. For smokers with additional tobacco-related illnesses, quitting smoking also has positive health effects. Quitting smoking for smokers with COPD lowers all-cause mortality, symptoms, and the likelihood of an exacerbation. It also slows the rate at which lung function declines. Quitting smoking can lower the risk of mortality, recurrence, and the development of a second primary cancer in smokers with lung cancer.

Reducing cigarette consumption without eventually giving up seems to have comparatively little health benefit, in contrast to the benefits of quitting. There is no correlation between reduced smoking and lower overall or tobacco-related disease mortality. A higher risk of CHD and stroke is linked to even one daily cigarette smoker. Therefore, giving up cigarettes should be the smokers' main objective if they want to improve their health.

6.2.4.2. Health Benefits of Reducing Second-Hand Tobacco Smoke Exposure

Governments and private-sector organizations have enacted several laws and policies banning smoking in public areas, workplaces, restaurants, bars, and other locations to protect nonsmokers from the health risks of secondhand tobacco smoke exposure. Comprehensive smoke-free regulations offer quantifiable health advantages. Reductions in hospitalizations or deaths from acute myocardial infarction (RR 0.85, 95% CI 0.82–0.88), other heart disease (0.61, 0.44–0.85), cerebrovascular accidents (0.84, 0.75–0.94), and respiratory disease (0.76, 0.68–0.85) were linked to comprehensive smoke-free laws in a 2012 meta-analysis. More comprehensive policies were also associated with greater risk reduction. In addition, a 2014 meta-analysis discovered that while there was no discernible difference in low birthweight, smoke-free laws were linked to fewer premature births and asthma-related hospital visits.

6.2.4.3. Evidence-Based Tobacco Control Policies

A strong body of evidence demonstrates the efficacy of public policies to reduce tobacco use. The majority of tobacco control laws work by lowering the market for tobacco goods. These include raising tobacco excise taxes to increase the cost of cigarettes, enacting smoke-free indoor policies, requiring health warning labels on tobacco packages, and endorsing public education and cessation campaigns through mass media. By increasing the legal age of tobacco purchase and strictly enforcing these laws, additional measures seek to decrease the availability of tobacco to teenagers.

The Framework Convention on Tobacco Control (FCTC), essentially a public health treaty, is a formal policy document that the World Health Organization created by compiling evidence-based tobacco control measures. The 181 nations that have ratified the FCTC have committed to implementing its set of tobacco control laws, which went into effect in 2005. To assist nations in putting these policies into practice, the acronym MPOWER was created (Table 6.2). Adoption of smoke-free laws and advertising bans has increased since the FCTC was put into effect. The prevalence of smoking has decreased in the nations that put the highest level of demand reduction measures into practice. However, a few nations have not yet put any of these policies into effect, and the U. S. The FCTC has not been ratified. Enhancing the uptake and efficient execution of tobacco control policies is a critical global public health priority. Cardiologists can act as tobacco control advocates to help reduce smoking initiation among youth and young adults and to encourage smoking cessation among adults at risk for or already affected by cardiovascular disease (CVD). This is because quitting smoking is crucial for cardiovascular health.

Table 6.2. *WHO MPOWER Measures*

Measure		Examples of Tobacco Control Actions
M	Monitor tobacco use and prevention policies	Conduct surveys to monitor tobacco use by adults and adolescents
P	Protect people from tobacco smoke	Enact smoke-free laws and policies in public places, workplaces, restaurants, bars
O	Offer help to quit tobacco use	Ensure that healthcare providers assess tobacco use, advise tobacco cessation, and offer behavioral and pharmacological assistance to quit.
W	Warn about the dangers of tobacco	Conduct mass media campaigns to educate children and adults about the health risks and addictiveness of tobacco, and promote the use of cessation resources. Require warning labels on tobacco packages.
E	Enforce bans on tobacco advertising, promotion, and sponsorship	Restrict tobacco industry sponsorship of events, and distribution of free samples.
R	Raise taxes on tobacco	Increase the tobacco excise tax rate to raise the price of tobacco products.
WHO, World Health Organization		

6.2.4.4. Harm Reduction

The best way for a current smoker to lower the risks associated with tobacco use is to achieve complete abstinence, especially from combustible tobacco products. However, not all tobacco users are willing or able to do so with current treatments.

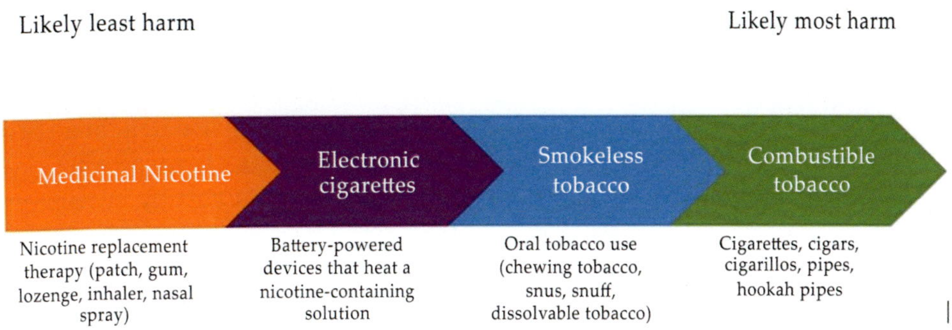

Figure 6.3. *Risk continuum of nicotine-containing products. Nicotine comes in many forms with varying degrees of potential harm to users. Medicinal nicotine, such as that contained in nicotine replacement therapy, is least likely to cause harm, while combustible tobacco, such as cigarettes, is most likely to cause harm. It is not known where heat-not-burn tobacco (also known as heated tobacco) products fall on this spectrum given the limited evidence on their health effects.*

Source: https://www.ncbi.nlm.nih.gov/pmc/articles/PMC6261256/bin/nihms-1506688-f0004.jpg.

Harm reduction is an alternative strategy for these people. This approach acknowledges that although nicotine keeps people smoking, other ingredients in tobacco smoke are primarily responsible for the health hazards associated with tobacco use. Products containing nicotine therefore fall on a risk continuum ranging from less hazardous to more hazardous (Figure 6.3). Shifting the population from higher-risk to lower-risk nicotine products could reduce harm. The U.S. This tactic was implemented by the Food and Drug Administration (FDA) in 2017 when it unveiled a plan to regulate tobacco and nicotine products to lower the use of combustible cigarettes and the related morbidity and mortality.

The FDA is considering mandating a decrease in cigarettes' nicotine levels to under 0.4 mg per gram of tobacco to make them minimally addictive. Smoking cigarettes with very low nicotine content has been shown to reduce smokers' nicotine intake, dependence, and daily cigarette consumption. There is concern that smokers may smoke more cigarettes to compensate for the lower nicotine levels, increasing their exposure to harmful toxins in cigarette smoke. However, studies have not found much evidence of compensation. Providing lower-risk nicotine products like nicotine replacement therapy or e-cigarettes to smokers of low-nicotine cigarettes will be crucial for the strategy to succeed. A simulation model predicts a significant decrease in tobacco-related deaths if cigarettes are made minimally addictive, despite uncertainty about the impact on smoking habits.

Determining the best regulatory strategy for substitute nicotine sources, like e-cigarettes, is a crucial part of the reduced nicotine approach. E-cigarettes should be safer for users than cigarette smoke because they don't burn tobacco. A 2018 study by the U.S. National Academies of Sciences, Engineering, and Medicine came to the conclusion that, while the long-term health effects of e-cigarettes are still unknown, using an aerosol from an e-cigarette exposes users to fewer toxicants than traditional cigarette smoke and is therefore probably less harmful than smoking cigarettes. According to the report, there is currently insufficient data to determine whether using e-cigarettes increases the risk of cardiovascular events or subclinical atherosclerosis. Policies that restrict access to e-cigarettes for young adults and nonsmokers must be weighed against those that promote access to them for smokers attempting to lessen the harm that comes with smoking cigarettes. Furthermore, as information about the long-term health effects of goods like e-cigarettes grows, these policies will need to be reviewed regularly.

6.2.5. Guidance for Healthcare Providers

6.2.5.1. Screening and Brief Clinical Interventions

Recent national surveys have shown that while many current smokers express a desire to quit smoking, their utilization of proven cessation methods and success rates with quit attempts are still relatively low. During outpatient visits, only 63% of patients are screened for tobacco use, and just 25% of identified smokers receive treatment in the form of medication or counselling. Healthcare providers who treat patients with cardiovascular disease can help bridge this gap by consistently screening for tobacco use, offering advice to quit, and supporting smokers in accessing evidence-based cessation treatments. Even brief interventions from clinicians have been shown to significantly increase the likelihood of successful smoking cessation. A Cochrane meta-analysis in 2015 revealed that psychosocial interventions for smokers with coronary heart disease led to a 22% increase in smoking abstinence after 6–12 months. Additionally, healthcare providers can protect nonsmokers from the dangers of secondhand smoke exposure on cardiovascular health by routinely screening for tobacco use and recommending the adoption of smoke-free home and car policies. Acute MI, acute coronary syndrome, a new diagnosis of CVD, or a cardiovascular procedure can all be considered "teachable moments" that can encourage a smoker to try quitting. A Cochrane meta-analysis of smokers admitted to hospitals for cardiovascular disease discovered that offering a smoking cessation intervention during hospitalization and continuing it after discharge improved the rate of smoking cessation (RR 1.42, 95% CI 1.29–1.56). However, a recent study found that just 7% of smokers with acute MI used smoking cessation drugs in the first post-discharge period.

6.2.5.2. Tobacco Cessation Treatment

Behavioral support and medication are two evidence-based smoking cessation treatments. The best strategy is to combine medication and counselling because it allows for the management of nicotine dependence as well as ingrained smoking behavior. The U.S. The 5As model from the Public Health Service offers a structure for short-term office-based tobacco treatment. Its actions include finding out about tobacco use, encouraging smokers to give up, determining when a person is ready to give up, helping people with their quit attempts by giving them medication or putting them in touch with counselling services, and setting up follow-up to track any progress or obstacles. For busy clinicians, an abridged 3-step model that acknowledges that care is increasingly provided by a healthcare team is beneficial. It consists of asking about tobacco use, supporting tobacco users in their attempts to quit, and referring them to the right resources to help them reach their cessation objectives (Figure 6.4).

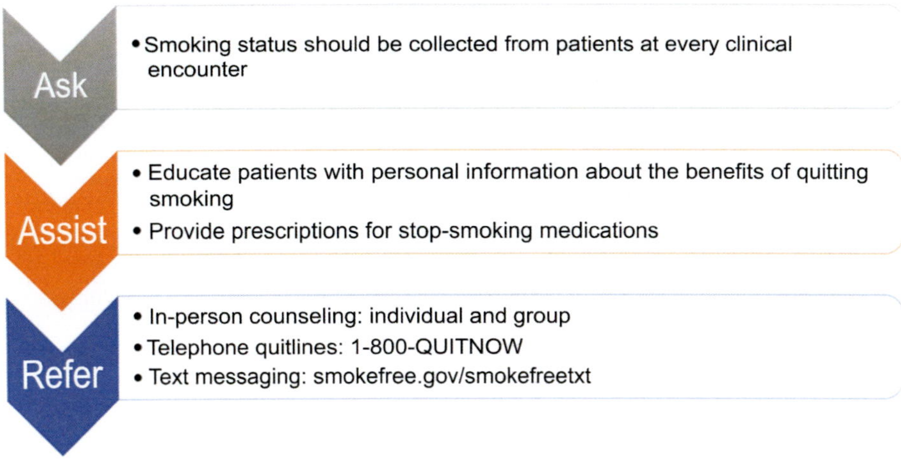

Figure 6.4. *The Ask, Assist, Refer tobacco cessation intervention. Providers can use this tool to screen for tobacco use among all patients, and refer them to appropriate resources to help with smoking cessation.*

Source: https://www.ncbi.nlm.nih.gov/pmc/articles/PMC6261256/bin/nihms-1506688-f0005.jpg.

Counselling for quitting smoking can take place in-person, over the phone, on a mobile device, or online. Individual or group settings are possible in in-person counselling. All U.S. states have phone quit lines available. S. States offer smoking individuals free services (1–800-QUIT-NOW). The success rate of smoking cessation is increased by proactive counselling, wherein counselors reach out to smokers over several sessions. Interventions using mobile phones have also proven successful in aiding smokers in quitting. Within the U. S, the Smoke freeTXT program is available from the National Cancer Institute at Smokefree, gov/smokefreetxt. On the other hand, there hasn't been any consistent evidence of acupuncture or hypnotherapy helping people stop smoking.

The drugs authorized by the U.S. NRT (five different products), varenicline, and bupropion are recommended by the FDA as smoking cessation aids (Table 6.3). Preferences and side effect profiles of the patient should be taken into consideration when choosing drugs, and drug combinations. By giving users nicotine in either a long-acting (patch) or short-acting (gum, lozenge, inhaler, nasal spray) form, NRT helps to prevent the symptoms of nicotine withdrawal. Throughout the day, transdermal nicotine is delivered by the nicotine patch, whereas short-acting nicotine replacement therapy acts faster but lasts shorter. When NRT is used in any form, smoking cessation increases by 60% when compared to a placebo (RR 1.60, 95% CI 1.53–1.68). It has been demonstrated that combining the nicotine patch with short-acting NRT increases its effectiveness compared to using just one type of NRT (RR 1.34, 95% CI 1.18–1.51).

Table 6.3. *Medications Approved by the U.S. Food and Drug Administration for Smoking Cessation*

Medication	**Dosing**	**Common Side Effects**	**Available Over the Counter?**
Nicotine patch	>10 cigarettes/day: 21mg to start, taper after 6 weeks ≤10 cigarettes/day: 14mg to start, taper after 6 weeks	Redness/irritation at patch site, sleep disturbance	Yes
Nicotine gum	Smokes first cigarette ≤30 minutes of waking: 4mg every 1–2 hours Smokes first cigarette >30 minutes of waking: 2mg every 1–2 hours	Oral issues, nausea, heartburn, hiccups	Yes
Nicotine lozenge	Smokes first cigarette ≤30 minutes of waking: 4mg every 1–2 hours Smokes first cigarette >30 minutes of waking: 2mg every 1–2 hours	Oral issues, nausea, heartburn, hiccups	Yes

Medication	Dosing	Common Side Effects	Available Over the Counter?
Nicotine inhaler	10mg cartridges 6–16 times per day	Oropharyngeal irritation, cough	No
Nicotine nasal spray	1–2 sprays per nostril per hour	Nasopharyngeal irritation, sneezing, coughing	No
Varenicline	0.5mg daily for 3 days, then 0.5mg twice daily for 4 days, then 1mg twice daily	Nausea, abnormal dreams	No
Bupropion	150mg daily for 3 days, then 150mg twice daily	Insomnia, dry mouth	No

Studies have looked into the safety of using NRT in patients with CVD because of the sympathomimetic effects of nicotine. NRT was linked to an increase in cardiovascular events relative to placebo in a network meta-analysis that included people with and without heart disease, but not major cardiovascular events. The use of nicotine patches as opposed to placebos did not significantly increase the risk of cardiovascular events, such as myocardial infarction, cardiac arrest, or hospital admission due to worsening angina, arrhythmia, or heart failure, according to a study that focused on outpatient smokers with CVD.

When compared to a placebo, the partial nicotinic receptor against varenicline more than doubles the rate of smoking cessation (RR 2.24, 95% CI 2.06–2.43). In the EAGLES trial, more than 8,000 smokers in 16 countries were randomized in a 1:1:1:1 ratio to receive varenicline, bupropion, nicotine patch, or placebo. The varenicline group had a significantly higher 6-month abstinence rate than the other groups. Treatment with varenicline increased the odds of continuous abstinence at one year over placebo in a randomized trial of smokers with stable cardiovascular disease (CVD) (OR 3.14, 95% 1.94–5.11). In a randomized study of smokers with acute coronary syndrome, those taking varenicline compared to those not taken showed higher rates of point-prevalence abstinence at 52 weeks and continuous abstinence at 24 weeks placebo.

Due to the nicotine-like effects of varenicline, questions have been raised regarding the drug's possible cardiovascular risk. The majority of the data does not point to an increased risk of CVD in smokers, whether or not they have the disease. When compared to bupropion, nicotine patches, or placebos, the CATS trial—which looked at cardiovascular events in over 8,000 smokers from the EAGLES trial—found no evidence of an increase in cardiovascular events. The trial's participants were middle-aged smokers, many of whom also had other risk factors for CVD. However, the trial was not restricted to smokers with CVD. Subsequent larger meta-analyzes and several large retrospective cohort studies found no evidence of a significantly increased CVD risk with varenicline use, despite one meta-analysis of earlier randomized trials reporting an increased risk of CVD events among smokers using the medication. There has been a recent observational study that used Canadian prescription and health outcome databases and found that smokers taking varenicline experienced more cardiovascular events than those who used a self-controlled time interval. However, the study design has limitations.

Similar to varenicline, the plant alkaloid cytisine is a partial agonist of the nicotinic receptor. For several decades, cytisine has been used in Eastern Europe as a smoking cessation aid due to its proven effectiveness in numerous clinical trials. The U.S. is working to develop cytisine as a smoking cessation aid. S. are in motion. Bupropion is licensed for use as an antidepressant and as a smoking cessation aid.

It raises dopamine and norepinephrine levels. Compared to a placebo or control group, bupropion increases the rate of smoking cessation. In two studies, smokers hospitalized for acute coronary events who received bupropion versus placebo did not show higher rates of smoking cessation. Treatment with bupropion does not seem to increase the risk of serious adverse cardiovascular events. Having a high risk of seizures or having a seizure disorder are contraindications to using bupropion.(Ambrose et al., 2004; Antonelli et al., 2016).

A Closer Look

Smokeless Tobacco

Smokeless tobacco, often overlooked in discussions of tobacco control, presents its own set of health risks and challenges. Unlike smoked tobacco products such as cigarettes, smokeless tobacco is used by placing the tobacco product inside the mouth, where it is chewed, sucked, or sniffed. Common forms of smokeless tobacco include chewing tobacco, snuff, and dissolvable tobacco products.

Despite perceptions of smokeless tobacco as a safer alternative to smoking, it poses significant health hazards. Smokeless tobacco contains numerous toxic chemicals, including nicotine, carcinogens, and other harmful substances that can lead to various health problems, including oral cancer, gum disease, and nicotine addiction. Additionally, smokeless tobacco use has been associated with an increased risk of cardiovascular diseases such as heart attacks and strokes.

Smokeless tobacco use is particularly prevalent in certain populations, including athletes, rural communities, and certain cultural groups. Marketing tactics by tobacco companies often target these populations, perpetuating misconceptions about the safety of smokeless tobacco products. Efforts to address smokeless tobacco use require comprehensive strategies that incorporate public education, regulatory policies, and targeted interventions. Increasing awareness of the health risks associated with smokeless tobacco, implementing regulations on advertising and promotion, and providing cessation support for smokeless tobacco users are essential components of tobacco control efforts aimed at reducing the prevalence of smokeless tobacco use and its associated health consequences.

Summary

- Tobacco control and prevention efforts are integral components of public health initiatives worldwide, aimed at reducing the prevalence of tobacco use and its associated health consequences.
- Tobacco control is a field of international public health science, policy, and practice dedicated to addressing tobacco use and thereby reducing the morbidity and mortality it causes.
- The origins of modern tobacco control can be traced back to the mid-20th century when scientific research began to uncover the severe health risks associated with tobacco use.
- Tobacco policies that limit the sale of cigarettes to minors and restrict smoking in public places are important strategies to deter youth from accessing and consuming cigarettes.
- The prevention and treatment of tobacco use remain critical public health priorities due to the significant health risks associated with tobacco consumption.
- Tobacco use is tenacious because it is both a physical dependence on nicotine and a deeply ingrained learned behavior. Nicotine binds to nicotinic acetylcholine receptors in the brain, leading to the release of neurotransmitters with rewarding and reinforcing effects.
- A substantial evidence base supports the effectiveness of public policies to reduce tobacco use. Most tobacco control policies act by reducing the demand for tobacco products.
- Evidence-based smoking cessation treatments include medications and behavioral support. The combination of medication and counselling is the most effective approach because it allows the management of both nicotine dependence and the conditioned behavior of smoking.

References

1. Ambrose, J. A., & Barua, R. S. (2004). The pathophysiology of cigarette smoking and cardiovascular disease: An update. *Journal of the American College of Cardiology, 43*(10), 1731–1737. https://doi.org/10.1016/j.jacc.2003.12.048.
2. Anthenelli, R. M., Benowitz, N. L., West, R., et al. (2016). Neuropsychiatric safety and efficacy of varenicline, bupropion, and nicotine patch in smokers with and without psychiatric disorders (EAGLES): A double-blind, randomized, placebo-controlled clinical trial. *Lancet, 387*(10037), 2507–2520. https://doi.org/10.1016/S0140-6736(16)30272-0.
3. Anthonisen, N. R., Skeans, M. A., Wise, R. A., Manfreda, J., Kanner, R. E., & Connett, J. E. (2005). The effects of a smoking cessation intervention on 14.5-year mortality: A randomized clinical trial. *Annals of Internal Medicine, 142*(4), 233–239. https://doi.org/10.7326/0003-4819-142-4-200502150-00004.
4. Apelberg, B. J., Feirman, S. P., Salazar, E., et al. (2018). Potential public health effects of reducing nicotine levels in cigarettes in the United States. *New England Journal of Medicine, 378*(17), 1725–1733. https://doi.org/10.1056/NEJMsa1716561.
5. Arefalk, G., Hambraeus, K., Lind, L., Michaelsson, K., Lindahl, B., & Sundström, J. (2014).

Discontinuation of smokeless tobacco and mortality risk after myocardial infarction. *Circulation, 130*(4), 325–332. https://doi.org/10.1161/CIRCULATIONAHA.114.009579.

6. Au, D. H., Bryson, C. L., Chien, J. W., et al. (2009). The effects of smoking cessation on the risk of chronic obstructive pulmonary disease exacerbations. *Journal of General Internal Medicine, 24*(5), 457–463. https://doi.org/10.1007/s11606-009-0940-0.
7. Babb, S., Malarcher, A., Schauer, G., Asman, K., & Jamal, A. (2017). Quitting smoking among adults—United States, 2000–2015. *MMWR Morbidity and Mortality Weekly Report, 65*(52), 1457–1464. https://doi.org/10.15585/mmwr.mm6552a1.
8. Bala, M. M., Strzeszynski, L., & Topor-Madry, R. (2017). Mass media interventions for smoking cessation in adults. *Cochrane Database of Systematic Reviews, 2017*(11), CD004704. https://doi.org/10.1002/14651858.CD004704.pub4.
9. Barbieri, S. S., Zacchi, E., Amadio, P., et al. (2011). Cytokines present in smokers' serum interact with smoke components to enhance endothelial dysfunction. *Cardiovascular Research, 90*(3), 475–483. https://doi.org/10.1093/cvr/cvr103.
10. Barnes, J., Dong, C. Y., McRobbie, H., Walker, N., Mehta, M., & Stead, L. F. (2010). Hypnotherapy for smoking cessation. *Cochrane Database of Systematic Reviews, 2010*(1), CD001008. https://doi.org/10.1002/14651858.CD001008.pub2.
11. Barnoya, J., & Glantz, S. A. (2005). Cardiovascular effects of secondhand smoke: Nearly as large as smoking. *Circulation, 111*(20), 2684–2698. https://doi.org/10.1161/CIRCULATIONAHA.104.510300.
12. Barth, J., Jacob, T., Daha, I., & Critchley, J. A. (2015). Psychosocial interventions for smoking cessation in patients with coronary heart disease. *Cochrane Database of Systematic Reviews, 2015*(4), CD006886. https://doi.org/10.1002/14651858.CD006886.pub3.
13. Bauer, J. E., Hyland, A., Li, Q., Steger, C., & Cummings, K. M. (2005). A longitudinal assessment of the impact of smoke-free worksite policies on tobacco use. *American Journal of Public Health, 95*(6), 1024–1029. https://doi.org/10.2105/AJPH.2004.051931.
14. Been, J. V., Nurmatov, U. B., Cox, B., Nawrot, T. S., van Schayck, C. P., & Sheikh, A. (2014). Effect of smoke-free legislation on perinatal and child health: A systematic review and meta-analysis. *Lancet, 383*(9928), 1549–1560. https://doi.org/10.1016/S0140-6736(13)62297-4.
15. Begh, R., Lindson-Hawley, N., & Aveyard, P. (2015). Does reduced smoking if you can't stop make any difference? *BMC Medicine, 13*, 257. https://doi.org/10.1186/s12916-015-0476-0.
16. Benowitz, N. L. (2003). Cigarette smoking and cardiovascular disease: Pathophysiology and implications for treatment. *Progress in Cardiovascular Diseases, 46*(1), 91–111. https://doi.org/10.1016/S0033-0620(03)00007-1.
17. Benowitz, N. L., Donny, E. C., & Hatsukami, D. K. (2017). Reduced nicotine content cigarettes, e-cigarettes, and the cigarette end game. *Addiction, 112*(6), 6–7. https://doi.org/10.1111/add.13770.
18. Benowitz, N. L., Pipe, A., West, R., et al. (2018). Cardiovascular safety of varenicline, bupropion, and nicotine patch in smokers: A randomized clinical trial. *JAMA Internal Medicine, 178*(5), 622–631. https://doi.org/10.1001/jamainternmed.2018.0048.

19. Boffetta, P., & Straif, K. (2009). Use of smokeless tobacco and risk of myocardial infarction and stroke: Systematic review with meta-analysis. *BMJ, 339*, b3060. https://doi.org/10.1136/bmj.b3060.

20. Botello-Harbaum, M. T., Haynie, D. L., Iannotti, R. J., Wang, J., Gase, L., & Simons-Morton, B. (2009). Tobacco control policy and adolescent cigarette smoking status in the United States. *Nicotine & Tobacco Research, 11*(7), 875–885. https://doi.org/10.1093/ntr/ntp085.

21. Brook, R. D., Rajagopalan, S., Pope, C. A., 3rd, et al. (2010). Particulate matter air pollution and cardiovascular disease: An update to the scientific statement from the American Heart Association. *Circulation, 121*(21), 2331–2378. https://doi.org/10.1161/CIR.0b013e3181dbece1.

22. Buchanan, D. M., Arnold, S. V., Gosch, K. L., et al. (2015). Association of smoking status with angina and health-related quality of life after acute myocardial infarction. *Circulation: Cardiovascular Quality and Outcomes, 8*(5), 493–500. https://doi.org/10.1161/CIRCOUTCOMES.114.001730.

23. Cahill, K., Lindson-Hawley, N., Thomas, K. H., Fanshawe, T. R., & Lancaster, T. (2016). Nicotine receptor partial agonists for smoking cessation. *Cochrane Database of Systematic Reviews, 2016*(5), CD006103. https://doi.org/10.1002/14651858.CD006103.pub7.

24. Cahill, K., Stead, L. F., & Lancaster, T. (2012). Nicotine receptor partial agonists for smoking cessation. *Cochrane Database of Systematic Reviews, 2012*(4), CD006103. https://doi.org/10.1002/14651858.CD006103.pub5.

25. Carter, B. D., Abnet, C. C., Feskanich, D., et al. (2015). Smoking and mortality—Beyond established causes. *New England Journal of Medicine, 372*(7), 631–640. https://doi.org/10.1056/NEJMsa1407211.

26. Chaiton, M. O., Cohen, J. E., O'Loughlin, J., & Rehm, J. (2009). A systematic review of longitudinal studies on the association between depression and smoking in adolescents. *BMC Public Health, 9*, 356. https://doi.org/10.1186/1471-2458-9-356.

27. Chaiton, M., Diemert, L., Cohen, J. E., et al. (2016). Estimating the number of quit attempts, it takes to quit smoking successfully in a longitudinal cohort of smokers. *BMJ Open, 6*(6), e010590. https://doi.org/10.1136/bmjopen-2015-010590.

28. Chaloupka, F. J., Straif, K., & Leon, M. E. (2011). Effectiveness of tax and price policies in tobacco control. *Tobacco Control, 20*(3), 235–238. https://doi.org/10.1136/tc.2010.037015.

29. Chamberlain, A. M., Agarwal, S. K., Folsom, A. R., et al. (2011). Smoking and incidence of atrial fibrillation: Results from the Atherosclerosis Risk in Communities (ARIC) study. *Heart Rhythm, 8*(8), 1160–1166. https://doi.org/10.1016/j.hrthm.2011.03.034.

30. Chandrupatla, S. G., Tavares, M., & Natto, Z. S. (2017). Tobacco use and effects of professional advice on smoking cessation among youth in India. *Asian Pacific Journal of Cancer Prevention, 18*(7), 1861–1867. https://doi.org/10.22034/APJCP.2017.18.7.1861.

31. Chapman, S. (2007). *Public Health Advocacy and Tobacco Control: Making Smoking History*. Wiley-Blackwell. ISBN 9781405161633.

32. Cheng, K. W., Okechukwu, C. A., McMillen, R., & Glantz, S. A. (2015). Association between clean indoor air laws and voluntary smokefree rules in homes and cars. *Tobacco Control, 24*(2), 168–174. https://doi.org/10.1136/tobaccocontrol-2013-051333.

33. Christakis, N. A., & Fowler, J. H. (2008). Quitting in droves: Collective dynamics of smoking behavior in a large social network. *New England Journal of Medicine, 358*(21), 2249–2258. https://doi.org/10.1056/NEJMsa0706154.

34. Critchley, J. A., & Capewell, S. (2003). Mortality risk reduction associated with smoking cessation in patients with coronary heart disease: A systematic review. *JAMA, 290*(1), 86–97. https://doi.org/10.1001/jama.290.1.86.

35. Czernin, J., & Waldherr, C. (2003). Cigarette smoking and coronary blood flow. *Progress in Cardiovascular Diseases, 45*(5), 395–404. https://doi.org/10.1016/S0033-0620(03)00019-9.

36. Dai, H., & Hao, J. (2018). Temporal trends of sources of cigarettes among U.S. high school students: 2001–2015. *Nicotine & Tobacco Research*. https://doi.org/10.1093/ntr/nty094.

37. DiFranza, J. R., Savageau, J. R., Rigotti, N. A., et al. (2002). Development of symptoms of tobacco dependence in youths: 30 month follow up data from the DANDY study. *Tobacco Control, 11*(3), 228–235. https://doi.org/10.1136/tc.11.3.228.

38. Donny, E. C., Denlinger, R. L., Tidey, J. W., et al. (2015). Randomized trial of reduced-nicotine standards for cigarettes. *New England Journal of Medicine, 373*(14), 1340–1349. https://doi.org/10.1056/NEJMsa1502403.

39. Doubeni, C. A., Reed, G., & DiFranza, J. R. (2010). Early course of nicotine dependence in adolescent smokers. *Pediatrics, 125*(6), 1127–1133. https://doi.org/10.1542/peds.2009-2534.

40. Drope, J., Schluger, N., Cahn, Z., et al. (2018). *The Tobacco Atlas*. American Cancer Society and Vital Strategies.

41. Duval, S., Long, K. H., Roy, S. S., et al. (2015). The contribution of tobacco use to high health care utilization and medical costs in peripheral artery disease: A state-based cohort analysis. *Journal of the American College of Cardiology, 66*(14), 1566–1574. https://doi.org/10.1016/j.jacc.2015.07.064.

42. Eisenberg, M. J., Grandi, S. M., Gervais, A., et al. (2013). Bupropion for smoking cessation in patients hospitalized with acute myocardial infarction: A randomized, placebo-controlled trial. *Journal of the American College of Cardiology, 61*(5), 524–532. https://doi.org/10.1016/j.jacc.2012.10.036.

43. Eisenberg, M. J., Windle, S. B., Roy, N., et al. (2015). Varenicline for smoking cessation in hospitalized patients with acute coronary syndrome. *Circulation*. https://doi.org/10.1161/CIRCULATIONAHA.114.014051.

44. Ellickson, P. L., Bird, C. E., Orlando, M., Klein, D. J., & McCaffrey, D. F. (2003). Social context and adolescent health behavior: Does school-level smoking prevalence affect students' subsequent smoking behavior? *Journal of Health and Social Behavior, 44*(4), 525–535. https://doi.org/10.2307/1519788.

45. Epstein, K. A., Viscoli, C. M., Spence, J. D., et al. (2017). Smoking cessation and outcome after ischemic stroke or TIA. *Neurology, 89*(17), 1723–1729. https://doi.org/10.1212/WNL.0000000000004598.

46. Fairchild, A. L., Lee, J. S., Bayer, R., & Curran, J. (2018). E-cigarettes and the harm-reduction continuum. *New England Journal of Medicine, 378*(3), 216–219. https://doi.org/10.1056/NEJMp1713791.

47. Farkas, A. J., Gilpin, E. A., White, M. M., & Pierce, J. P. (2000). Association between household and workplace smoking restrictions and adolescent smoking. *JAMA, 284*(6), 717–722. https://doi.org/10.1001/jama.284.6.717.

48. Fiore, M. C., Bailey, W. C., Cohen, S. J., et al. (2000). *Treating Tobacco Use and Dependence: Clinical Practice Guideline*. Rockville, MD: US Department of Health and Human Services. https://doi.org/10.1.1.452.5012.

49. Fiore, M. C., Jaen, C. R., Baker, T. B., et al. (2008). *Treating Tobacco Use and Dependence: 2008 Update*. Rockville, MD: US Department of Health and Human Services. https://doi.org/10.1.1.452.5012.

50. Gershon, A. S., Campitelli, M. A., Hawken, S., et al. (2017). Cardiovascular and neuropsychiatric events following varenicline use for smoking cessation. *American Journal of Respiratory and Critical Care Medicine*. https://doi.org/10.1164/rccm.201701-0165OC.

51. Global Burden of Disease Study 2015. (2017). Smoking prevalence and attributable disease burden in 195 countries and territories, 1990–2015: A systematic analysis. *Lancet, 389*(10082), 1885–1906. https://doi.org/10.1016/S0140-6736(17)30819-X.

52. Godtfredsen, N. S., Holst, C., Prescott, E., Vestbo, J., & Osler, M. (2002). Smoking reduction, smoking cessation, and mortality: A 16-year follow-up of 19,732 men and women from The Copenhagen Centre for Prospective Population Studies. *American Journal of Epidemiology, 156*(10), 994–1001. https://doi.org/10.1093/aje/kwf128.

53. Goette, A., Lendeckel, U., Kuchenbecker, A., et al. (2007). Cigarette smoking induces atrial fibrosis in humans via nicotine. *Heart, 93*(9), 1056–1063. https://doi.org/10.1136/hrt.2007.122785.

54. Goldenberg, I., Jonas, M., Tenenbaum, A., et al. (2003). Current smoking, smoking cessation, and the risk of sudden cardiac death in patients with coronary artery disease. *Archives of Internal Medicine, 163*(19), 2301–2305. https://doi.org/10.1001/archinte.163.19.2301.

55. Goldenberg, I., Moss, A. J., McNitt, S., et al. (2006). Cigarette smoking and the risk of supraventricular and ventricular tachyarrhythmias in high-risk cardiac patients with implantable cardioverter defibrillators. *Journal of Cardiovascular Electrophysiology, 17*(9), 931–936. https://doi.org/10.1111/j.1540-8167.2006.00536.x.

56. Goodwin, R. D., Pagura, J., Spiwak, R., Lemeshow, A., & Sareen, J. (2011). Predictors of persistent nicotine dependence among adults in the United States. *Drug and Alcohol Dependence, 118*(1), 127–133. https://doi.org/10.1016/j.drugalcdep.2011.03.013.

57. Gopal, D. M., Kalogeropoulos, A. P., Georgiopoulou, V. V., et al. (2012). Cigarette smoking exposure and heart failure risk in older adults: The Health, Aging, and Body Composition Study. *American Heart Journal, 164*(2), 236–242. https://doi.org/10.1016/j.ahj.2012.05.008.

58. Gottlieb, S., & Zeller, M. (2017). A nicotine-focused framework for public health. *New England Journal of Medicine, 377*(11), 1111–1114. https://doi.org/10.1056/NEJMp1707610.

59. Gravely, S., Giovino, G. A., Craig, L., et al. (2017). Implementation of key demand-reduction measures of the WHO Framework Convention on Tobacco Control and change in smoking prevalence in 126 countries: An association study. *The Lancet Public Health, 2*(4), e166–e174. https://doi.org/10.1016/S2468-2667(17)30045-7.

60. Hackshaw, A., Morris, J. K., Boniface, S., Tang, J. L., & Milenkovic, D. (2018). Low cigarette consumption and risk of coronary heart disease and stroke: Meta-analysis of 141 cohort studies in 55 study reports. *BMJ, 360*, j5855. https://doi.org/10.1136/bmj.j5855.

61. Hatsukami, D. K., Donny, E. C., Koopmeiners, J. S., & Benowitz, N. L. (2015). Compensatory smoking from gradual and immediate reduction in cigarette nicotine content. *Cancer Epidemiology, Biomarkers & Prevention, 24*(3), 472–476. https://doi.org/10.1158/1055-9965.EPI-14-0635.

62. Hatsukami, D. K., Kotlyar, M., Hertsgaard, L. A., et al. (2010). Reduced nicotine content cigarettes: Effects on toxicant exposure, dependence and cessation. *Addiction, 105*(2), 343–355. https://doi.org/10.1111/j.1360-0443.2009.02721.x.

63. Hatsukami, D. K., Luo, X., Dick, L., et al. (2017). Reduced nicotine content cigarettes and use of alternative nicotine products: Exploratory trial. *Addiction, 112*(1), 156–167. https://doi.org/10.1111/add.13600.

64. Herd, N., & Borland, R. (2009). The natural history of quitting smoking: Findings from the International Tobacco Control (ITC) Four Country Survey. *Addiction, 104*(12), 2075–2087. https://doi.org/10.1111/j.1360-0443.2009.02731.x.

65. Hiilamo, H., & Glantz, S. (2017). FCTC followed by accelerated implementation of tobacco advertising bans. *Tobacco Control, 26*(4), 428–433. https://doi.org/10.1136/tobaccocontrol-2016-053007.

66. Hitchman, S. C., Fong, G. T., Zanna, M. P., Thrasher, J. F., & Laux, F. L. (2014). The relation between number of smoking friends, and quit intentions, attempts, and success: Findings from the International Tobacco Control (ITC) Four Country Survey. *Psychology of Addictive Behaviors, 28*(4), 1144–1152. https://doi.org/10.1037/a0036483.

67. Hughes, J. R., Solomon, L. J., Naud, S., Fingar, J. R., Helzer, J. E., & Callas, P. W. (2014). Natural history of attempts to stop smoking. *Nicotine & Tobacco Research, 16*(9), 1190–1198. https://doi.org/10.1093/ntr/ntu052.

68. Hughes, J. R., Stead, L. F., Hartmann-Boyce, J., Cahill, K., & Lancaster, T. (2014). Antidepressants for smoking cessation. *Cochrane Database of Systematic Reviews, 2014*(1), CD000031. https://doi.org/10.1002/14651858.CD000031.pub4.

69. Institute of Medicine Committee on the Public Health Implications of Raising the Minimum Age for Purchasing Tobacco Products, Bonnie, R. J., Kwan, L. Y., & Stratton, K. R. (2015). *Public Health Implications of Raising the Minimum Age of Legal Access to Tobacco Products*. National Academies Press. https://doi.org/10.17226/18997.

70. Jamal, A., Dube, S. R., & King, B. A. (2015). Tobacco use screening and counseling during hospital outpatient visits among US adults, 2005–2010. *Preventing Chronic Disease, 12*, E132. https://doi.org/10.5888/pcd12.150020.

71. Jamal, A., Gentzke, A., Hu, S. S., et al. (2017). Tobacco use among middle and high school students—United States, 2011–2016. *MMWR Morbidity and Mortality Weekly Report, 66*(23), 597–603. https://doi.org/10.15585/mmwr.mm6623a1.

72. Jamal, A., Phillips, E., Gentzke, A. S., et al. (2018). Current cigarette smoking among adults—United States, 2016. *MMWR Morbidity and Mortality Weekly Report, 67*(2), 53–59. https://doi.org/10.15585/mmwr.mm6702a1.

73. Jha, P., Ramasundarahettige, C., Landsman, V., et al. (2013). 21st-century hazards of smoking and benefits of cessation in the United States. *New England Journal of Medicine, 368*(4), 341–350. https://doi.org/10.1056/NEJMsa1211128.

74. Kalhan, R., Wilkins, J. T., & Hitsman, B. L. (2017). Tobacco smoking is a medical problem: We ought to treat it like one. *American Journal of Respiratory and Critical Care Medicine*. https://doi.org/10.1164/rccm.201702-0391ED.

75. Kasza, K. A., Ambrose, B. K., Conway, K. P., et al. (2017). Tobacco-product use by adults and youths in the United States in 2013 and 2014. *New England Journal of Medicine, 376*(4), 342–353. https://doi.org/10.1056/NEJMsa1607538.

76. Kotz, D., Viechtbauer, W., Simpson, C., van Schayck, O. C., West, R., & Sheikh, A. (2015). Cardiovascular and neuropsychiatric risks of varenicline: A retrospective cohort study. *Lancet Respiratory Medicine, 3*(10), 761–768. https://doi.org/10.1016/S2213-2600(15)00229-9.

77. Lancaster, T., & Stead, L. F. (2017). Individual behavioral counselling for smoking cessation. *Cochrane Database of Systematic Reviews, 2017*(3), CD001292. https://doi.org/10.1002/14651858.CD001292.pub3.

78. Lederle, F. A., Johnson, G. R., Wilson, S. E., et al. (2000). The aneurysm detection and management study screening program: Validation cohort and final results. *Archives of Internal Medicine, 160*(10), 1425–1430. https://doi.org/10.1001/archinte.160.10.1425.

79. Levitzky, Y. S., Guo, C. Y., Rong, J., et al. (2008). Relation of smoking status to a panel of inflammatory markers: The Framingham Offspring. *Atherosclerosis, 201*(1), 217–224. https://doi.org/10.1016/j.atherosclerosis.2008.02.019.

80. Lu, L., Mackay, D. F., & Pell, J. P. (2014). Meta-analysis of the association between cigarette smoking and peripheral arterial disease. *Heart, 100*(5), 414–423. https://doi.org/10.1136/heartjnl-2013-304082.

81. Matetzky, S., Tani, S., Kangavari, S., et al. (2000). Smoking increases tissue factor expression in atherosclerotic plaques: Implications for plaque thrombogenicity. *Circulation, 102*(6), 602–604. https://doi.org/10.1161/01.CIR.102.6.602.

82. Mayne, S. L., Auchincloss, A. H., Stehr, M. F., et al. (2017). Longitudinal associations of local cigarette prices and smoking bans with smoking behavior in the Multi-Ethnic Study of Atherosclerosis. *Epidemiology, 28*(6), 863–871. https://doi.org/10.1097/EDE.0000000000000713.

83. McEvoy, J. W., Nasir, K., DeFilippis, A. P., et al. (2015). Relationship of cigarette smoking with inflammation and subclinical vascular disease: The Multi-Ethnic Study of Atherosclerosis. *Arteriosclerosis, Thrombosis, and Vascular Biology, 35*(4), 1002–1010. https://doi.org/10.1161/ATVBAHA.114.304960.

84. Messner, B., & Bernhard, D. (2014). Smoking and cardiovascular disease: Mechanisms of endothelial dysfunction and early atherogenesis. *Arteriosclerosis, Thrombosis, and Vascular Biology, 34*(3), 509–515. https://doi.org/10.1161/ATVBAHA.113.302951.

85. Mills, E. J., Thorlund, K., Eapen, S., Wu, P., & Prochaska, J. J. (2014). Cardiovascular events associated with smoking cessation pharmacotherapies: A network meta-analysis. *Circulation, 129*(1), 28–41. https://doi.org/10.1161/CIRCULATIONAHA.113.003961.

86. Monarrez-Espino, J., Galanti, M. R., Hansson, J., Janszky, I., Soderberg, K., & Moller, J. (2017). Treatment with bupropion and varenicline for smoking cessation and the risk of acute cardiovascular events and injuries: A Swedish case-crossover study. *Nicotine & Tobacco Research*. https://doi.org/10.1093/ntr/ntx100.

87. Nash, S. H., Liao, L. M., Harris, T. B., & Freedman, N. D. (2017). Cigarette smoking and mortality in adults aged 70 years and older: Results from the NIH-AARP cohort. *American Journal of Preventive Medicine, 52*(3), 276–283. https://doi.org/10.1016/j.amepre.2016.11.019.

88. National Academies of Sciences, Engineering, and Medicine. (2018). *Public Health Consequences of E-Cigarettes*. The National Academies Press. https://doi.org/10.17226/24952.

89. Newby, D. E., McLeod, A. L., Uren, N. G., et al. (2001). Impaired coronary tissue plasminogen activator release is associated with coronary atherosclerosis and cigarette smoking: Direct link between endothelial dysfunction and atherothrombosis. *Circulation, 103*(15), 1936–1941. https://doi.org/10.1161/01.CIR.103.15.1936.

90. Oono, I. P., Mackay, D. F., & Pell, J. P. (2011). Meta-analysis of the association between secondhand smoke exposure and stroke. *Journal of Public Health, 33*(4), 496–502. https://doi.org/10.1093/pubmed/fdr025.

91. Pagidipati, N. J., Hellkamp, A., Thomas, L., Gulati, M., Peterson, E. D., & Wang, T. Y. (2017). Use of prescription smoking cessation medications after myocardial infarction among older patients in community practice. *JAMA Cardiology, 2*(9), 1040–1042. https://doi.org/10.1001/jamacardio.2017.2307.

92. Parsons, A., Daley, A., Begh, R., & Aveyard, P. (2010). Influence of smoking cessation after diagnosis of early-stage lung cancer on prognosis: Systematic review of observational studies with meta-analysis. *BMJ, 340*, b5569. https://doi.org/10.1136/bmj.b5569.

93. Patton, G. C., Carlin, J. B., Coffey, C., Wolfe, R., Hibbert, M., & Bowes, G. (1998). Depression, anxiety, and smoking initiation: A prospective study over 3 years. *American Journal of Public Health, 88*(10), 1518–1522. https://doi.org/10.2105/AJPH.88.10.1518.

94. Peers, K., & Kobus, K. (2003). Adolescent smoking. *Addiction, 98*(Supplement 1), 37–55. https://doi.org/10.1046/j.1360-0443.98.s1.4.x.

95. Peto, R., Darby, S., Deo, H., Silcocks, P., Whitley, E., & Doll, R. (2000). Smoking, smoking cessation, and lung cancer in the UK since 1950: Combination of national statistics with two case-control studies. *BMJ, 321*(7257), 323–329. https://doi.org/10.1136/bmj.321.7257.323.

96. Phillips, E., Wang, T. W., Husten, C. G., et al. (2017). Tobacco product use among adults—United States, 2015. *MMWR Morbidity and Mortality Weekly Report, 66*(44), 1209–1215. https://doi.org/10.15585/mmwr.mm6644a2.

97. Piano, M. R., Benowitz, N. L., Fitzgerald, G. A., et al. (2010). Impact of smokeless tobacco products on cardiovascular disease: Implications for policy, prevention, and treatment: A policy statement from the American Heart Association. *Circulation, 122*(15), 1520–1540. https://doi.org/10.1161/CIR.0b013e3181f432c3.

98. Planer, D., Lev, I., Elitzur, Y., et al. (2011). Bupropion for smoking cessation in patients with acute coronary syndrome. *Archives of Internal Medicine, 171*(12), 1055–1060. https://doi.org/10.1001/archinternmed.2011.199.

99. Primatesta, P., Falaschetti, E., Gupta, S., Marmot, M. G., & Poulter, N. R. (2001). Association between smoking and blood pressure: Evidence from the Health Survey for England. *Hypertension, 37*(2), 187–193. https://doi.org/10.1161/01.hyp.37.2.187.

100. Prochaska, J. J., & Hilton, J. F. (2012). Risk of cardiovascular serious adverse events associated with varenicline use for tobacco cessation: Systematic review and meta-analysis. *BMJ, 344*, e2856. https://doi.org/10.1136/bmj.e2856.

101. Rea, T. D., Heckbert, S. R., Kaplan, R. C., Smith, N. L., Lemaitre, R. N., & Psaty, B. M. (2002). Smoking status and risk for recurrent coronary events after myocardial infarction. *Annals of Internal Medicine, 137*(6), 494–500. https://doi.org/10.7326/0003-4819-137-6-200209170-00007.

102. Regalado, M., Yang, S., & Wesson, D. E. (2000). Cigarette smoking is associated with augmented progression of renal insufficiency in severe essential hypertension. *American Journal of Kidney Diseases, 35*(4), 687–694. https://doi.org/10.1016/s0272-6386(00)70018-0.

103. Rigotti, N. A., Clair, C., Munafo, M. R., & Stead, L. F. (2012). Interventions for smoking cessation in hospitalized patients. *Cochrane Database of Systematic Reviews, 2012*(5), CD001837. https://doi.org/10.1002/14651858.CD001837.pub3.

104. Rigotti, N. A., Pipe, A. L., Benowitz, N. L., Arteaga, C., Garza, D., & Tonstad, S. (2010). Efficacy and safety of varenicline for smoking cessation in patients with cardiovascular disease: A randomized trial. *Circulation, 121*(2), 221–229. https://doi.org/10.1161/CIRCULATIONAHA.109.869008.

105. Ross, H., & Chaloupka, F. J. (2003). The effect of cigarette prices on youth smoking. *Health Economics, 12*(3), 217–230. https://doi.org/10.1002/hec.709.

106. Saleheen, D., Zhao, W., Young, R., et al. (2017). Loss of cardioprotective effects at the ADAMTS7 locus as a result of gene-smoking interactions. *Circulation, 135*(24), 2336–2353. https://doi.org/10.1161/CIRCULATIONAHA.116.025568.

107. Singh, S., Loke, Y. K., Spangler, J. G., & Furberg, C. D. (2011). Risk of serious adverse cardiovascular events associated with varenicline: A systematic review and meta-analysis. *CMAJ, 183*(12), 1359–1366. https://doi.org/10.1503/cmaj.110218.

108. Song, A. V., Dutra, L. M., Neilands, T. B., & Glantz, S. A. (2015). Association of smoke-free laws with lower percentages of new and current smokers among adolescents and young adults: An 11-year longitudinal study. *JAMA Pediatrics, 169*(7), e152285. https://doi.org/10.1001/jamapediatrics.2015.2285.

109. Stead, L. F., & Lancaster, T. (2005). Interventions for preventing tobacco sales to minors. *Cochrane Database of Systematic Reviews, 2005*(1), CD001497. https://doi.org/10.1002/14651858.CD001497.pub2.

110. Stead, L. F., & Lancaster, T. (2012). Combined pharmacotherapy and behavioral interventions for smoking cessation. *Cochrane Database of Systematic Reviews, 2012*(10), CD008286. https://doi.org/10.1002/14651858.CD008286.pub2.

111. Stead, L. F., Buitrago, D., Preciado, N., Sanchez, G., Hartmann-Boyce, J., & Lancaster, T. (2013). Physician advice for smoking cessation. *Cochrane Database of Systematic Reviews, 2013*(5), CD000165. https://doi.org/10.1002/14651858.CD000165.pub4.

112. Stead, L. F., Carroll, A. J., & Lancaster, T. (2017). Group behavior therapy programmers for smoking cessation. *Cochrane Database of Systematic Reviews, 2017*(3), CD001007. https://doi.org/10.1002/14651858.CD001007.pub3.

113. Stead, L. F., Hartmann-Boyce, J., Perera, R., & Lancaster, T. (2013). Telephone counselling for smoking cessation. *Cochrane Database of Systematic Reviews, 2013*(8), CD002850. https://doi.org/10.1002/14651858.CD002850.pub3.

114. Stead, L. F., Perera, R., Bullen, C., et al. (2012). Nicotine replacement therapy for smoking

cessation. *Cochrane Database of Systematic Reviews, 2012*(11), CD000146. https://doi.org/10.1002/14651858.CD000146.pub4.

115. Sterling, L. H., Windle, S. B., Filion, K. B., Touma, L., & Eisenberg, M. J. (2016). Varenicline and adverse cardiovascular events: A systematic review and meta-analysis of randomized controlled trials. *Journal of the American Heart Association, 5*(2), e002849. https://doi.org/10.1161/JAHA.115.002849.

116. Substance Abuse and Mental Health Services Administration, Center for Behavioral Health Statistics and Quality. (2017). *The NSDUH Report: Adults with Mental Illness or Substance Use Disorder Account for 40% of All Cigarettes Smoked.* Retrieved from: https://www.samhsa.gov/data/sites/default/files/spot104-cigarettes-mental-illness-substance-use-disorder/spot104-cigarettes-mental-illness-substance-use-disorder.pdf (accessed on 3 September 2024).

117. Suskin, N., Sheth, T., Negassa, A., & Yusuf, S. (2001). Relationship of current and past smoking to mortality and morbidity in patients with left ventricular dysfunction. *Journal of the American College of Cardiology, 37*(6), 1677–1682. https://doi.org/10.1016/S0735-1097(01)01258-2.

118. Svanström, H., Pasternak, B., & Hviid, A. (2012). Use of varenicline for smoking cessation and risk of serious cardiovascular events: Nationwide cohort study. *BMJ, 345*, e7176. https://doi.org/10.1136/bmj.e7176.

119. Sweeting, M. J., Thompson, S. G., Brown, L. C., & Powell, J. T. (2012). Meta-analysis of individual patient data to examine factors affecting growth and rupture of small abdominal aortic aneurysms. *British Journal of Surgery, 99*(5), 655–665. https://doi.org/10.1002/bjs.8707.

120. Tabuchi, T., Kiyohara, K., Hoshino, T., Bekki, K., Inaba, Y., & Kunugita, N. (2016). Awareness and use of electronic cigarettes and heat-not-burn tobacco products in Japan. *Addiction, 111*(4), 706–713. https://doi.org/10.1111/add.13231.

121. Tan, C. E., & Glantz, S. A. (2012). Association between smoke-free legislation and hospitalizations for cardiac, cerebrovascular, and respiratory diseases: A meta-analysis. *Circulation, 126*(18), 2177–2183. https://doi.org/10.1161/CIRCULATIONAHA.112.121301.

122. Tate, C. (2000). *Cigarette Wars: The Triumph of "The Little White Slaver"*. Oxford University Press, USA.

123. Teo, K. K., Ounpuu, S., Hawken, S., et al. (2006). Tobacco use and risk of myocardial infarction in 52 countries in the INTERHEART study: A case-control study. *Lancet, 368*(9536), 647–658. https://doi.org/10.1016/S0140-6736(06)69249-0.

124. Thun, M. J., Carter, B. D., Feskanich, D., et al. (2013). 50-year trends in smoking-related mortality in the United States. *New England Journal of Medicine, 368*(4), 351–364. https://doi.org/10.1056/NEJMsa1211127.

125. Tomiyama, H., Hashimoto, H., Tanaka, H., et al. (2010). Continuous smoking and progression of arterial stiffening: A prospective study. *Journal of the American College of Cardiology, 55*(18), 1979–1987. https://doi.org/10.1016/j.jacc.2009.11.089.

126. Tverdal, A., & Bjartveit, K. (2006). Health consequences of reduced daily cigarette consumption. *Tobacco Control, 15*(6), 472–480. https://doi.org/10.1136/tc.2006.016246.

127. Tyas, S. L., & Pederson, L. L. (1998). Psychosocial factors related to adolescent smoking: A critical review of the literature. *Tobacco Control, 7*(4), 409–420. https://doi.org/10.1136/tc.7.4.409.

128. U.S. Department of Health and Human Services. (2010). *How Tobacco Smoke Causes Disease: The Biology and Behavioral Basis for Smoking-Attributable Disease: A Report of the Surgeon General.* U.S. Department of Health and Human Services, Centers for Disease Control and Prevention, National Center for Chronic Disease Prevention and Health Promotion, Office on Smoking and Health.

129. U.S. Department of Health and Human Services. (2012). *Preventing Tobacco Use Among Youth and Young Adults: A Report of the Surgeon General.* U.S. Department of Health and Human Services, Centers for Disease Control and Prevention, National Center for Chronic Disease Prevention and Health Promotion, Office on Smoking and Health.

130. U.S. Department of Health and Human Services. (2014). *The Health Consequences of Smoking—50 Years of Progress: A Report of the Surgeon General.* U.S. Department of Health and Human Services, Centers for Disease Control and Prevention, National Center for Chronic Disease Prevention and Health Promotion, Office on Smoking and Health.

131. Uang, R., Hiilamo, H., & Glantz, S. A. (2016). Accelerated adoption of smoke-free laws after ratification of the World Health Organization Framework Convention on Tobacco Control. *American Journal of Public Health, 106*(1), 166–171. https://doi.org/10.2105/AJPH.2015.302872.

132. van Domburg, R. T., Meeter, K., van Berkel, D. F., Veldkamp, R. F., van Herwerden, L. A., & Bogers, A. J. (2000). Smoking cessation reduces mortality after coronary artery bypass surgery: A 20-year follow-up study. *Journal of the American College of Cardiology, 36*(3), 878–883. https://doi.org/10.1016/S0735-1097(00)00858-0.

133. Vink, J. M., Willemsen, G., & Boomsma, D. I. (2005). Heritability of smoking initiation and nicotine dependence. *Behavior Genetics, 35*(4), 397–406. https://doi.org/10.1007/s10519-004-1327-8.

134. Ware, J. H., Vetrovec, G. W., Miller, A. B., et al. (2013). Cardiovascular safety of varenicline: Patient-level meta-analysis of randomized, blinded, placebo-controlled trials. *American Journal of Therapeutics, 20*(3), 235–246. https://doi.org/10.1097/MJT.0b013e31825ff1de.

135. Wellman, R. J., Sugarman, D. B., DiFranza, J. R., & Winickoff, J. P. (2006). The extent to which tobacco marketing and tobacco use in films contribute to children's use of tobacco: A meta-analysis. *Archives of Pediatrics & Adolescent Medicine, 160*(12), 1285–1296. https://doi.org/10.1001/archpedi.160.12.1285.

136. White, A. R., Rampes, H., Liu, J. P., Stead, L. F., & Campbell, J. (2014). Acupuncture and related interventions for smoking cessation. *Cochrane Database of Systematic Reviews, 2014*(1), CD000009. https://doi.org/10.1002/14651858.CD000009.pub4.

137. Whittaker, R., McRobbie, H., Bullen, C., Rodgers, A., & Gu, Y. (2016). Mobile phone-based interventions for smoking cessation. *Cochrane Database of Systematic Reviews, 2016*(4), CD006611. https://doi.org/10.1002/14651858.CD006611.pub4.

138. Willi, C., Bodenmann, P., Ghali, W. A., Faris, P. D., & Cornuz, J. (2007). Active smoking and the risk of type 2 diabetes: A systematic review and meta-analysis. *JAMA, 298*(22), 2654–2664. https://doi.org/10.1001/jama.298.22.2654.

139. Wilson, K., Gibson, N., Willan, A., & Cook, D. (2000). Effect of smoking cessation on mortality after myocardial infarction: Meta-analysis of cohort studies. *Archives of Internal Medicine, 160*(7), 939–944. https://doi.org/10.1001/archinte.160.7.939.

140. Windle, S. B., Dehghani, P., Roy, N., et al. (2018). Smoking abstinence 1 year after acute coronary syndrome: Follow-up from a randomized controlled trial of varenicline in patients admitted to hospital. *CMAJ, 190*(12), E347–E354. https://doi.org/10.1503/cmaj.170377.

141. Winickoff, J. P., Hippie, B., Drehmer, J., et al. (2012). The Clinical Effort Against Secondhand Smoke Exposure (CEASE) intervention: A decade of lessons learned. *Journal of Clinical Outcomes Management: JCOM, 19*(9), 414–419.

142. World Health Organization. (2003). *WHO Framework Convention on Tobacco Control*. World Health Organization. https://apps.who.int/iris/handle/10665/42811 (accessed on 3 September 2024).

143. World Health Organization. (2017). *WHO Report on the Global Tobacco Epidemic 2017: Monitoring Tobacco Use and Prevention Policies*. https://apps.who.int/iris/handle/10665/255874 (accessed on 3 September 2024).

144. World Health Organization. (2018). *Tobacco*. http://www.who.int/mediacentre/factsheets/fs339/en/ (accessed on 3 September 2024).

145. Wu, Y., Song, P., Zhang, W., et al. (2015). Activation of AMPKalpha2 in adipocytes is essential for nicotine-induced insulin resistance *in vivo*. *Nature Medicine, 21*(4), 373–382. https://doi.org/10.1038/nm.3815.

146. Young, T. K. (2005). *Population Health: Concepts and Methods* (2nd ed.). Oxford University Press. ISBN: 0-19-515854-7.

147. Yusuf, S., Hawken, S., Ounpuu, S., et al. (2004). Effect of potentially modifiable risk factors associated with myocardial infarction in 52 countries (the INTERHEART study): Case-control study. *The Lancet, 364*(9438), 937–952. https://doi.org/10.1016/S0140-6736(04)17018-9.

Chapter

7

MENTAL HEALTH AND COMMUNITY WELL-BEING

Contents

Introduction

Mental health encompasses our emotional, psychological, and social well-being, influencing how we think, feel, and act. It's an integral aspect of our overall health, just as important as physical well-being. Good mental health allows us to cope with the stresses of life, maintain fulfilling relationships, and make meaningful contributions to our communities. However, mental health issues can arise due to various factors, including biological factors, life experiences, and genetic predispositions.

Mental health is not solely an individual concern; it's intricately linked to the well-being of communities. A community's collective mental health is shaped by various factors, including social relationships, economic stability, access to healthcare, and the physical environment. When individuals within a community experience good mental health, it contributes to a positive social fabric characterized by resilience, empathy, and support.

Community well-being encompasses the mental, emotional, and social health of its members. It thrives when people feel connected, valued, and supported within their social networks and environments. Strong community bonds and a sense of belonging are vital for promoting mental health and resilience, providing a buffer against stressors and adversity. Conversely, when communities face challenges such as poverty, discrimination, or social isolation, it can have detrimental effects on mental health outcomes for individuals within that community.

Promoting mental health within communities involves creating inclusive environments that prioritize empathy, understanding, and support. It requires addressing social determinants of health, such as poverty, housing instability, and access to education and healthcare. Community-based interventions, including mental health education programs, support groups, and outreach initiatives, play a crucial role in raising awareness, reducing stigma, and providing resources for individuals facing mental health challenges.

Orientation and Directional Terms

Term	Definition	Illustration
Bipolar disorder	Bipolar disorder (formerly called manic-depressive illness or manic depression) is a mental illness that causes unusual shifts in a person's mood, energy, activity levels, and concentration.	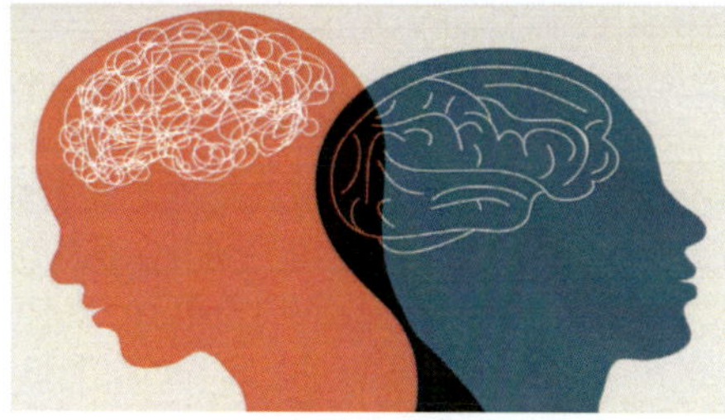
Schizophrenia	Schizophrenia is a serious mental illness that affects how a person thinks, feels, and behaves. People with schizophrenia may seem like they have lost touch with reality, which can be distressing for them and their family and friends.	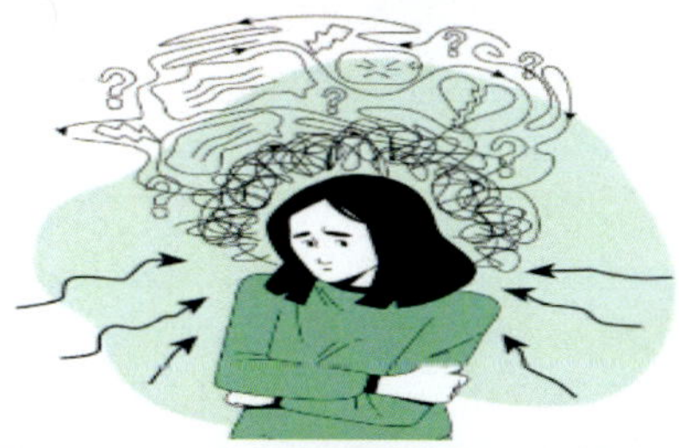
Autism Spectrum Disorder (ASD)	Autism spectrum disorder (ASD) is a neurological and developmental disorder that affects how people interact with others, communicate, learn, and behave.	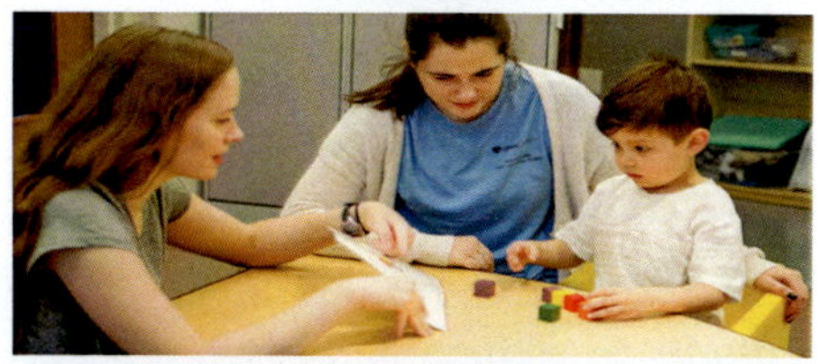
Panic Disorder	People with panic disorder have frequent and unexpected panic attacks. These attacks are characterized by a sudden wave of fear or discomfort or a sense of losing control even when there is no clear danger or trigger. Not everyone who experiences a panic attack will develop panic disorder.	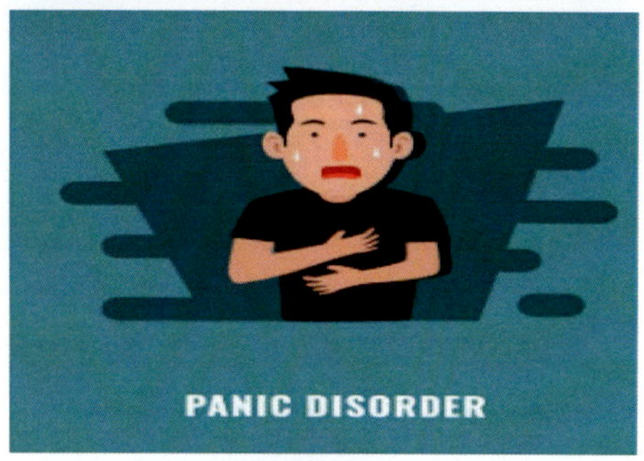
STIGMA	Stigma is something about a person that causes her or him to have a deeply compromised social standing, a mark of shame or discredit. Many persons with serious mental disorders appear to be different because of their symptoms or the side effects of their medication.	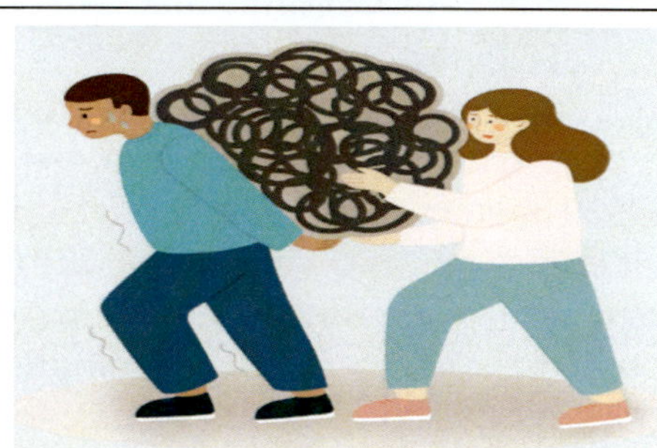

7.1. Mental Health

A person in a state of mental health is able to manage life's stresses, reach their full potential, learn and work effectively, and give back to their community. It is a vital aspect of health and well-being that supports our capacity as individuals and as a society to make choices, form bonds with others, and influence the environment in which we live. A fundamental human right is mental health. Furthermore, it is essential for socioeconomic, communal, and personal growth.

Mental health is more than the absence of mental disorders. It exists on a complex continuum, which is experienced differently from one person to the next, with varying degrees of difficulty and distress and potentially very different social and clinical outcomes.

Mental health conditions include mental disorders and psychosocial disabilities as well as other mental states associated with significant distress, impairment in functioning, or risk of self-harm. People with mental health conditions are more likely to experience lower levels of mental well-being, but this is not always or necessarily the case (Sullivan & Neale, 2000).

7.1.1. Risk Factors for Mental Health Conditions

Mental health conditions are influenced by a complex interplay of various risk factors. Understanding these factors is crucial for prevention, early intervention, and effective treatment. This essay delves into the major risk factors for mental health conditions, which can be broadly categorized into genetic and biological factors, environmental factors, psychological factors, and social and cultural factors. Each category encompasses numerous elements that contribute to the development and progression of mental health issues.

7.1.1.1. Genetic and Biological Factors

1. **Genetic Predisposition:** One of the most significant risk factors for mental health conditions is genetic predisposition. Numerous studies have shown that mental illnesses tend to run in families, suggesting a hereditary component. For instance, conditions such as schizophrenia, bipolar disorder, and major depressive disorder have higher concordance rates among monozygotic (identical) twins compared to dizygotic (fraternal) twins. The heritability of schizophrenia is estimated to be around 80%, indicating a strong genetic influence.
2. **Neurochemical Imbalances:** The brain's neurochemical environment plays a crucial role in mental health. Imbalances in neurotransmitters such as serotonin, dopamine, and norepinephrine are implicated in various mental health disorders. For example, depression has been associated with low levels of serotonin and norepinephrine, while schizophrenia is linked to excessive dopamine activity in certain brain regions.
3. **Brain Structure and Function:** Abnormalities in brain structure and function are also significant risk factors. Neuroimaging studies have revealed differences in brain areas such as the prefrontal cortex, hippocampus, and amygdala in individuals with mental health conditions. For instance, reduced hippocampal volume is commonly observed in people with depression and PTSD (post-traumatic stress disorder), whereas individuals with schizophrenia often exhibit enlarged ventricles and reduced gray matter.

7.1.1.2. Environmental Factors

1. **Early Life Stress and Trauma:** Early life stress and trauma, including physical, emotional, and sexual abuse, significantly increase the risk of developing mental health conditions. Adverse childhood experiences (ACEs) have a profound impact on brain development and stress response systems. Children who have experienced trauma are more likely to develop disorders such as PTSD, anxiety, depression, and substance abuse in later life.
2. **Prenatal Exposure:** Prenatal exposure to harmful substances and stress can predispose individuals to mental health conditions. Maternal smoking, alcohol consumption, and drug use during pregnancy are linked to developmental and behavioral problems in children. Additionally, high levels of maternal stress and malnutrition can negatively affect fetal brain development, increasing the risk of disorders such as ADHD (attention-deficit/hyperactivity disorder) and autism spectrum disorder (ASD).
3. **Environmental Toxins:** Exposure to environmental toxins, such as lead, mercury, and pesticides, can adversely affect mental health. For example, lead exposure is associated with cognitive deficits, behavioral problems, and an increased risk of neurodevelopmental disorders. Similarly, prolonged exposure to air pollution has been linked to higher rates of depression and anxiety.

7.1.1.3. Psychological Factors

1. **Personality Traits:** Certain personality traits can predispose individuals to mental health conditions. Traits such as high neuroticism, low self-esteem, and poor coping mechanisms are commonly associated with increased vulnerability to anxiety and depression. High neuroticism, characterized by emotional instability and negative affectivity, is a well-documented risk factor for a range of mental health disorders.
2. **Cognitive Patterns:** Negative cognitive patterns, including pessimism, rumination, and distorted thinking, contribute to the development and maintenance of mental health issues. Cognitive distortions such as all-or-nothing thinking, overgeneralization, and catastrophizing are frequently observed in individuals with depression and anxiety disorders. Cognitive-behavioral therapy (CBT) often targets these maladaptive thought patterns to alleviate symptoms.
3. **Stress Response:** An individual's response to stress plays a critical role in mental health. Chronic stress and maladaptive stress responses can lead to the development of mental health conditions. The hypothalamic-pituitary-adrenal (HPA) axis, which regulates stress responses, is often dysregulated in individuals with mental health disorders. Prolonged activation of the HPA axis can result in elevated cortisol levels, contributing to conditions such as depression, anxiety, and PTSD.

7.1.1.4. Social and Cultural Factors

1. **Socioeconomic Status:** Socioeconomic status (SES) is a significant determinant of mental health. Low SES is associated with increased stress, limited access to healthcare, poor nutrition, and inadequate living conditions, all of which contribute to mental health

problems. Children and adults from low-income families are at higher risk for developing anxiety, depression, and substance abuse disorders.

2. **Social Support:** The presence or absence of social support profoundly impacts mental health. Strong social networks and supportive relationships act as protective factors, reducing the risk of mental health conditions. Conversely, social isolation, loneliness, and lack of support can exacerbate mental health issues. Individuals with robust social connections are better able to cope with stress and are less likely to experience severe mental health problems.

3. **Cultural Factors:** Cultural beliefs and practices influence the perception and management of mental health. The stigma associated with mental illness can prevent individuals from seeking help and accessing treatment. Cultural norms and values can also affect the expression of symptoms and the types of coping strategies used. For example, in some cultures, mental health issues may be somatized, leading to physical rather than psychological complaints.

4. **Discrimination and Social Inequality:** Experiencing discrimination and social inequality significantly impacts mental health. Marginalized groups, including racial and ethnic minorities, LGBTQ+ individuals, and people with disabilities, often face systemic discrimination and prejudice. These experiences can lead to chronic stress, low self-esteem, and increased vulnerability to mental health conditions. Discrimination and social inequality can also limit access to resources and support, exacerbating mental health issues.

5. **Interaction of Risk Factors**: Mental health conditions often result from the interaction of multiple risk factors. For instance, genetic predisposition may make an individual more susceptible to the effects of environmental stressors. A person with a family history of depression might be more vulnerable to developing the condition if they experience significant life stressors, such as trauma or chronic stress. This interplay underscores the importance of considering the cumulative and interactive effects of various risk factors.

6. **Gene-Environment Interaction:** Gene-environment interaction (G×E) refers to the dynamic interplay between genetic predispositions and environmental influences. For example, individuals with a specific genetic variant related to the serotonin transporter gene may be more likely to develop depression following exposure to stressful life events. This interaction highlights the complexity of mental health etiology and the need for personalized approaches to prevention and treatment.

7. **Epigenetics:** Epigenetics involves changes in gene expression without altering the DNA sequence, often in response to environmental factors. Epigenetic modifications can be influenced by stress, diet, and exposure to toxins, among other factors. These changes can have long-lasting effects on brain function and behavior, contributing to the risk of mental health conditions. Understanding epigenetic mechanisms offers potential for new therapeutic targets and interventions.

7.1.2. Types of Mental Health Disorders

7.1.2.1. Anxiety Disorders

Anxiety disorders are among the most common mental health conditions, affecting millions of individuals worldwide. These disorders encompass a range of conditions characterized by excessive fear, worry, and related behavioral disturbances. While anxiety is a normal and often beneficial response to stress, anxiety disorders represent pathological levels of fear and worry that significantly impair daily functioning. This comprehensive overview delves into the various types of anxiety disorders, their symptoms, causes, and treatment options, highlighting the profound impact these conditions can have on individuals and society. (Robinson et al., 2009).

7.1.2.1.1. Types of Anxiety Disorders

1. **Generalized Anxiety Disorder (GAD):** Generalized Anxiety Disorder is characterized by persistent and excessive worry about various aspects of daily life. Individuals with GAD often anticipate disaster and may be overly concerned about health, finances, work, or other issues. This anxiety is difficult to control and can be accompanied by physical symptoms such as restlessness, fatigue, muscle tension, and sleep disturbances. The worry in GAD is often disproportionate to the actual situation and is pervasive, affecting multiple areas of the individual's life.
2. **Panic Disorder:** Panic Disorder involves recurrent, unexpected panic attacks—sudden periods of intense fear or discomfort that peak within minutes. These attacks are often accompanied by physical symptoms like palpitations, sweating, trembling, shortness of breath, and a sense of impending doom. Individuals with Panic Disorder may develop a fear of having future attacks, leading to significant behavioral changes and avoidance of certain situations or activities.
3. **Social Anxiety Disorder (SAD):** Social Anxiety Disorder, also known as social phobia, is characterized by a significant fear of social or performance situations in which the individual may be scrutinized by others. This fear often leads to avoidance of social interactions, which can severely impact personal and professional relationships. Symptoms include intense fear of embarrassment, humiliation, or rejection, and physical symptoms such as blushing, sweating, and trembling in social settings.
4. **Specific Phobias:** Specific phobias involve an intense, irrational fear of a particular object or situation, such as heights, animals, or flying. The fear is out of proportion to the actual danger posed and leads to avoidance behaviors that can interfere with daily functioning. Individuals with specific phobias may experience panic attacks or severe anxiety when confronted with the phobic stimulus.
5. **Obsessive-Compulsive Disorder (OCD):** Obsessive-Compulsive Disorder is characterized by the presence of obsessions (intrusive, unwanted thoughts) and/or compulsions (repetitive behaviors or mental acts performed to reduce anxiety). Common obsessions include fears of contamination, harming others, or needing things to be symmetrical. Compulsions may involve excessive cleaning, checking, or arranging items

in a specific order. The behaviors associated with OCD are time-consuming and cause significant distress and impairment.

6. **Post-Traumatic Stress Disorder (PTSD):** Post-Traumatic Stress Disorder can develop after exposure to a traumatic event, such as a natural disaster, accident, or violence. Individuals with PTSD experience intrusive memories, flashbacks, and nightmares related to the trauma. They may also exhibit avoidance behaviors, hyperarousal (such as being easily startled), and negative changes in mood and cognition. PTSD can severely impact an individual's ability to function in daily life and maintain relationships.
7. **Separation Anxiety Disorder:** Separation Anxiety Disorder involves excessive fear or anxiety about being separated from attachment figures, such as parents or caregivers. This disorder is most common in children but can also occur in adults. Symptoms include distress when anticipating or experiencing separation, excessive worry about losing the attachment figure, and reluctance or refusal to go out because of fear of separation.

7.1.2.1.2. Causes and Risk Factors

1. **Genetic Factors:** Research has shown that genetics play a significant role in the development of anxiety disorders. Family studies indicate that these disorders tend to run in families, suggesting a hereditary component. Twin studies further support this, showing higher concordance rates for anxiety disorders among monozygotic twins compared to dizygotic twins. Specific genetic variations, such as those affecting serotonin and other neurotransmitter systems, have been implicated in increasing susceptibility to anxiety disorders.
2. **Environmental Factors:** Environmental factors also contribute significantly to the onset and progression of anxiety disorders. Traumatic experiences, such as abuse, neglect, or witnessing violence, are strong risk factors. Chronic stressors, such as financial difficulties, relationship problems, and major life changes, can exacerbate anxiety. Additionally, upbringing and parenting styles, particularly those involving overprotection or lack of emotional support, can influence the development of anxiety disorders.
3. **Biological Factors:** Biological factors, including brain chemistry and structure, are crucial in understanding anxiety disorders. Dysregulation of neurotransmitters such as serotonin, norepinephrine, and gamma-aminobutyric acid (GABA) is associated with increased anxiety. Functional and structural abnormalities in brain regions involved in fear processing and emotional regulation, such as the amygdala and prefrontal cortex, have been observed in individuals with anxiety disorders.
4. **Psychological Factors:** Certain personality traits and cognitive patterns can predispose individuals to anxiety disorders. Traits such as neuroticism and a tendency towards negative thinking increase vulnerability. Cognitive theories suggest that maladaptive thought patterns, such as overestimating danger and underestimating coping abilities, play a critical role in the development and maintenance of anxiety disorders.

Additionally, individuals with low self-esteem and poor stress management skills are at higher risk.

7.1.2.1.3. Symptoms and Diagnosis

1. **Common Symptoms:** While each anxiety disorder has specific criteria, they share several common symptoms. These include excessive fear and worry, physical symptoms such as palpitations, sweating, and trembling, and behavioral changes like avoidance of feared situations. Cognitive symptoms, such as difficulty concentrating and intrusive thoughts, are also prevalent. The severity and combination of symptoms vary, but they all contribute to significant distress and impairment in daily functioning.
2. **Diagnostic Criteria:** The diagnosis of anxiety disorders is based on criteria outlined in the Diagnostic and Statistical Manual of Mental Disorders (DSM-5). Clinicians assess the duration, intensity, and impact of symptoms on the individual's life. A thorough clinical interview, including a detailed medical and psychological history, is essential for accurate diagnosis. In some cases, standardized assessment tools and questionnaires may be used to aid in diagnosis and measure symptom severity.

7.1.2.1.4. Treatment Options

1. Psychotherapy

- **Cognitive Behavioral Therapy (CBT):** Cognitive Behavioral Therapy is the most widely used and empirically supported treatment for anxiety disorders. CBT focuses on identifying and challenging maladaptive thoughts and behaviors that contribute to anxiety. Through techniques such as cognitive restructuring, exposure therapy, and relaxation training, individuals learn to manage their anxiety more effectively. CBT is typically structured and time-limited, with patients often seeing significant improvements within 12–20 sessions.
- **Exposure Therapy:** Exposure Therapy, a key component of CBT, involves gradually and systematically exposing individuals to feared situations or objects. This exposure helps to reduce anxiety over time by allowing individuals to confront their fears in a controlled and safe environment. Through repeated exposure, the individual learns that the feared outcomes are unlikely or manageable, which diminishes the anxiety response.
- **Acceptance and Commitment Therapy (ACT):** Acceptance and Commitment Therapy emphasizes accepting anxiety-related thoughts and feelings rather than fighting them. ACT encourages individuals to focus on their values and commit to actions that align with those values, despite the presence of anxiety. This approach helps individuals to develop a more flexible and compassionate relationship with their anxiety, reducing its impact on their lives.

2. Pharmacotherapy

- **Antidepressants:** Selective serotonin reuptake inhibitors (SSRIs) and serotonin-norepinephrine reuptake inhibitors (SNRIs) are commonly prescribed for anxiety disorders. These medications help to regulate neurotransmitter levels, reducing symptoms of anxiety. They are often used as a first-line treatment due to their efficacy and relatively favorable side effect profile. Examples include fluoxetine, sertraline, and venlafaxine.

- **Benzodiazepines:** Benzodiazepines, such as diazepam and lorazepam, are effective for short-term relief of acute anxiety symptoms. They work by enhancing the effect of GABA, a neurotransmitter that inhibits brain activity, producing a calming effect. However, due to their potential for dependence and withdrawal issues, they are typically prescribed for short durations and in specific situations.

3. Complementary and Alternative Treatments

- **Mindfulness and Meditation:** Mindfulness and meditation practices can be beneficial in managing anxiety. These practices involve focusing on the present moment and developing an awareness of thoughts and feelings without judgment. Techniques such as mindfulness-based stress reduction (MBSR) and mindfulness-based cognitive therapy (MBCT) have been shown to reduce anxiety symptoms and improve overall well-being.
- **Exercise:** Regular physical activity has been found to reduce anxiety symptoms and improve mood. Exercise promotes the release of endorphins and other neurotransmitters that have calming effects on the brain. Activities such as aerobic exercise, yoga, and tai chi can be particularly effective in managing anxiety.
- **Nutritional Interventions:** Diet and nutrition can also play a role in managing anxiety. Certain foods and nutrients, such as omega-3 fatty acids, magnesium, and probiotics, have been linked to reduced anxiety symptoms. Maintaining a balanced diet and avoiding excessive caffeine and sugar can help stabilize mood and reduce anxiety.

7.1.2.1.5. Impact of Anxiety Disorders

- **Personal Impact:** Anxiety disorders can profoundly impact an individual's quality of life. The constant fear and worry can lead to significant emotional distress, impairing the ability to enjoy life and engage in daily activities. Physical symptoms can further exacerbate this distress, leading to chronic health problems such as gastrointestinal issues, cardiovascular diseases, and weakened immune function. Social isolation and strained relationships are common as individuals may avoid social situations to prevent anxiety triggers.
- **Professional Impact:** In the workplace, anxiety disorders can lead to decreased productivity, increased absenteeism, and difficulties in maintaining employment. Individuals may

struggle with concentration, decision-making, and meeting deadlines. The stigma associated with mental health issues can further hinder career advancement and job satisfaction. Employers and colleagues may misinterpret anxiety-related behaviors as a lack of commitment or competence, leading to further stress and isolation.

- **Economic Impact:** The economic burden of anxiety disorders is substantial. Direct costs include medical expenses for treatment and medication, while indirect costs arise from lost productivity, absenteeism, and disability claims. The societal cost is significant, with billions of dollars lost annually due to reduced workforce participation and increased healthcare utilization. Investing in effective treatments and workplace accommodations can mitigate these economic impacts and improve overall productivity.
- **Social Impact:** Anxiety disorders can strain personal relationships and social interactions. The avoidance behaviors common in anxiety disorders can lead to social isolation, reducing opportunities for support and connection. Family members and friends may feel helpless or frustrated, impacting their well-being and the overall family dynamic. Educating loved ones about anxiety disorders and encouraging open communication can help alleviate some of these social challenges.

7.1.2.2. Mood Disorders

Mood disorders encompass a wide range of mental health conditions characterized by disturbances in a person's emotional state. These disorders can significantly impair an individual's ability to function in daily life, affecting their thoughts, behavior, and physical well-being (Sapolsky, 2004).

7.1.2.2.1. Types of Mood Disorders

1. **Major Depressive Disorder (MDD):** Major Depressive Disorder, often referred to as depression, is characterized by persistent and intense feelings of sadness, hopelessness, and a lack of interest or pleasure in nearly all activities. Symptoms must last for at least two weeks and represent a change from previous functioning. Additional symptoms may include changes in appetite and weight, sleep disturbances, fatigue, difficulty concentrating, feelings of worthlessness or excessive guilt, and recurrent thoughts of death or suicide. MDD can vary in severity and duration, significantly impairing social, occupational, and educational functioning.
2. **Bipolar Disorder:** Bipolar Disorder is characterized by alternating episodes of mania (or hypomania) and depression. There are several subtypes of bipolar disorder:

- **Bipolar I Disorder:** Bipolar I Disorder involves episodes of mania that last at least seven days or are so severe that immediate hospital care is required, usually alternating with depressive episodes. Mania is characterized by an abnormally elevated or irritable mood, increased activity or energy, grandiosity, decreased need for sleep, talkativeness, racing thoughts, distractibility, and impulsive or risky behavior.

- **Bipolar II Disorder:** Bipolar II Disorder involves a pattern of depressive episodes and hypomanic episodes, but not the full-blown manic episodes typical of Bipolar I Disorder. Hypomania includes similar symptoms to mania but is less severe and does not cause significant impairment in social or occupational functioning.
- **Cyclothymic Disorder:** Cyclothymic Disorder is a milder form of bipolar disorder characterized by chronic fluctuating moods involving periods of hypomania and depressive symptoms that do not meet the criteria for major depressive episodes. These symptoms persist for at least two years in adults or one year in children and adolescents.

3. **Persistent Depressive Disorder (Dysthymia):** Persistent Depressive Disorder, also known as dysthymia, involves chronic depression that lasts for at least two years in adults (or one year in children and adolescents). While the symptoms are less severe than those of Major Depressive Disorder, they are more enduring. Individuals with dysthymia may experience low energy, poor self-esteem, difficulty concentrating, and feelings of hopelessness. The persistent nature of the symptoms often leads to significant impairment in daily functioning and quality of life.
4. **Disruptive Mood Dysregulation Disorder (DMDD):** Disruptive Mood Dysregulation Disorder is a condition that typically begins in childhood and involves severe and recurrent temper outbursts that are out of proportion to the situation. These outbursts occur three or more times a week, and the child remains irritable or angry between episodes. DMDD is diagnosed in children between the ages of 6 and 18 and is intended to address concerns about overdiagnosis and treatment of bipolar disorder in children.

7.1.2.2.2. Causes and Risk Factors

1. **Genetic Factors:** Mood disorders often run in families, suggesting a significant genetic component. Studies indicate that individuals with a first-degree relative who has a mood disorder are at higher risk of developing a similar condition. Twin studies have shown higher concordance rates for mood disorders among monozygotic twins compared to dizygotic twins, reinforcing the role of heredity. Specific genes related to neurotransmitter function, such as those affecting serotonin and dopamine, have been implicated in mood disorders.
2. **Biological Factors:** Biological factors play a crucial role in the development of mood disorders. Neurotransmitter imbalances, particularly involving serotonin, norepinephrine, and dopamine, are associated with depression and bipolar disorder. Structural and functional abnormalities in brain regions involved in mood regulation, such as the prefrontal cortex, amygdala, and hippocampus, have been observed in individuals with mood disorders. Hormonal imbalances, such as those related to

thyroid function and the hypothalamic-pituitary-adrenal (HPA) axis, can also contribute to these conditions.

3. **Psychological Factors:** Certain personality traits and cognitive patterns can predispose individuals to mood disorders. Traits such as neuroticism, low self-esteem, and a tendency toward negative thinking are linked to an increased risk of depression. Cognitive theories suggest that maladaptive thought patterns, such as rumination, catastrophizing, and self-criticism, play a critical role in the development and maintenance of mood disorders. Additionally, poor coping skills and high levels of stress can exacerbate these conditions.
4. **Environmental Factors:** Environmental factors, including stressful life events, trauma, and chronic stress, can trigger or worsen mood disorders. Experiences such as the loss of a loved one, relationship problems, financial difficulties, and exposure to violence or abuse are significant risk factors. Social support, or lack thereof, also influences the onset and course of mood disorders. Individuals with weak social networks and poor family relationships are more vulnerable to these conditions.

7.1.2.2.3. Symptoms and Diagnosis

1. **Common Symptoms:** Mood disorders share several common symptoms, though their presentation may vary depending on the specific condition:

- **Emotional Symptoms:** Persistent sadness, hopelessness, irritability, and feelings of emptiness or worthlessness.
- **Cognitive Symptoms:** Difficulty concentrating, indecisiveness, and intrusive negative thoughts.
- **Behavioral Symptoms:** Withdrawal from social activities, changes in sleep patterns, and alterations in appetite and weight.
- **Physical Symptoms:** Fatigue, changes in energy levels, and unexplained aches and pains.

2. **Diagnostic Criteria:** The diagnosis of mood disorders is based on criteria outlined in the Diagnostic and Statistical Manual of Mental Disorders (DSM-5). A comprehensive clinical evaluation, including a detailed medical and psychological history, is essential for accurate diagnosis. Clinicians assess the duration, intensity, and impact of symptoms on the individual's life. Standardized assessment tools and questionnaires, such as the Hamilton Depression Rating Scale (HDRS) and the Mood Disorder Questionnaire (MDQ), may be used to aid in diagnosis and measure symptom severity.

7.1.2.2.4. Treatment Options

1. Psychotherapy

- **Cognitive Behavioral Therapy (CBT):** Cognitive Behavioral Therapy is a widely used and effective treatment for mood disorders. CBT focuses on identifying and changing maladaptive thought patterns and behaviors that contribute to depressive and manic symptoms. Techniques such as cognitive restructuring, behavioral activation, and problem-solving skills are employed to help individuals manage their mood and improve functioning. CBT is typically structured and time-limited, with patients often seeing significant improvements within 12–20 sessions.

- **Interpersonal Therapy (IPT):** Interpersonal Therapy is a time-limited psychotherapy that focuses on resolving interpersonal problems and improving communication skills. IPT is based on the idea that mood disorders are linked to relationship issues and social functioning. Treatment involves identifying and addressing problematic relationships, improving social support, and developing healthier ways to deal with conflict and stress. IPT is particularly effective for individuals with depression who have significant interpersonal difficulties.
- **Psychodynamic Therapy:** Psychodynamic Therapy explores the underlying psychological roots of mood disorders, often focusing on unconscious processes and early life experiences. This therapy aims to help individuals gain insight into their emotional conflicts and develop healthier ways of coping with distress. Psychodynamic therapy is typically longer-term and can be particularly beneficial for individuals with chronic or complex mood disorders.

2. Pharmacotherapy

- **Antidepressants:** Antidepressants are commonly prescribed to treat depressive symptoms in mood disorders. Selective serotonin reuptake inhibitors (SSRIs) and serotonin-norepinephrine reuptake inhibitors (SNRIs) are often the first-line treatment due to their efficacy and relatively favorable side effect profile. Examples include fluoxetine, sertraline, and venlafaxine. Other classes of antidepressants, such as tricyclic antidepressants (TCAs) and monoamine oxidase inhibitors (MAOIs), may be used when other treatments are ineffective.
- **Mood Stabilizers:** Mood stabilizers are primarily used to treat bipolar disorder and prevent mood swings. Lithium is one of the most effective mood stabilizers and has been used for decades. Anticonvulsant medications, such as valproate, carbamazepine, and lamotrigine, are also used to stabilize mood and prevent manic and depressive episodes.
- **Antipsychotics:** Atypical antipsychotic medications, such as olanzapine, quetiapine, and aripiprazole, are often used to treat bipolar disorder, particularly during manic episodes. These medications can also be used as adjunctive treatments for major depressive disorder, especially in cases where individuals do not respond adequately to antidepressants alone.

3. Complementary and Alternative Treatments

- **Electroconvulsive Therapy (ECT):** Electroconvulsive Therapy is a highly effective treatment for severe and treatment-resistant mood disorders. ECT involves inducing controlled seizures through electrical stimulation of the brain. It is typically used when other treatments have failed or when rapid symptom relief is necessary, such as in cases of severe depression with suicidal ideation. ECT is performed under general anesthesia and has been shown to produce significant improvements in mood.

- **Transcranial Magnetic Stimulation (TMS):** Transcranial Magnetic Stimulation is a non-invasive treatment that uses magnetic fields to stimulate nerve cells in the brain. TMS is primarily used for individuals with depression who have not responded to other treatments. It involves delivering repetitive magnetic pulses to specific areas of the brain associated with mood regulation. TMS has been shown to reduce depressive symptoms and improve overall functioning.

7.1.2.3. Psychotic Disorders

Psychotic disorders represent a group of severe mental health conditions characterized by disruptions in thought processes, perception, emotions, and behavior. These disorders profoundly impact an individual's ability to interpret reality, often leading to hallucinations, delusions, disorganized thinking, and impaired social functioning.

7.1.2.3.1. Classification of Psychotic Disorders

Psychotic disorders encompass a diverse range of conditions characterized by the presence of psychosis, which involves a loss of contact with reality. The fifth edition of the Diagnostic and Statistical Manual of Mental Disorders (DSM-5) classifies psychotic disorders into several primary categories, including:

1. **Schizophrenia Spectrum and Other Psychotic Disorders:** This category includes schizophrenia, schizoaffective disorder, schizophreniform disorder, brief psychotic disorder, delusional disorder, unspecified schizophrenia spectrum and other psychotic disorder disorders.
2. **Bipolar and Related Disorders:** While bipolar disorder primarily involves episodes of mood disturbance, individuals may also experience psychotic symptoms during manic or depressive episodes, leading to classification within the psychotic disorders spectrum.
3. **Substance/Medication-Induced Psychotic Disorder:** Psychotic symptoms may arise as a result of substance intoxication or withdrawal, as well as medication side effects. This category encompasses a range of substances, including drugs of abuse, medications, and toxins.
4. **Psychotic Disorder Due to Another Medical Condition:** Some medical conditions, such as neurological disorders, infections, and metabolic imbalances, can precipitate psychotic symptoms. This category includes conditions where psychosis is directly attributable to a specific medical condition.

7.1.2.3.2. Epidemiology of Psychotic Disorders

Psychotic disorders are relatively rare compared to other mental health conditions but can have profound and debilitating effects on affected individuals. The prevalence and incidence of psychotic disorders vary across populations, with schizophrenia being the most well-known and extensively studied condition within this spectrum. Key epidemiological findings include:

- **Prevalence:** Schizophrenia affects approximately 0.3% to 0.7% of the global population, with slight variations observed across regions and demographics.
- **Age of Onset:** The onset of psychotic disorders typically occurs in late adolescence or early adulthood, although some conditions may manifest at different stages of life.
- **Gender Differences:** Certain psychotic disorders, such as schizophrenia, tend to have an earlier age of onset in males compared to females. However, the overall prevalence does not differ significantly between genders.
- **Socioeconomic Factors:** Psychotic disorders are associated with socioeconomic disparities, with higher rates observed in socioeconomically disadvantaged populations.

7.1.2.3.3. Etiology of Psychotic Disorders

The etiology of psychotic disorders is multifactorial and involves complex interactions between genetic, neurobiological, environmental, and psychosocial factors. While the exact mechanisms underlying these conditions remain incompletely understood, several key contributors have been identified, including:

1. **Genetic Factors:** Genetic predisposition plays a significant role in the development of psychotic disorders, particularly schizophrenia. Family studies, twin studies, and genome-wide association studies (GWAS) have provided compelling evidence of genetic contributions to these conditions.
2. **Neurobiological Abnormalities:** Dysregulation of neurotransmitter systems, particularly dopamine and glutamate, is implicated in the pathophysiology of psychotic disorders. Structural and functional abnormalities in brain regions involved in perception, cognition, and emotion regulation have also been identified.
3. **Environmental Stressors:** Environmental factors, such as prenatal exposure to maternal infections, obstetric complications, childhood trauma, urban upbringing, and substance abuse, contribute to the risk of developing psychotic disorders. These stressors can interact with genetic vulnerabilities to increase susceptibility.
4. **Psychosocial Factors:** Social adversity, including social isolation, poverty, discrimination, and lack of access to education or employment opportunities, is associated with an increased risk of psychosis. Psychosocial stressors can exacerbate symptoms and contribute to poor outcomes in affected individuals.

7.1.2.3.4. Clinical Presentation of Psychotic Disorders

Psychotic disorders manifest through a wide array of symptoms, which can vary in severity, duration, and impact on daily functioning. The hallmark features of psychosis include:

1. **Hallucinations:** Perceptual disturbances involving sensory experiences in the absence of external stimuli. Common types of hallucinations include auditory (e.g., hearing voices), visual, tactile, olfactory, and gustatory hallucinations.
2. **Delusions:** Fixed, false beliefs that

are resistant to evidence or logical reasoning. Delusions may involve themes of persecution, grandiosity, reference, control, or nihilism.

3. **Disorganized Thinking:** Impaired thought processes characterized by tangentiality, derailment, incoherence, or loosening of associations. Disorganized thinking contributes to difficulties in communication and goal-directed behavior.
4. **Negative Symptoms:** Deficits in emotional expression, motivation, social engagement, and cognitive functioning. Negative symptoms may include affective flattening, anhedonia, avolition, and social withdrawal.
5. **Impaired Reality Testing:** Difficulty distinguishing between internal experiences (e.g., thoughts, feelings, perceptions) and external reality. Impaired reality testing contributes to the formation and persistence of psychotic symptoms.

7.1.2.3.5. Diagnosis of Psychotic Disorders

The diagnosis of psychotic disorders relies on comprehensive clinical assessment, including detailed history-taking, mental status examination, collateral information from family members or caregivers, and appropriate laboratory and imaging studies to rule out medical or substance-induced causes. Key diagnostic criteria include:

1. **Duration and Severity:** Symptoms must persist for a specified duration (e.g., at least six months for schizophrenia) and significantly impair social, occupational, or other areas of functioning.
2. **Exclusion of Other Causes:** Psychotic symptoms should not be attributable to substance intoxication or withdrawal, medication side effects, or another medical condition.
3. **Presence of Psychotic Features:** The presence of hallucinations, delusions, disorganized thinking, or grossly disorganized or catatonic behavior is essential for the diagnosis of psychotic disorders.
4. **Subtypes and Specifiers:** Subtypes of psychotic disorders, such as paranoid, disorganized, catatonic, and undifferentiated schizophrenia, may be specified based on predominant symptomatology and clinical presentation.

7.1.2.3.6. Treatment Approaches for Psychotic Disorders

The management of psychotic disorders typically involves a multimodal approach incorporating pharmacological, psychosocial, and supportive interventions tailored to the individual's needs and preferences. Key treatment modalities include:

1. **Antipsychotic Medications:** Antipsychotic drugs are the cornerstone of pharmacological treatment for psychotic disorders. First-generation (typical) and second-generation (atypical) antipsychotics are prescribed to alleviate psychotic symptoms and prevent relapse.
2. **Psychosocial Interventions:** Psychosocial interventions, such as cognitive-behavioral therapy (CBT), family therapy, supportive therapy, and social skills training, can help individuals cope with symptoms, improve functional outcomes, and enhance quality of life.
3. **Rehabilitation Services:** Rehabilitation services, including

vocational rehabilitation, supported employment, housing assistance, and assertive community treatment (ACT), aim to promote recovery, independence, and community integration in individuals with psychotic disorders.

4. **Hospitalization and Crisis Intervention:** In cases of severe symptom exacerbation, suicidal ideation, or impairment in reality testing, hospitalization may be necessary to ensure safety, stabilize acute symptoms, and initiate appropriate treatment interventions.

7.2. Mental Health Stigma

Mental health stigma is a pervasive social issue that affects millions of people worldwide. It refers to the negative attitudes, beliefs, and stereotypes surrounding mental illness, which often lead to discrimination, prejudice, and marginalization of individuals experiencing mental health challenges. Despite significant progress in understanding and treating mental health conditions, stigma remains a significant barrier to seeking help, accessing treatment, and achieving recovery for those affected.

7.2.1. Origins and Evolution of Mental Health Stigma

Mental health stigma has deep historical roots, dating back centuries when mental illness was often misunderstood and attributed to supernatural causes or moral failings. Throughout history, individuals with mental health conditions were often ostracized, feared, or subjected to inhumane treatments, reinforcing negative perceptions and attitudes toward mental illness.

The institutionalization of people with mental illness during the 19th and early 20th centuries further perpetuated stigma by segregating individuals from society and labeling them as "insane" or "unfit." This segregation reinforced the perception of mental illness as something to be hidden or ashamed of, contributing to the development of pervasive societal attitudes that continue to influence perceptions of mental health today.

7.2.2. Manifestations of Mental Health Stigma

Mental health stigma manifests in various forms, including:

1. **Social Stigma:** Social stigma involves negative attitudes and beliefs held by society towards individuals with mental illness. This stigma can lead to social exclusion, discrimination, and the perpetuation of stereotypes that portray those with mental health conditions as dangerous, unpredictable, or incompetent.
2. **Self-Stigma:** Self-stigma occurs when individuals internalize negative stereotypes and beliefs about mental illness, leading to feelings of shame, low self-esteem, and reluctance to seek help. Self-stigma can significantly impact an individual's willingness to engage in treatment and recovery efforts, perpetuating cycles of distress and avoidance.
3. **Structural Stigma:** Structural stigma refers to systemic barriers within institutions and policies that contribute to the marginalization of individuals with mental health conditions. This can include limited access to healthcare services, discriminatory practices in employment and housing, and inadequate funding for mental health programs and initiatives.

7.2.3. Impact of Mental Health Stigma

The impact of mental health stigma is profound and far-reaching, , communities, and society as a whole. Some of the key impacts include: affecting individuals, families

1. **Barriers to Treatment:** Stigma creates significant barriers to accessing mental health treatment and support services. Many individuals delay or avoid seeking help due to fear of judgment, rejection, or discrimination, leading to untreated mental health conditions and exacerbation of symptoms.
2. **Reduced Quality of Life:** Stigma contributes to social isolation, loneliness, and diminished quality of life for individuals with mental illness. The fear of being judged or misunderstood can lead to withdrawal from social activities, strained relationships, and feelings of alienation and despair.
3. **Economic Burden:** Stigma imposes a substantial economic burden on individuals, families, and society. The costs associated with untreated mental illness, including healthcare expenses, lost productivity, and unemployment, place strain on healthcare systems and contribute to socioeconomic disparities.
4. **Negative Health Outcomes:** Stigma has been linked to negative health outcomes for individuals with mental illness, including higher rates of substance abuse, suicide, and chronic physical health conditions. The stress of stigma can exacerbate symptoms of mental illness and undermine efforts towards recovery and well-being.
5. **Cultural and Intersectional Factors:** Stigma intersects with cultural, racial, and identity-related factors, leading to unique experiences of discrimination and marginalization for certain groups. Cultural beliefs, language barriers, and systemic inequalities can further exacerbate stigma and limit access to culturally competent care and support.

7.2.4. Strategies for Combating Mental Health Stigma

Addressing mental health stigma requires a multifaceted approach that involves individuals, communities, institutions, and policymakers. Some effective strategies for combating stigma include:

1. **Education and Awareness:** Increasing public education and awareness about mental health is essential for challenging stereotypes, dispelling myths, and fostering greater understanding and empathy. Educational initiatives in schools, workplaces, and communities can help promote mental health literacy and reduce stigma.
2. **Media Representation:** Media plays a powerful role in shaping public perceptions of mental health. Encouraging accurate and empathetic portrayals of mental illness in the media can help challenge stereotypes and promote positive representations of individuals living with mental health conditions.
3. **Language and Communication:** Language plays a crucial role in shaping attitudes towards mental health. Encouraging the use of person-first language and avoiding stigmatizing terms can help promote respectful and inclusive communication about mental illness.
4. **Peer Support and Advocacy:** Peer support groups and advocacy organizations play a vital role in

empowering individuals with lived experience to challenge stigma, share their stories, and advocate for change. Peer support networks provide validation, connection, and encouragement for individuals navigating their mental health journey.

5. **Policy and Legal Reform:** Addressing structural stigma requires policy and legal reform to ensure equitable access to mental health services, protect the rights of individuals with mental illness, and dismantle discriminatory practices in healthcare, employment, and housing. Advocating for policy changes at the local, national, and international levels is essential for promoting systemic change.
6. **Cultural Competence:** Recognizing and addressing cultural factors in mental health stigma is critical for ensuring that services and supports are accessible and responsive to the needs of diverse communities. Culturally competent care involves understanding and respecting the cultural beliefs, values, and experiences of individuals and tailoring services accordingly.(Barbui et al., 2010; Bora et al., 2011).

7.3. Advocacy in Mental Health

Advocacy in mental health is a crucial component of promoting awareness, challenging stigma, and advancing policies and practices that support the well-being of individuals with mental illness. Mental health advocacy encompasses a range of activities aimed at influencing public attitudes, shaping policies, and improving access to care and support services.

7.3.1. What Is Advocacy?

The concept of mental health advocacy has been developed to promote the human rights of persons with mental disorders and to reduce stigma and discrimination. It consists of various actions aimed at changing the major structural and attitudinal barriers to achieving positive mental health outcomes in populations.

Advocacy in this field began more than 30 years ago when the families of people with mental disorders first made their voices heard. People with mental disorders then added their contributions. Gradually, these people and their families were joined and supported by a range of organizations, many mental health workers and their associations, and some governments. Recently, the concept of advocacy has been broadened to include the needs and rights of persons with mild mental disorders and the mental health needs and rights of the general population.

Advocacy is considered to be one of the 11 areas for action in any mental health policy because of the benefits that it produces for people with mental disorders and their families. The advocacy movement has substantially influenced mental health policy and legislation in some countries and is believed to be a major force behind the improvement of services in others (World Health Organization).

7.3.2. Importance of Mental Health Advocacy

Mental health advocacy is of paramount importance for several reasons, each contributing to the well-being of individuals, communities, and society as a whole. Here are some key reasons highlighting the significance of mental health advocacy:

1. **Reducing Stigma and Discrimination:** Mental health advocacy helps challenge the stigma and discrimination

surrounding mental illness. By raising awareness, sharing personal stories, and promoting understanding, advocates work to break down stereotypes and misconceptions that contribute to discrimination and social exclusion.

2. **Promoting Access to Care:** Advocacy efforts play a critical role in advocating for policies, funding, and resources that improve access to mental health care and support services. This includes advocating for parity in insurance coverage, expanding community-based services, and addressing barriers to care for marginalized populations.
3. **Empowering Individuals:** Mental health advocacy empowers individuals with lived experience to share their stories, access support, and advocate for their rights. By amplifying the voices of those affected by mental illness, advocacy creates opportunities for empowerment, validation, and self-advocacy.
4. **Influencing Policy and Legislation:** Advocacy in mental health contributes to shaping policies and legislation that support mental health promotion, prevention, and treatment. Advocates engage with policymakers, participate in legislative processes, and advocate for changes that prioritize mental health as a public health priority.
5. **Improving Quality of Life:** Mental health advocacy efforts contribute to improving the quality of life for individuals with mental illness by advocating for services and supports that meet their needs. This includes promoting recovery-oriented approaches, advocating for housing and employment opportunities, and addressing social determinants of health.
6. **Addressing Structural Inequities:** Mental health advocacy addresses structural inequities and systemic barriers that contribute to disparities in mental health outcomes. By advocating for social justice, equity, and inclusion, advocates work to dismantle systems of oppression and promote health equity for all.
7. **Fostering Community Support:** Advocacy efforts build community support and solidarity around mental health issues, fostering a culture of empathy, understanding, and support. By engaging with communities, educating the public, and promoting dialogue, advocates create environments that promote mental health and well-being.
8. **Preventing Suicide and Mental Health Crises:** Mental health advocacy plays a crucial role in suicide prevention and crisis intervention by promoting awareness, reducing stigma, and advocating for accessible and effective mental health services. By advocating for early intervention, support networks, and crisis response systems, advocates help prevent tragedies and save lives.
9. **Promoting Research and Innovation:** Advocacy in mental health contributes to advancing research, innovation, and evidence-based practices in the field. By advocating for funding, collaboration, and support for research initiatives, advocates drive progress toward better understanding, treatment, and prevention of mental illness.
10. **Creating Social Change:** Mental health advocacy contributes to broader social change by challenging systems of oppression, promoting human rights, and advocating for policies and practices that promote social justice

and equity. By advocating for a more inclusive and compassionate society, advocates contribute to creating environments that support mental health and well-being for all.

7.3.3. Roles of Different Groups in Advocacy

1. Patients and Families – Patients have played various roles in advocacy, ranging from influencing policies and legislation to providing concrete help for persons with mental disorders. The provision of care for persons with mental disorders is a distinctive role for families, particularly in developing countries. In many places, they are the primary care providers and their organizations are fundamental as support networks. In addition to providing mutual support and services, many family groups have become advocates, educating the community, increasing the support obtained from policy-makers, denouncing stigma and discrimination, and fighting for improved services
2. Nongovernmental organizations involving mental health professionals, or people from diverse fields fulfil many of the advocacy roles described for patients and families. Their distinctive contribution to the advocacy movement is that they support and empower patients and families
3. General health workers and mental health workers have taken a more active role in protecting patients' rights and raising awareness for improved services, where care has been shifted from psychiatric hospitals to community services. Some specific advocacy roles for mental health workers relate to clinical work from a patient and family perspective and planning and participation in the activities of patients and family groups
4. Policy-makers and planners in the ministries of health play an important role in advocacy either by direct actions to influence the mental health of populations or working indirectly through supporting advocacy groups (patients, families, nongovernmental organizations, mental health workers), convincing other policy-makers and planners, e.g., the executive branch of government, the ministry of finance and other ministries, the judiciary, the legislature, and political parties, to focus on and invest in mental health.

7.3.4. Mental Health Advocacy Examples

There are many instances of advocacy programs for mental health that aim to lower stigma, raise awareness, and provide more people with access to mental health services. Public health leaders are better equipped to address the mental health needs of their communities and create successful mental health policies and programs when they are aware of pertinent organizations and initiatives.

Reducing stigma and increasing public awareness of mental health issues are frequently achieved through the work of mental health advocacy groups and initiatives. Together with these groups and programs, public health leaders can lower barriers to care and raise mental health awareness. Public health leaders can also help individuals and families get the support they need by connecting them with these organizations' and initiatives' services and resources.

7.3.4.1. Mental Health Advocacy Organizations

The following mental health advocacy organizations and initiatives serve as a great place to start for public health leaders exploring the resources that can support their advocacy efforts.

1. **National Alliance on Mental Illness (NAMI):** NAMI is a grassroots mental health advocacy organization that works to enhance the lives of people with mental illness and their families. They provide advocacy campaigns, support groups, and educational programs to broaden access to high-quality mental health care. These include:

- The Mental Health Advocate Program trains volunteers to advocate for individuals and families affected by mental illness and help them navigate the mental healthcare system.
- NAMI Basics provides a free six-week education program for parents and caregivers of children and adolescents with mental illness. The program provides information on mental illness, treatment options, communication strategies, and advocacy.

2. **Mental Health America (MHA):** Mental Health America, a prominent mental health advocacy group in the United States, works to advance mental health and wellness, prevent mental illnesses, and enhance access to mental health services. The organization provides individuals and communities with a range of resources, tools, and information to aid them in their mental health endeavors. Two MHA initiatives include:

- **B4Stage4** strives to change how people think about mental health by promoting early identification and intervention for mental health conditions and emphasizing that, like other chronic illnesses, mental health conditions are easier to manage when identified and treated early. The initiative provides tools for individuals and organizations that support early intervention efforts.
- **Screening to Supports (S2S)** offers free, confidential mental health screenings to individuals online. The initiative aims to make it easy and accessible for individuals to assess their mental health and find support and resources. S2S also provides referral resources for individuals seeking treatment.

7.3.4.2. Active Minds

Active Minds is a nonprofit organization dedicated to combating the stigma surrounding mental health and encouraging young adults to seek help when needed. They provide mental health education and advocacy programs led by peers on college campuses and in high schools.

Their initiatives include:

- **Send Silence Packing:** It features an exhibit of 1,100 backpacks, representing the number of college students who die by suicide each year. The exhibit travels to college campuses across the country and serves as a starting point for conversations about mental health and stigma.
- **Active Minds @Work:** It focuses on mental health and support in the workplace. The program provides

employers with resources including webinars, tool kits, and workshops designed to help organizations develop policies and practices that prioritize employee mental health and well-being. It also offers training to create a mental health-friendly workplace culture and to support employees in managing their mental health.

7.3.4.3. American Foundation for Suicide Prevention (AFSP)

AFSP aims to save lives and bring hope to those affected by suicide. They offer education, support groups, and resources for individuals and families affected by suicide. The organization also lobbies for suicide prevention legislation and policies that prioritize mental health and suicide prevention at the local, state, and federal levels. Their initiatives include:

- **Out of the Darkness Walks** serve as fundraising events in hundreds of communities across the U.S. each year. The walks raise awareness about suicide prevention and support AFSP's research and advocacy initiatives.
- **Interactive Screening Program** is a web-based mental health screening tool used at many organizations including universities, hospitals, and law enforcement agencies. It allows individuals to complete a self-assessment and receive personalized feedback, as well as referrals to resources if needed.

7.3.4.4. Black Mental Health Alliance (BMHA)

BMHA focuses on developing and supporting culturally relevant education, training, and referral services that support the health and well-being of Black individuals and other underserved communities. The organization aims to increase awareness and access to mental health services, promoting the development of social and emotional intelligence, as well as the health and well-being of Black communities. BMHA initiatives include:

- **The Black Mental Health Provider Directory:** It helps people locate Black therapists, psychologists, psychiatrists, and other mental health providers. The directory includes professionals trained in cultural competency and with experience working with Black communities. The initiative works to address the underrepresentation of Black mental health providers and the unique challenges faced by Black individuals seeking mental health care.
- **Emotional Emancipation Circles**: It is created by the Community Healing Network, are community healing circles that BMHA sponsors. The program involves group discussions and activities designed to help participants understand the various forms of racism and their impact on mental health, including racial stress and historical trauma. The groups also focus on internalized racism — ways in which individuals may internalize negative messages and beliefs about their own racial identity.

7.4. Community Mental Health Care Worldwide

The majority of individuals with mental illnesses worldwide do not receive treatment (Wang PS, Aguilar-Gaxiola S, Alonso J, et al., 2007).

The "treatment gap" is becoming more widely recognized globally. The first edition of the Mental Health Gap Action Program (mhGAP) Implementation Guide, which provides case finding and treatment guidelines for nine categories of mental and neurological disorders that have a significant impact on global public health, was published by the World Health Organization (WHO) in 2010.

This evidence-based approach is currently being implemented in more than 90 countries across the globe. This paper addresses the question of which pattern of services and systems of care are most effective in supporting the delivery of quality treatment and care for individuals with mental illnesses in various scenarios. This includes not only comparing high-income countries to low-income countries but also examining high-resource areas versus low-resource areas within countries. The paper focuses on the current status and innovative advancements in community mental health care on a global scale.

7.4.1. Defining Community Mental Health Care

Our definition of community mental health care highlights several fundamental issues.

First, Community mental health care involves: a) focusing on the population as a whole, b) considering patients within their socio-economic circumstances, c) preventive measures for individuals and the population, d) a comprehensive approach to service delivery, e) providing easy access to services, f) offering services as part of a team, g) taking a long-term perspective on mental health needs, and h) ensuring cost-effective care for the population. Additionally, it emphasizes social justice by addressing the needs of marginalized populations, such as ethnic minorities, homeless individuals, children and adolescents, and immigrants, by providing services that are accessible and acceptable to those in need (Thornicroft et al., 2010).

Second, community mental health care strives to not only address individuals' weaknesses and limitations from an illness perspective, but also to recognize and enhance their strengths, abilities, and goals from a recovery perspective. Services are designed to help individuals build a positive self-concept, understand their illness, effectively manage it, and pursue meaningful social roles that align with their values.

Third, the community is encompassed by community mental health care in a wide sense. As a logical extension of the second point, it highlights the assets of the communities, organizations, and social networks that support those with mental illnesses in addition to the mitigation or management of environmental adversity.

Fourth, evidence-based medicine and practical ethics are combined in community mental health care. Using the best data on intervention effectiveness that is currently available is prioritized in a scientific approach to services. Simultaneously, individuals with mental illnesses have the right to comprehend their conditions (to the extent that medical professionals comprehend them), weigh their options for interventions and any available data on their benefits and drawbacks, and have their preferences taken into account during a shared decision-making process.

Community mental health care is the set of principles and practices that aim to improve mental health within a specific population by (1) addressing the needs of the population in accessible and acceptable ways, (2) leveraging the strengths and goals of individuals with mental illnesses, (3) creating a broad network of support, services, and resources that are sufficient in capacity, and (4) prioritizing evidence-based and recovery-oriented services.

7.4.2. A Conceptual Framework for Community Mental Health Care

Based on the current evidence, a care model that only includes hospital-based services (usually inpatient and outpatient care) will not be adequate to give people who face care barriers access and continuity of follow-up for those with longer-term disabilities. However, there is insufficient proof that community-based services by themselves can provide the short bursts of intensive care that are occasionally required during mental health emergencies. to provide hospital-based and community-based services, a conceptual framework known as the balanced care model was developed.

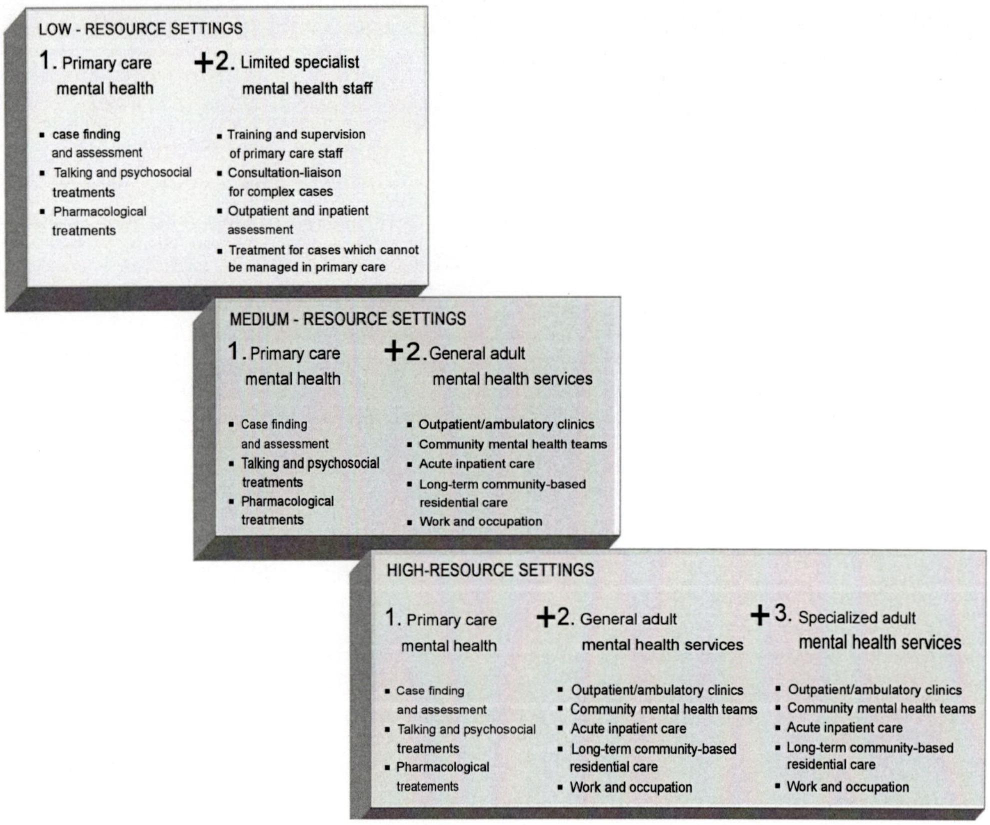

Figure 7.1. *Balanced care model in relation to high-, middle- and low-income countries.*

Source: https://www.ncbi.nlm.nih.gov/pmc/articles/PMC5032514/figure/wps20349-fig-0001/.

However, it is evident that high-income nations have roughly 200 times more financial resources available to them for mental health services than do low-income nations. In contrast to the US, which has 137 psychiatrists per million, many low-income countries in sub-Saharan Africa, such as Chad, Eritrea, and Liberia, have only one psychiatrist per million people. Therefore, a single global model of care is just not applicable. As a result, the balanced care model applies somewhat differently to nations that the World Bank Group classifies as high-, middle-, or low-income (see Figure 7.1). If the balanced care model is used, it must be carefully considered for any major or minor adaptation in any given site or nation.

According to the balanced care model, the majority of mental health resources in low-income nations or locations should go toward hiring staff for community settings and primary healthcare. These employees' responsibilities also include conducting assessments and case findings, providing brief psychosocial counselling, administering medication, and more. Only training and supervision for primary care staff, consultation liaison for complex cases, and outpatient and inpatient assessment and treatment for cases that cannot be managed in primary care are provided by the extremely small number of specialist mental health care staff (usually in the capital city and occasionally also in regional centers).

Although there is still a lack of evidence regarding several aspects of inpatient care or highly supported alternative settings, the balanced care model in middle-income settings suggests investing in five essential components of general adult mental health services: (a) outpatient/ambulatory clinics; (b) community mental health teams; (c) acute inpatient care; (d) long term community-based residential care, with an appropriate range of support; and (e) options for work and occupation.

The balanced care model suggests that, in high-income settings, a range of specialized services should be offered, as resources permit, in addition to primary care and general adult mental health services (see Figure 7.1). The same five categories that are specified for middle-income nations must apply to these services.

7.4.3. Community Services Provided Across Wider Platforms of Care

Some mental health interventions may be more effective if provided by entities outside of traditional health services, as outlined in the Disease Control Priorities Manual (DSP-3). These wider interventions, known as "platforms," include population-level initiatives such as legislation and public information campaigns, as well as community-level initiatives in schools, workplaces, and community groups. A recent review of evidence from low- and middle-income settings has identified the most cost-effective interventions in these areas.

Evidence-based interventions at the population level include laws and regulations that restrict access to means of self-harm/suicide, child protection laws, laws promoting conditional cash transfers to alleviate poverty, and widespread public awareness campaigns. Laws and regulations to reduce demand for alcohol use include those that enforce blood alcohol limits for drivers, alcohol taxes, advertising bans, and minimum drinking age.

Interventions with proven efficacy at the community level include incorporating mental health promotion techniques (e.g., integration of stress reduction and education about alcohol and drug abuse) into occupational health and safety policies; broad and focused socio-emotional learning school programs for children at risk; mental health awareness school programs; strategies for identifying and detecting mental health disorders in children attending school; early childhood enrichment/preschool educational programs; parenting programs for children between the ages of two and fourteen; gender equity and/or economic empowerment programs for vulnerable groups; and training for gatekeepers (such as community health workers, police, and social workers) in the identification of youth with mental disorders, including self-harm. (Chibanda et al., 2011).

7.4.4. The Extent of Community Mental Health Service Development

Globally, there is a great deal of variation in how community mental health services are developed. The WHO World Mental Health Atlas, which enumerates the salient features of national mental health systems worldwide and is updated regularly, is the most comprehensive global source of information in this regard. In the most recent edition (2014), data from 171 of the 194 United Nations members are included.

The proportionate spending on mental hospitals, other inpatient and day care facilities, as well as outpatient and primary care services, is displayed in Figure 7.2 for lower middle-income, upper middle-income, and high-income nations. The stark differences in absolute spending and the varying relative spending across the three service categories are demonstrated by this, further supporting the idea that a comparatively small portion of the meager mental health budgets in low- and middle-income nations is allocated to outpatient care.

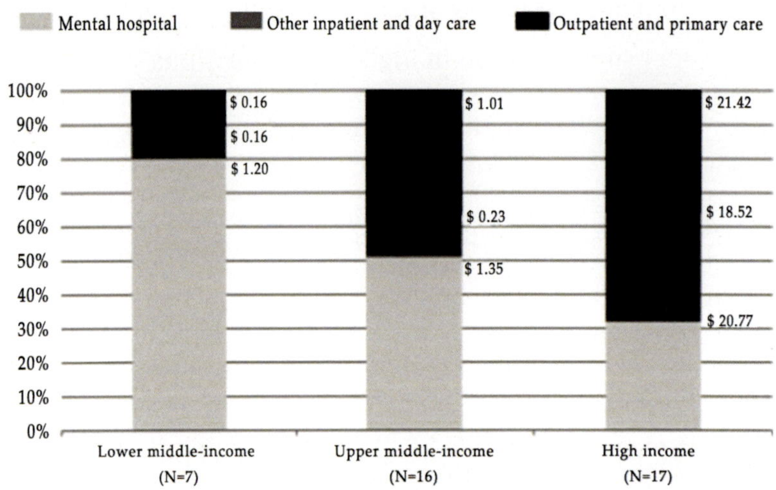

Figure 7.2. *Global distribution of mental health expenditure per capita, by health setting.*

Source: https://www.ncbi.nlm.nih.gov/pmc/articles/PMC5032514/Figure/wps20349-fig-0002/.

The WHO Atlas reveals several noteworthy trends. In comparison to the findings of the 2011 survey, there was a minor (5%) decline in the total number of mental hospitals worldwide, and a more significant (nearly 30%) decline in the number of mental hospital beds, with the Region of the Americas experiencing the largest decline (45%). Concurrently, there was a notable rise of more than 20% in the number of admissions to mental health facilities, suggesting a rising rate of bed turnover and a declining average duration of stay.

On a worldwide scale, the amount of beds in psychiatric units in mainstream hospitals grew by 60% from 2011 to 2014. Specifically in the Western Pacific Region, the number of psychiatric beds in mainstream hospitals increased over 8 times since 2011. The information provided by the WHO Atlas lacks sufficient data to determine if decreasing the number of beds in psychiatric hospitals correlates with increased spending on community services.

7.4.5. Developing Community Mental Health Models in Low and Middle Income Countries

More specific patterns in the evolution of community mental health services in recent years can be found in the work of the WPA Task Force on the Steps, Obstacles, and Mistakes to Avoid in the Implementation of Community Mental Health Care. The present study integrated an examination of pertinent literature with comprehensive consultation procedures across multiple global locations to pinpoint obstacles and remedies in the execution of community-based mental health care models. Table 7.1 enumerates the primary obstacles that were found and provides instances of strategies that have occasionally led to advancements.

Table 7.1. *Obstacles, Challenges, Lessons Learned and Solutions in Implementing Community-Oriented Mental Health Care*

Obstacles and Challenges		**Examples of Lessons Learned and Solutions**
Society	Disregard for, or violation of, human rights of people with mental illness	• Oversight by: civil society and service user groups, government inspectorates, international non-governmental organizations (NGOs), professional associations
	Stigma and discrimination, reflected in negative attitudes of health staff	• Encourage consumer family and carer involvement in policy-making, medical training, service provision (e.g., board member, consumer provider), service evaluation (consumer satisfaction survey)
	Need to address different models of abnormal behavior	• Traditional and faith-based paradigms need to be amalgamated, blended, or aligned as much as possible with medical paradigms
Government	The low priority given by the government to mental health	• Government task force on mental illness • Establish cross-party political support for the national policy and implementation • Effective advocacy on the mental health gap, global burden of disease, impact of mental health conditions, cost-effectiveness of interventions
	Absence or inappropriate mental health policy	• Advocate for and formulate policy based upon widespread consultation with the full range of stakeholder groups
	Old or inappropriate mental health legislation	• Create a powerful lobby and rationale for mental health law
	Inadequate financial resources to population-level needs	• Recruit key political and governance champions to advocate for adequate funding of initiatives

	Lack of alignment between payment methods, services, and outcomes	• Provide small financial incentives for valued outcomes • Create categories of reimbursement consistent with system strategy
	Need to address infrastructure	• Government to plan and finance efficient use of buildings, essential supplies, and electronic information systems
	Need to address the structure of community-oriented service system	• Design the mental health system from local primary care to regional care to central specialty care and fill in gaps with new resources as funding grows
	Inadequate human resources for delivery of mental health care	• Task sharing with non-traditional staff cadres such as community health workers and health extension workers
	Brain drain and failure to retain staff	• United Nations agencies/international NGOs to optimize the sustainability of their projects
	Non-sustainable, parallel programs by international NGOs	• Close relations with ministries and other stakeholders and international NGOs • Mental health plan in place so NGOs can help achieve these goals sustainably
Organization of the Health System	Need to design, monitor, and adjust the organization of the mental health system	• Set an implementation plan with clear coordination between services • Prioritization of target groups, especially people with severe mental illness
	Lack of a feasible mental health program or non-implementation of a mental health program	• Make the program highly practical by identifying resources available, tasks to be completed, allocation of responsibilities, timescales, reporting and accountability arrangements, progress monitoring/evaluation systems
	Need to specify developmental phases	• Planners and professional leaders to design five- and ten-year plans
	Poor utilization of existing mental health facilities	• Improve awareness of the benefits of facilities and services • Inbuilt monitoring of quality of care, especially process and outcome phases
	Need to include non-medical services	• Include families, faith-based social services, NGOs, housing services, vocational services, peer-support services, and self-help services. All stakeholders involved in designing the system
	Lack of multi-sectoral collaboration, e.g., including traditional healers, housing, criminal justice, or education sectors	• Development of a clear policy/implementation plan by all stakeholders • Collaborate with other local service to identify and help people with mental illness • Familiarization sessions between practitioners in the Western and local traditions

	Poor availability of psychotropic medication	• Drug revolving funds, public-private partnerships
Professionals and Practitioners	Need for leadership	• Psychiatrists and other professionals need to be involved as experts in planning, education, research, and overcoming inertia and resistance in the current environment
	Difficulty sustaining in-service training/adequate supervision	• Training of the trainers by staff from other regions or countries • Shifting of some psychiatric functions to trained and available practitioners
	High staff turnover and burnout, or low staff morale	• Emphasize career-long continuing training programs • Training of supervisors
	Poor quality of care/concern about staff skills	• Ongoing training and supervision • Encourage and reward quality by awards and similar processes
	Professional resistance, e.g., to community-oriented care and service user involvement	• Government and professional societies promote the importance of community-oriented care and service user involvement • Develop training in recovery-oriented psychosocial rehabilitation as part of training of new psychiatrists, including at medical schools in low- and middle-income countries
	Dearth of relevant research to inform cost-effective services and lack of data on mental health service evaluation	• More funding on research, for both qualitative and quantitative evidence of successfully implemented examples of community-oriented care
	Failure to address disparities (e.g., by ethnic, and economic groups)	• All key stakeholders involved; advocacy for under-represented groups to develop policies and implementation plans
Users, Families, and Other Advocates	Need for advocacy	• Users and other advocates may be involved in all aspects of social change, planning, lobbying the government, monitoring the development and functioning of the service system, and improving the service system
	Need for self-help and peer support services	• Users to lead these movements
	Need for shared decision-making	• Users and other advocates must demand at all levels that the system shift to value the goals of users and families and that shared decision-making become the norm

Source: https://www.ncbi.nlm.nih.gov/pmc/articles/PMC5032514/#wps20349-bib-0001.

One major problem that impacts most countries in the world is the persistent shortage of mental health professionals with training. As a result, different strategies have been put into place that assign non-specialized employees to tasks that were previously performed by psychiatrists or psychiatric nurses. Usually referred to as task shifting or task sharing, this reallocation of clinical tasks has been used to treat a variety of illnesses, such as diabetes, HIV/AIDS, epilepsy, surgery, and hypertension.

Emerging data suggests that this approach may be a financially viable way to treat and care for individuals with psychosis, depression, and perinatal mental health issues. As part of this new strategy, staff members will receive training utilizing tools like the WHO mhGAP Intervention Guide, which offers pertinent and lucid guidance that they can immediately apply in clinical settings. However, training on its own is insufficient, and it is becoming more and more obvious that continuing supervision is probably required to help staff start implementing the guidelines and develop and maintain clinical competence. Therefore, the costs of this kind of supervision must be factored into the core resources required to ensure the sustainability of community care.

Front-line healthcare providers like community health workers and positions in between the traditional roles of doctor and nurse, like clinical officer or medical officer, make up the new cadre of employees. These employees are frequently hired from the neighborhood and have extensive knowledge of the sociocultural setting.

First and foremost, a new training program that highlights the public health necessity of psychiatrists working directly in secondary and tertiary services as well as serving as multipliers by enhancing primary care staff's ability to identify and treat patients with mental illness is needed to rethink the role of the psychiatrist. It has been proposed that in high-income nations, modifications to the structure and operations of healthcare teams—such as those already in place to enhance outcomes in other chronic diseases—may well improve this capacity, particularly in the treatment of individuals with major depressive disorder. Active follow-up should be left to a case manager (like a practice nurse); treatment plans should be frequently modified when patients do not improve; adherence to treatment and patient outcomes should be routinely monitored; and the primary care physician and case manager should have the option to consult and refer to a psychiatrist when needed.

To enable the majority of patients with mental disorders to receive more effective treatment in primary care and to identify and refer the minority who require ongoing specialist care, it is thought that flexible and accessible working relationships between the primary care physician, the case manager, and a mental health specialist are essential. Further research is needed to determine how the concepts behind this model can be applied to low- and middle-income nations (Bora et al., 2011; Chibanda et al., 2011).

A Closer Look

Community Factors on Mental Health Outcomes

Community factors play a significant role in shaping mental health outcomes, often influencing an individual's well-being in profound ways. One crucial aspect is the availability and accessibility of mental health services within a community. Communities with well-established mental health support systems tend to have better outcomes as individuals can easily access resources such as therapy, counselling, and support groups. Conversely, in communities where mental health services are scarce or stigmatized, individuals may face barriers in seeking help, leading to untreated mental health issues and poorer outcomes.

Social support networks within a community also play a vital role in mental health. Strong social connections can provide emotional support, reduce feelings of loneliness and isolation, and buffer against stressors that contribute to mental health problems. Communities that foster a sense of belonging and interconnectedness tend to have better mental health outcomes as individuals feel supported and valued by those around them. On the other hand, communities characterized by social fragmentation or isolation may experience higher rates of mental health issues due to the lack of support networks and meaningful social interactions.

Furthermore, socioeconomic factors significantly impact mental health within communities. Poverty, unemployment, and inadequate housing can create chronic stressors that contribute to the development of mental health disorders such as depression and anxiety. Additionally, disparities in access to education, healthcare, and economic opportunities can exacerbate mental health inequalities within communities, disproportionately affecting marginalized populations. Addressing socioeconomic inequities and ensuring access to essential resources and opportunities is crucial for promoting positive mental health outcomes within communities.

Environmental factors also play a role in mental health. Communities with safe and supportive physical environments, including access to green spaces, recreational facilities, and safe neighborhoods, tend to have better mental health outcomes. Conversely, communities plagued by crime, pollution, and environmental hazards can contribute to feelings of insecurity, stress, and anxiety, negatively impacting mental well-being. Promoting environmental sustainability and creating safe, healthy community environments are essential for fostering positive mental health outcomes.

Summary

- Mental health is about how people think, feel, and behave. Mental health care professionals can help people manage conditions such as depression, anxiety, bipolar disorder, addiction, and other disorders that affect their thoughts, feelings, and behaviors.
- Mental health conditions encompass mental disorders, psychosocial disabilities, and other mental states that may cause significant distress, impair functioning, or pose a risk of self-harm.
- People with mental health conditions are more likely to experience lower levels of mental well-being, but this is not always or necessarily the case.
- Anxiety is a normal stress reaction. Mild levels of anxiety can be beneficial in some situations. It can alert us to dangers and help us prepare and pay attention. Anxiety disorders differ from normal feelings of nervousness or anxiousness and involve excessive fear or anxiety. Anxiety disorders are the most common mental disorders. They affect nearly 30% of adults at some point in their lives. However, anxiety disorders are treatable with many psychotherapeutic treatments. Treatment helps most people lead normal productive lives.
- A mood disorder is a mental health condition that primarily affects your emotional state. It's a disorder in which you experience long periods of extreme happiness, extreme sadness, or both. Certain mood disorders involve other persistent emotions, such as anger and irritability.
- Schizophrenia is a psychiatric condition that has severe effects on your physical and mental well-being. It disrupts how your brain works, interfering with things like your thoughts, memory, senses and behaviors.

References

1. American Psychiatric Association. (2013). *Diagnostic and Statistical Manual of Mental Disorders* (5th ed.). Arlington, VA: American Psychiatric Publishing.
2. Barbui, C., Dua, T., Van Ommeren, M., et al. (2010). Challenges in developing evidence-based recommendations using the GRADE approach: The case of mental, neurological, and substance use disorders. *PLoS Medicine, 7*(8), e1000322. https://doi.org/10.1371/journal.pmed.1000322.
3. Bora, E., Fornito, A., Radua, J., et al. (2011). Neuroanatomical abnormalities in schizophrenia: A multimodal voxelwise meta-analysis and meta-regression analysis. *Schizophrenia Research, 127*(1–3), 46–57. https://doi.org/10.1016/j.schres.2010.12.020.
4. Chibanda, D., Mesu, P., Kajawu, L., et al. (2011). Problem-solving therapy for depression and common mental disorders in Zimbabwe: Piloting a task-shifting primary mental health care intervention in a population with a high prevalence of people living with HIV. *BMC Public Health, 11*(1), 828. https://doi.org/10.1186/1471-2458-11-828.
5. Clark, L. A., & Watson, D. (1991). Tripartite model of anxiety and depression: Psychometric evidence and taxonomic implications. *Journal of Abnormal Psychology, 100*(3), 316–336. https://doi.org/10.1037/0021-843X.100.3.316.

6. Collins, P. Y., & Saxena, S. (2016). Action on mental health needs global cooperation. *Nature, 532*(7597), 25–27. https://doi.org/10.1038/532025a.

7. Collins, P. Y., Patel, V., Joestl, S. S., et al. (2011). Grand challenges in global mental health. *Nature, 475*(7354), 27–30. https://doi.org/10.1038/475027a.

8. Correll, C. U., & Schooler, N. R. (2020). Negative symptoms in schizophrenia: A review and clinical guide for recognition, assessment, and treatment. *Neuropsychopharmacology, 45*(2), 168–177. https://doi.org/10.1038/s41386-019-0461-1.

9. Demyttenaere, K., Bruffaerts, R., Posada-Villa, J., et al. (2004). Prevalence, severity, and unmet need for treatment of mental disorders in the World Health Organization World Mental Health Surveys. *JAMA, 291*(21), 2581–2590. https://doi.org/10.1001/jama.291.21.2581.

10. Dua, T., Barbui, C., Clark, N., et al. (2011). Evidence-based guidelines for mental, neurological, and substance use disorders in low- and middle-income countries: Summary of WHO recommendations. *PLoS Medicine, 8*(11), e1001122. https://doi.org/10.1371/journal.pmed.1001122.

11. Felitti, V. J., Anda, R. F., Nordenberg, D., et al. (1998). Relationship of childhood abuse and household dysfunction to many of the leading causes of death in adults. *American Journal of Preventive Medicine, 14*(4), 245–258. https://doi.org/10.1016/S0749-3797(98)00017-8.

12. Fusar-Poli, P., Borgwardt, S., Bechdolf, A., et al. (2013). The psychosis high-risk state: A comprehensive state-of-the-art review. *JAMA Psychiatry, 70*(1), 107–120. https://doi.org/10.1001/jamapsychiatry.2013.269.

13. Heim, C., & Nemeroff, C. B. (2001). The role of childhood trauma in the neurobiology of mood and anxiety disorders: Preclinical and clinical studies. *Biological Psychiatry, 49*(12), 1023–1039. https://doi.org/10.1016/S0006-3223(01)01157-X.

14. Howes, O. D., & Murray, R. M. (2014). Schizophrenia: An integrated sociodevelopmental-cognitive model. *The Lancet, 383*(9929), 1677–1687. https://doi.org/10.1016/S0140-6736(13)62036-X.

15. Kahn, R. S., Sommer, I. E., Murray, R. M., et al. (2015). Schizophrenia. *Nature Reviews Disease Primers, 1*(1), 15067. https://doi.org/10.1038/nrdp.2015.67.

16. Kendler, K. S., & Eaves, L. J. (1986). Models for the joint effect of genotype and environment on liability to psychiatric illness. *American Journal of Psychiatry, 143*(3), 279–289. https://doi.org/10.1176/ajp.143.3.279.

17. Kendler, K. S., Gatz, M., Gardner, C. O., & Pedersen, N. L. (2006). A Swedish national twin study of lifetime major depression. *American Journal of Psychiatry, 163*(1), 109–114. https://doi.org/10.1176/appi.ajp.163.1.109.

18. McGrath, J., Saha, S., Chant, D., et al. (2008). Schizophrenia: A concise overview of incidence, prevalence, and mortality. *Epidemiologic Reviews, 30*(1), 67–76. https://doi.org/10.1093/epirev/mxn001.

19. Mueser, K. T., Deavers, F., Penn, D. L., & Cassisi, J. E. (2013). Psychosocial treatments for schizophrenia. *Annual Review of Clinical Psychology, 9*(1), 465–497. https://doi.org/10.1146/annurev-clinpsy-050212-185620.

20. National Institute for Health and Care Excellence (NICE). (2014). *Psychosis and Schizophrenia in Adults: Treatment and Management.* Clinical guideline [CG178]. London: NICE.

21. Nestler, E. J., & Hyman, S. E. (2010). Animal models of neuropsychiatric disorders. *Nature Neuroscience, 13*(10), 1161–1169. https://doi.org/10.1038/nn.2647.

22. Owen, M. J., Sawa, A., & Mortensen, P. B. (2016). Schizophrenia. *The Lancet, 388*(10039), 86–97. https://doi.org/10.1016/S0140-6736(15)01121-6.

23. Robinson, M., Mattes, E., Oddy, W. H., et al. (2009). Prenatal stress and risk of behavioral morbidity from age 2 to 14 years: The influence of the number, type, and timing of stressful life events. *Development and Psychopathology, 21*(1), 271–287. https://doi.org/10.1017/S0954579409000153.

24. Sapolsky, R. M. (2004). *Why Zebras Don't Get Ulcers: The Acclaimed Guide to Stress, Stress-Related Diseases, and Coping*. Holt Paperbacks.

25. Saxena, S., Thornicroft, G., Knapp, M., & Whiteford, H. (2007). Resources for mental health: Scarcity, inequity, and inefficiency. *The Lancet, 370*(9590), 878–889. https://doi.org/10.1016/S0140-6736(07)61239-2.

26. Sullivan, P. F., Neale, M. C., & Kendler, K. S. (2000). Genetic epidemiology of major depression: Review and meta-analysis. *American Journal of Psychiatry, 157*(10), 1552–1562. https://doi.org/10.1176/appi.ajp.157.10.1552.

27. Taylor, S. E. (2011). Social support: A review. In M. S. Friedman (Ed.), *The Handbook of Health Psychology* (pp. 189–214). Oxford University Press.

28. Thornicroft, G. (2007). Most people with mental illness are not treated. *The Lancet, 370*(9590), 807–808. https://doi.org/10.1016/S0140-6736(07)61392-0.

29. Thornicroft, G., & Tansella, M. (2009). *Better Mental Health Care*. Cambridge University Press.

30. Thornicroft, G., Alem, A., Antunes Dos Santos, R., et al. (2010). WPA guidance on steps, obstacles, and mistakes to avoid in the implementation of community mental health care. *World Psychiatry, 9*(2), 67–77. https://doi.org/10.1002/j.2051-5545.2010.tb00276.x.

31. Wang, P. S., Aguilar-Gaxiola, S., Alonso, J., et al. (2007). Use of mental health services for anxiety, mood, and substance disorders in 17 countries in the WHO World Mental Health Surveys. *The Lancet, 370*(9590), 841–850. https://doi.org/10.1016/S0140-6736(07)61414-7.

32. World Health Organization. (2010). *mhGAP Intervention Guide for Mental, Neurological, and Substance Use Disorders in Non-Specialized Health Settings*. Geneva: World Health Organization.

33. Wright, R. J., & Subramanian, S. V. (2007). Advancing a multilevel framework for epidemiologic research on asthma disparities. *Chest, 132*(5), 757S–769S. https://doi.org/10.1378/chest.07-1904.

Chapter 8

PREVENTION OF SEXUALLY TRANSMITTED DISEASES AND HIV

Contents

Introduction

The prevention of sexually transmitted diseases (STDs) and HIV is a critical public health priority aimed at reducing the incidence and impact of these infections. STDs, including chlamydia, gonorrhea, syphilis, herpes, human papillomavirus (HPV), and HIV, can lead to serious health complications if left untreated, such as infertility, chronic pain, and increased susceptibility to other infections. Effective prevention strategies are multifaceted, involving education, behavioral interventions, and medical measures.

Education plays a foundational role in STD and HIV prevention. Comprehensive sex education programs that start early and are age-appropriate provide individuals with the knowledge needed to make informed decisions about their sexual health. These programs emphasize the importance of safe sex practices, such as consistent and correct condom use, regular testing, and mutual monogamy. They also address myths and misconceptions about STDs and HIV, fostering a better understanding of how these infections are transmitted and prevented.

Behavioral interventions focus on reducing risky behaviors associated with the transmission of STDs and HIV. Encouraging open communication between sexual partners about sexual history and testing can reduce the likelihood of infection. Additionally, promoting the use of barrier methods like condoms and dental dams during all forms of sexual activity significantly decreases the risk of transmission. Pre-exposure prophylaxis (PrEP) is a highly effective medication that, when taken consistently, can prevent HIV infection in high-risk populations.

Medical interventions are also crucial in preventing the spread of STDs and HIV. Regular screening and early treatment of STDs can prevent complications and reduce transmission rates. Vaccinations for HPV and hepatitis B are effective preventive measures that can protect against these infections. For HIV, antiretroviral therapy (ART) not only improves the health outcomes of those living with the virus but also reduces their viral load to undetectable levels, effectively preventing transmission (U=U: undetectable equals untransmittable).

Orientation and Directional Terms

Term	**Definition**	**Illustration**
HIV	HIV is a sexually transmitted infection and occurs by contact with or transfer of blood, pre-ejaculate, semen, and vaginal fluids.	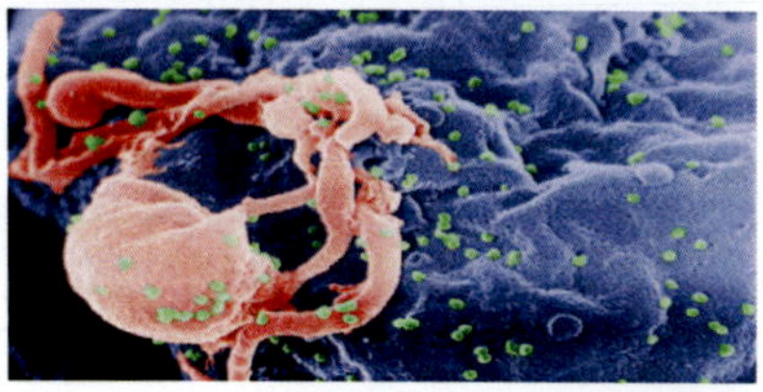
Donovanosis	Donovanosis, also known as granuloma inguinale, is a chronic, progressive, sexually transmitted bacterial infection (STI) that causes genital ulcers.	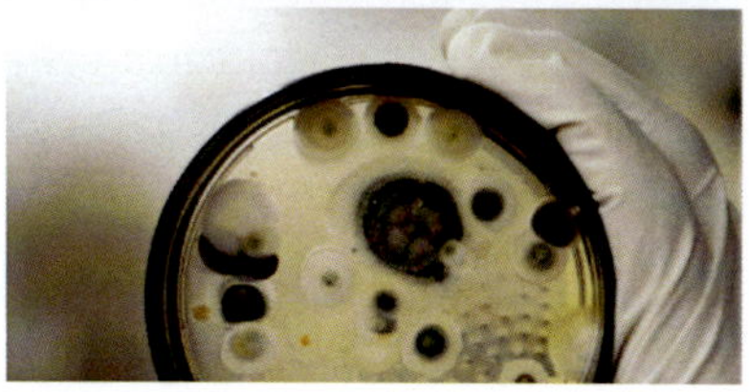
Lymphogranuloma	Lymphogranuloma venereum (LGV) is a sexually transmitted disease (STD) caused by infection with chlamydia trachomati bacteria.	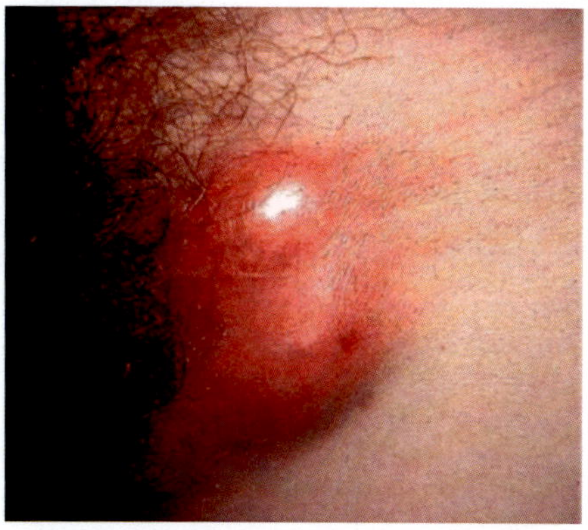
Trichomoniasis	Trichomoniasis is a sexually transmitted infection (STI) which is most often spread through vaginal, oral, or anal sex.	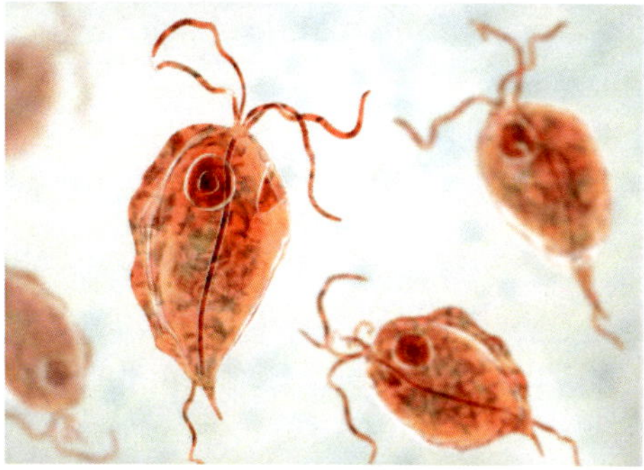

8.1. Etiology

STIs are a global health concern that every public health organization needs to be aware of. STIs are more often underdiagnosed and more common in populations with limited access to healthcare. The particular organism, route, signs, and symptoms all influence the presenting condition or disease. A history of STIs, prostitution, unprotected sexual contact with multiple partners, sexual assault, having a partner with multiple concurrent sexual contacts or a history of STIs, and alcohol or recreational drug use are risk factors that increase the transmission of STIs. Below is a list of specific causative organisms.

Some sexually transmitted infections (STIs), such as genital herpes, human papillomavirus, and particularly HIV, where the infective risk drops by 50–60%, appear to be considerably decreased by male circumcision. (Farley et al., 2020). The seven most common sexually transmitted infections (STIs) consist of three incurable but treatable conditions (herpes simplex virus, HIV, and human papillomavirus (HPV)) and five curable infections (chlamydia, gonorrhea, syphilis, and trichomonas). Interestingly, although they can also be spread sexually, hepatitis B and hepatitis C are more frequently contracted through other exposures.

The most common and relevant STIs include the following:

8.1.1. Chancroid

- *Haemophilus ducreyi* is the causative organism of chancroid.
- This fastidious Gram-negative coccobacillus (very short rod) requires special media and environmental conditions to grow in the culture.
- Microscopically, the organism will tend to form long strands, forming a pattern described as "railroad tracks" or "a school of fish."
- The organism significantly increases the risk and transmissibility of HIV.
- This infection is exceedingly rare in the United States (US) and developed countries globally.

8.1.2. Chlamydia

- Gram-negative obligate, nonmotile intracellular bacteria known as *Chlamydia trachomatis* (*C. trachomatis*).
- Typically, serotypes D-K.
- The most common curable sexually transmitted infection in the United States, according to the Centers for Disease Control (CDC) and the World Health Organization (WHO).
- Two infectious forms exist: the elementary (EB) and reticulate body (RB).
- The EB form invades the cell, and the RB form will produce other infectious EB that will infect other non-infectious forms.

8.1.3. Genital Herpes

- Genital herpes is caused by the herpes simplex virus 1 (HSV-1) or herpes simplex virus 2 (HSV-2).
- HSV is a double-stranded DNA virus coated by a lipoglycoprotein with an affinity to infect target cells.
- HSV-1 is usually associated with orolabial infections, but according to the CDC, HSV-1 is now leading in the cause of genital herpes in young and homosexual patients.

- There is an estimation that 50 million people in the US are infected with HSV.

8.1.4. Gonorrhea

- This condition is caused by Gram-negative diplococci bacteria *Neisseria gonorrhoeae. (N gonorrhoeae).*
- This is the second most common sexually transmitted infection in the US (the first is *C. trachomatis.*).
- Gonorrhea uses glucose to invade mucus epithelial cells.
- Gonorrhea modifies cellular proteins that allow further penetration of other organisms.
- The proliferation of gonorrhea leads to a localized inflammatory reaction, leading to signs and symptoms of an STI.

8.1.5. Granuloma Inguinale

- This is caused by Gram-negative intracellular *Klebsiella granulomatis,* formerly known as *Calymmatobacterium granulomatis.* (This is also referred to as Donovanosis.).
- Rarely found in the US, granuloma inguinale is seen mostly in developing countries, especially in the tropics.
- This condition is most commonly found in the Caribbean, southern Africa, South America, New Guinea, and India.

8.1.6. Human Immunodeficiency Virus and Acquired Immunodeficiency Syndrome

- These are enveloped retroviruses encapsulated with 2 single-stranded ribonucleic acids.
- Primary HIV signs and symptoms are described as flu-like and often diagnosed as an acute viral syndrome.
- The duration of onset of symptoms ranges from 4 to 10 weeks.
- Most HIV infections in the US are HIV1.
- Acquired immunodeficiency syndrome (AIDS) is described as the late stage of HIV disease.
- The median time to progression from HIV to AIDS is about 11 years but is highly variable.
- The risk of syphilis in patients infected with HIV is 77 times greater than in the general population.

8.1.7. Human Papillomavirus

- HPV is a double-stranded deoxyribonucleic acid virus that replicates in the basal cell layer of the stratified squamous epithelial cells. This replication cycle induces hyperplasia and possible conversion carcinoma.
- HPV types 16 and 18 are oncogenic strains that induce malignant transformation.
- Types 6 and 11 are common strains that induce anogenital warts, known as condyloma acuminata.

- By far, HPV is the most common sexually transmitted infectious organism in the US and worldwide.

8.1.8. Lymphogranuloma venereum

- This condition is caused by *Chlamydia trachomatis,* a Gram-negative obligate, nonmotile intracellular bacteria but a different serotype from the more common chlamydial infections.
- The bacteria are serotypes or serovars L1, L2, and L3.
- This infection is rare in the US but common in tropical and subtropical regions.
- Lymphogranuloma venereum is most frequently found in men who have sex with other men.
- Closely associated with HIV infections.

8.1.9. Mycoplasma genitalium

- *Mycoplasma genitalium* is the second most common cause of nongonococcal urethritis after chlamydia and a common cause of female cervicitis and resistant or recurrent urethritis.
- Mycoplasma is very slow growing in a culture, which can take up to 6 months.
- Since it lacks a cell wall, it cannot be gram-stained.
- Risk factors include young age (<25 years), smoking, frequent sexual contact, and a large number of sexual partners.
- This condition is closely associated with HIV infections.

8.1.10. Syphilis

- This illness is caused by a spirochete bacterium, *Treponema pallidum* (*T. pallidum*).
- *T. pallidum* is very slow-growing and cannot be cultured nor seen on standard light microscopy.
- The initial immune response is muted because *T. pallidum* has few exposed proteins and no lipopolysaccharides in its outer membrane.
- According to the CDC, infections of this type are increasing compared to previous reports.
- Syphilis is far more common in the developing world, particularly among the poorest populations with the most limited access to healthcare.
- This condition presents with a painless chancre, a well-demarcated lesion at the inoculation site.
- Syphilis presents in various forms and, depending on the duration, is classified as primary, secondary, or tertiary.

- Globally, this condition affects about 12% of men who have sex with men.

8.1.11. Trichomoniasis

- This condition is caused by single-celled flagellated anaerobic protozoa known as *Trichomonas vaginalis.*
- Trichomoniasis causes direct damage to the epithelium. The injuries lead to microulcerations primarily in the vagina, cervix, urethra, and paraurethral glands.

8.2. Epidemiology of STI

The human papillomavirus, or HPV, is the most prevalent STI in the United States. An estimated 80% of sexually active individuals are thought to be infected at any given time, with 42% of adults between the ages of 18 and 59 being among them. Oral HPV will affect 7% of those infected, and an estimated 14 million new cases of this illness are reported each year. Because HPV is so widespread, almost everyone who engages in sexual activity and is not vaccinated will contract the virus at some point in their lives, according to CDC estimates. At least 291 million women have HPV infections worldwide.

Roughly 24.4 million STIs unrelated to HPV were reported in the US in 2020, according to data from the CDC. Out of all of these, chlamydia was the most prevalent with 1.6 million cases. Subsequently, 133,945 cases of primary and secondary syphilis, up 52% over the same period, and 677,769 cases of gonorrhea, up 45% from 2016, were reported in 2020. *Congenital syphilis* was found in 2148 babies in 2020, a 235% increase from 2016.

Men account for more than 80% of primary and secondary syphilis cases that are reported. Nearly half (47%) of cases of men that are reported involve men having sex with other men. According to CDC estimates, 44% of men who test positive for syphilis and bisexual men who have sex with men will also test positive for HIV. In the US, the prevalence of STIs is generally rising.

According to the WHO, global epidemiological data for STIs indicates the following:

- Worldwide, over 1 million new potentially curable STIs are acquired daily, most of which are asymptomatic.
- There is an estimation that 376 million new infections occur annually, with one of the four curable STIs (chlamydia, gonorrhea, syphilis, and trichomoniasis).
- Of these, trichomonas is the most common globally, with 156 million new cases yearly, followed by chlamydia at 127 million, gonorrhea at 87 million, and syphilis at 6.3 million.
- The US incidence of STIs is rising; there was close to a 30% increase in reportable STIs between 2015 and 2019.
- About 12% of the US population between 14 and 49 years is estimated to be infected with herpes currently.
- Herpes simplex virus type 2 has a global prevalence estimated at over 500 million people.
- About one million pregnant women were estimated to have an STI in 2016, causing over 350,000 birthing or neonatal complications.
- HPV infections have been linked to over 310,000 cervical cancer deaths annually.

- Syphilis is the second leading cause of stillbirths worldwide.
- HIV/AIDS affected about 37 million people worldwide in 2016.
- About 15% of HIV-infected individuals in the US are unaware they have the infection and are responsible for 40% of all new HIV infections.
- According to the CDC, there are approximately 35,000 new cases of HIV in the US annually.
- *Mycoplasma genitalium* causes 15% to 20% of all non-gonococcal urethritis (NGU), 20% to 25% of all non-chlamydial NGU cases, and 40% of all recurrent or persistent urethritis infections.

A centralized data collection system would be ideal for analyzing and thoroughly assessing the incidence, distribution, progression, and treatment of all sexually transmitted infections (STIs). This would include physicians, public health officials, political leaders, international and regional healthcare organizations, and other healthcare professionals. As medical professionals, the most reliable sources are a variety of published studies as well as official government agencies and healthcare organizations that evaluate the statistical significance of sexually transmitted infections (STIs), taking into account factors like geographic regions with rising incidence or specific demographics of impacted populations. Most nations have high STI rates, particularly for those between the ages of 15 and 50. Infertility in women is thought to result from undiagnosed sexually transmitted infections in 20,000 cases per year in the US. (Fleming et al., 1999; Hayes et al., 1995).

8.3. Pathophysiology of STI

This review aims to provide a general overview of sexually transmitted infections (STIs), encompassing the most prevalent infections like gonorrhea, chlamydia, genital herpes, HPV, trichomoniasis, and syphilis. Bacterial, viral, or parasitic infections can result from sexual activity. Through microscopic abrasions in the mucosal membranes of the penis, vagina, anus, or any other mucosal surface, STIs enter the human body. STIs can spread through intravenous drug use, as well as through contact with the body during childbirth or nursing. Typical disease signs and symptoms are produced when organisms overburden the immune system and infiltrate normal cells.

The fundamental symptomatology, encompassing genital, extragenital, or disseminated, will be examined along with a physical examination and history to aid in differential diagnosis and suggested interventions. The presentation will include an overview of all common sexually transmitted infections and updated treatment guidelines from the WHO and CDC. Healthcare professionals, including physicians, need to be aware of the differences between treatable and incurable sexually transmitted infections. Infertility, scarring, chronic pain, sexual dysfunction, and cancers are just a few of the serious, lifelong health issues that can result from untreated STIs.

8.3.1. History and Physical of STI

To identify the main complaints of their patients and create a useful differential diagnosis, medical professionals are trained in effective communication with patients, partners, and families. Either in an emergency room or a primary clinic, obtaining a thorough medical history is a requirement. When a patient exhibits symptoms and signs that point to an undiagnosed STD, the clinician's job is to effectively communicate with the patient. Clinicians need to know that in the US, all adolescents under the age of 18 are entitled to an STI screening and treatment without their parents' permission.

Clinicians should be aware that there is a strong correlation between STIs and patient behavior. During the clinical evaluation, this relationship should be addressed in a polite, diplomatic, and nonjudgmental manner. The duties of healthcare providers include assisting, treating, and educating patients about their conditions as well as encouraging and recommending healthy behaviors that reduce the risk of re-infections.

While performing the sexual history collection, an easy mnemonic that can help guide clinical questions can be remembered as the "other 5 Ps":

1. Partners;
2. Practices;
3. Prevention against pregnancy;
4. Prior history of STIs; and
5. Protection against STIs.

The chief complaint that is currently presenting as well as the symptoms gathered during the system review should direct the physical examination. A chaperone should be present at the patient's bedside during the private examination, and their name should be recorded in the patient's medical file. Ask the patient an open-ended question after the examination to foster a candid discussion and find out if they have any additional information about their sexual behavior that has not yet been brought up. The most typical signs and symptoms, physical exam results, and diagnosis will be used to break down the physical examination.

8.3.1.1. Chancroid

- Women and Men
  - **Signs and Symptoms:** This condition often occurs in the 20 to 30-year-old age group, frequently among sex workers and their clients. The areas most often affected include the distal portion of the penis in men, while in women, the vagina, labia, and perianal regions are involved. The most significant symptom is the extremely high pain level noted when the lesion reaches the ulcerative stage.
  - **Physical Exam:** The lesion starts as a reddish papule, rapidly progressing to a pustule, followed by an extremely painful ulcer. The ulcer, sometimes called a "soft chancre," will have soft and irregular margins with a friable base and a grayish-yellowish exudate; the ulcer tends to bleed easily. The ulcers are typically 1 to 2 cm in diameter and usually resolve spontaneously within 3 months, even if left untreated. Close to half of the affected individuals will develop regional lymphadenopathy, which may be tender. A minority (about 25%) of these patients will progress to infected bulla or abscesses that can rupture and become superinfected, leading to significant tissue destruction and damage to the genitalia. There is an estimation that 10% of affected individuals will also have syphilis or genital herpes.

8.3.1.2. Chlamydia

- Women
  - **Signs and Symptoms**: Most infections can be asymptomatic but may present with vaginal discharge, abnormal vaginal bleeding, lower pelvic pain, urinary frequency, or dysuria. If systemic infection is present, the patient may be febrile, with abdominal pain, nausea, vomiting, fatigue, and malaise.
  - **Physical Exam:** Inflammation of the cervix with mucopurulent discharge can be seen, and ectropion, vaginal discharge, increased sensitivity of the cervix, and tenderness of the adnexal regions and abdomen are present. If systemic infection or Fitz-Hugh-Curtis syndrome is considered in the differential, right upper quadrant tenderness may be secondary to perihepatitis.
- Men
  - **Signs and Symptoms:** The most common presenting symptoms are dysuria, testicular pain, and pain with defecation secondary to inflammation of the rectal area and prostate. This common cause of male urethral discharge is typically beige or yellowish.
  - **Physical Exam:** Tenderness to the testicles (specifically over the epididymis) or discomfort with palpation to the prostate or rectum.

8.3.1.3. Genital Herpes

- Women and Men
  - **Signs and Symptoms:** Primary infections tend to induce systemic symptoms, including painful vesicular lesions over affected areas, pruritus, dysuria, fever, headaches, malaise, and lymphadenopathy. Initial infections typically resolve spontaneously, starting at about 2 weeks. Reactivation usually presents with a prodromal phase, including tingling, itching, and rash consistent with vesicular lesions. Recurrent infections tend to be less intense and have a shorter duration.
  - **Physical Exam:** The affected area may be localized or systemic. A primary herpes infection tends to be worse with diffuse symptomatically involving various systems, possibly resulting in pneumonitis, hepatitis, meningitis, and encephalitis. Women may have diffuse vesicular lesions in the internal and external vaginal areas. Men may have diffuse vesicular lesions to the glans of the penis, penile shaft, scrotum, perineal/perianal area, and rectum, both internally and externally. Recurrent herpes infections may cause isolated vesicular lesions over a neuronal tract where the virus is dormant.

8.3.1.4. Gonorrhea

- Women

- **Genitourinary Exam:** This may include inflammation of the external vagina, causing excoriations from pruritus, mucopurulent discharge, and friable inflamed mucosal tissue of the cervix.
- **Signs and Symptoms:** Patients may present with dysuria, urgency, urinary frequency, lower pelvic pain, and abnormal vaginal bleeding.
- **Physical Exam:** A thorough physical exam should be performed if you suspect systemic infection.

- Men
  - **Signs and Symptoms:** Patients may present with testicular pain, dysuria, purulent discharge from the meatus, and pain with defecation secondary to inflammation of the rectum or prostate. The clinician should also observe carefully for systemic signs and symptoms consistent with disseminated gonococcal infection, i.e., sore throat, redness of the eyes, joint pain, and cutaneous lesions.
  - **Physical Exam:** There may be palpable tenderness over the epididymis, purulent discharge from the meatus, or palpable tenderness to the prostate or rectum. A thorough general physical examination is required due to concerns about disseminated gonococcal infections, particularly in the joints.

8.3.1.5. Granuloma Inguinale

- Women and Men
- **Signs and Symptoms**: Patients will present with highly vascularized lesions over the genitals and perineum that tend to be painless but can cause severe scarring.
- **Physical Exam:** Typical findings include beefy, red ulcer-like lesions consistent with high vascularization that bleeds easily with manipulation. Subcutaneous granulomas may be present, but lymphadenopathy is uncommon. The lesions are relatively large and irregular and often associated with secondary infections.
- Four Main Lesions Can Be Seen on Examination
  1. Ulcer vegetative: Large painless ulcer on the patient's physical exam
  2. Nodular: Soft and erythematous that tend to ulcerate throughout the infectious process
  3. Cicatricial: Dry ulcerations that tend to transition into plaques.
  4. Hypertrophic: Lesions are thick and painless

8.3.1.6. HIV

- Women and Men
  - **Signs and Symptoms:** Patients may be asymptomatic or present with an acute viral syndrome, including systemic symptoms: malaise, fatigue, anorexia, fever, chills, arthralgias, myalgias,

or cutaneous presentations. Signs of a more advanced infection include fever, diarrhea, shortness of breath, cough, and oral candidiasis. Acute retroviral syndrome may occur with non-specific symptoms, including fatigue, muscle pain, skin rash, headache, sore throat, swollen lymph nodes, arthralgia, night sweats, and diarrhea. Acute retroviral syndrome will occur early in 50% to 90% of new HIV-infected individuals, usually before their antibody tests turn positive.

- **Physical Exam:** The chief complaint will guide the physical exam. The patient should have a thorough history and physical exam to rule out a broad differential diagnosis. Secondary and opportunistic infections are common, especially with AIDS.

8.3.1.7. HPV and Genital Warts

- Women and Men
    - **Signs and Symptoms:** Most complaints are cosmetic or incidental findings due to the asymptomatic nature of common HPV types 6 and 11. These are usually asymptomatic but are responsible for most (90%) venereal and anogenital warts. Patients may also present with ulcerative lesions secondary to oncogenic HPV types 16 and 18, which can progress to malignancies when triggered or stimulated by folate deficiency, ultraviolet light exposure, pregnancy, immunosuppression, or smoking.
    - **Physical Exam:** On exam, an exophytic lesion may be described as a cauliflower-like growth known as condylomata acuminata. Lesions can be observed over the external genital region, perineum, or perianal area. An examination for women includes a speculum exam with screening to rule out cervical cancer.

8.3.1.8. Lymphogranuloma Venereum

- Women and Men
- **Signs and Symptoms:** Patients will present with painful lymphadenopathy localized to the inguinal area. Patients may note the initial presentation of a pustule that gradually progresses to extensive painful ulceration. Men present with early or acute stages, while women present much later.
- **Physical Exam:** Lymphogranuloma venereum presents with two stages. The primary phase is a small, painless papule/pustule that will ulcerate and can be visualized throughout the affected genital area. During the secondary phase, patients present with unilateral lymphadenopathy that is fluctuant with palpation or may be suppurative in a presentation known as buboes. Buboes tend to rupture in the acute phase and progress to a thickened mass.

8.3.1.9. *Mycoplasma genitalium*

- Women
  - **Signs and Symptoms:** Patients may present with pelvic pain, dysuria, and similar type symptoms to gonorrhea or chlamydia infection, including vaginal irritation, discharge, foul odor, or even pelvic inflammatory disease.
  - **Physical Exam:** Common findings would be irritation of the external and internal vagina, vaginal discharge, cervical tenderness, cervicitis, adnexal tenderness, or abnormal vaginal spotting.
- Men
  - **Signs and Symptoms:** Patients may present with suprapubic pain, dysuria, urinary frequency, urgency, or testicular pain. This is a common cause (40%) of persistent or recurrent urethritis.
  - **Physical Exam:** The examination may be painless and benign, or there may be tenderness to the epididymis with palpation or discomfort from the prostate on the rectal exam.

8.3.1.10. Pelvic Inflammatory Disease in Women

- Pelvic inflammatory disease (PID) is a sexually transmitted infection that involves the upper female genital tract and can affect long-term fertility, and the infections can be serious.
- Risk factors include multiple sexual partners, prior episodes of pelvic inflammatory disease, intrauterine device implants, history of tubal ligation, and younger age.
- The most common causative organisms are chlamydia and gonorrhea, but *Mycoplasma genitalium* can also cause PID. There is no specific test for pelvic inflammatory disease, as the diagnosis is primarily clinical.
- The typical physical finding is tenderness on cervical motion or pain on palpation of the pelvic area.
- Other findings include cervical friability or discharge and increased white blood cells on wet prep.
- Typical symptoms include the following:
  - Abdominal tenderness.
  - Adnexal tenderness.
  - Cervical motion tenderness.
  - Fever (>38°C or >100.4°F).
  - Increased vaginal discharge.
  - Irregular menstrual bleeding.
  - Lower abdominal pain.
  - Mild pelvic pain.
  - Pain with intercourse.
  - Painful and frequent urination.
  - Uterine tenderness.

8.3.1.11. Syphilis

- Women and Men
  - **Primary:** The patient presents with a painless, well-demarcated lesion/ ulcer known as a chancre at the inoculation site. This is typically within 3 months of the inoculating event. If

untreated, the lesions will heal on their own in 3 to 8 weeks, but 30% will progress to tertiary syphilis.

- **Secondary:** Presents 2 to 4 weeks after initial chancre with systemic symptoms involving a cutaneous lesion and characteristic maculopapular rash. Cutaneous wart-like lesions known as condylomata lata may present and resolve during this phase. The rash does not itch and specifically includes mucus membranes as well as the palmar regions of the hands and soles of the feet, which are generally spared in other disorders.
- **Latent:** No clinical signs or symptoms are present, but serological tests are positive.
- **Tertiary:** About 33% of untreated patients will show tertiary symptoms presenting months, years, or decades after the original inoculation. Systemic symptoms can range from cardiovascular and neurologic to cutaneous gummatous lesions. Neurosyphilis can present with stroke-like symptoms, cranial nerve deficits, a change in mental status, general paresis, or tabes dorsalis. (See the companion StatPearls reference reviews on "*Neurosyphilis*" and "*Tabes dorsalis.*").
- **Signs and Symptoms:** Presenting symptoms of a syphilis infection depends on the phase of the infection at the time of evaluation. Symptoms can be categorized into primary, secondary, latent, and tertiary phases, which are best detailed and discussed in the companion StatPearls reference review on "Syphilis."
- **Physical Exam:** The physical exam depends on the presenting phase of the syphilis infection.

8.3.1.12. Trichomoniasis

- Women
    - **Signs and Symptoms:** Women can remain asymptomatic or may present with a complaint of foul-smelling discharge, pruritus, dyspareunia, dysuria, and vaginal spotting.
    - **Physical Exam:** The exam will show irritation of the external and internal vagina, including classic physical findings of "strawberry cervix," known as colpitis macularis. A foul frothy vaginal discharge may be present on exam.
- Men
    - **Signs and Symptoms:** Men can remain asymptomatic with a trichomonas vaginalis infection but can also present with testicular pain, dysuria, or rectal pain.
    - **Physical Exam:** Tenderness will be present, with palpation of the epididymis and prostate on rectal exam. No overlying skin lesions or inflammatory processes will be seen.

8.3.2. Evaluation

A comprehensive presentation of the CDC's "Sexually Transmitted Disease Treatment Guidelines 2021" includes screening and evaluation recommendations."

The following information has been extrapolated from the guidelines and should be used at the patient's and physician's discretion. Generally speaking, all patients who exhibit STI symptoms ought to get tested for HIV as well as any other STIs that are common in the community.

8.3.2.1. Chancroid

- **Women/Men:** Diagnosis is by clinical history and examination, together with the exclusion of alternative ulcerative infections such as herpes and syphilis. One or more deep, relatively large, painful ulcers on the genitalia associated with inguinal adenopathy that are tender and suppurative are highly suggestive of chancroid. (Herpetic ulcers are usually smaller, and chancres from syphilis are typically painless.).
- Gram stain may show a typical "school of fish" pattern, but this is only 80% sensitive. The definitive diagnosis requires growing Haemophilus ducreyi in culture; this is difficult and requires using specially enriched media grown under conditions of high humidity and high CO_2, which is not generally available to most clinical laboratories. No Food and Drug Administration (FDA)-approved polymerase chain reaction (PCR) serological test is available for *H ducreyi.*
  - The CDC recommends using the following clinical criteria:
  - One or more painful genital ulcers.
  - Clinical findings, such as the appearance of genital ulcers and regional lymphadenopathy consistent with chancroid.
  - No evidence of *Treponema pallidum* infection by darkfield microscopy of the exudate or by serologic testing within 1 week after the onset of ulcers.
  - A negative Herpes simplex virus culture or PCR test was performed on the exudate.

8.3.2.2. Chlamydia

- **Women:** Diagnosis is made by using a nucleic acid amplification test (NAAT) on a vaginal swab, first-catch urine sample, or self-endocervical swab.
- **Men:** Diagnosis is made using NAAT of a first-catch urine or urethral sample.

8.3.2.3. Genital Herpes

- Women/Men: Diagnosis is by clinical examination, NAAT from genital ulceration, or viral culture.
- Fluorescein-labeled monoclonal antibodies are available using a direct immunofluorescence assay for herpes simplex virus antibodies, but this is not currently recommended due to the test's insensitivity.
- Cellular changes on cytologic examination associated with HSV infections are also not recommended for diagnosis. They are considered too nonspecific and insensitive.

- HIV testing is recommended in all patients who test positive for genital herpes.

8.3.2.4. Gonorrhea

- **Women:** Diagnosis is made using a NAAT vulvovaginal or endocervical swab.
- **Men:** Diagnosis is made using NAAT of a first-catch urine or urethral sample.

8.3.2.5. Granuloma inguinale

- Women/Men: The diagnosis is primarily clinical, based on the gross appearance of the lesions and microscopic findings of intracellular Donovan bodies on a scraping, tissue, or biopsy specimen.
- Donovan bodies are rod or oval-shaped intracellular inclusions in the cytoplasm of histiocytes or mononuclear phagocytes of infected patients, which stain dark purple with Wright stain.
- The infecting organism is difficult to culture, and no FDA-approved molecular diagnostic laboratory test is currently available.

8.3.2.6. HIV

- Women/Men: Diagnosis involves using a blood sample or saliva for antibodies as a preliminary test, followed by more specific tests, including PCR or specific immunoassays.
- The CDC recommends at least one HIV test for all adults from 15 to 65.
- High-risk individuals (e.g., multiple sexual partners, sex workers, men who have sex with multiple men) should be tested at least annually.
- PCR testing is essentially diagnostic of an HIV infection.
- The CDC recommends HIV1/HIV2 antigen-antibody immunoassay.
- Patients who are unlikely to return for follow-up should be offered a rapid point-of-care HIV test. Results are available in less than 20 minutes but may be negative in early infections.
- A reverse transcriptase (RT)-PCR-based viral load test is also recommended.
- HIV ribonucleic acid testing is best for acute HIV infections.
- An HIV1/HIV2 antibody differentiation assay is confirmatory.
- HIV-infected individuals should be screened for chlamydia, gonorrhea, and syphilis when diagnosed and at least annually afterward.
- Individual assays to isolate specific antibodies or viral antigens can be used for confirmation. (See the companion StatPearls reference review on "HIV Testing.").

8.3.2.7. HPV and Genital Warts

- Women/Men: Diagnosis is primarily clinical, based on the gross appearance of any cutaneous or other lesions discovered on the physical examination.
- A biopsy can be performed for confirmation, but this is usually reserved for the following situations:
- Patients who are immunocompromised patients (cancer risk is highest).

  - Diagnosis is uncertain.
  - Atypical lesions.
  - Lesions that do not respond to standard therapy.
- Women: Reflex HPV testing can be done on cervical cells from a Pap smear to identify HPV subtypes.
- Suspicious Pap smear results can be further evaluated by colposcopy using acetic acid to highlight specific white-colored areas that can be biopsied.

8.3.2.8. Lymphogranuloma venereum

- Women/Men: Initial diagnosis is primarily by clinical suspicion in regions where this infection is common and by eliminating other causes of genital ulcerations with inguinal lymphadenopathy.
- Ulcerative infections of the genitalia to exclude, which also cause inguinal lymphadenopathy, would be chancroid, herpes, granuloma inguinale, and syphilis.
- Lymphoma, penile cancer, and HIV are additional causes of lymphadenopathy.
- Serological testing with complement fixation, micro-immunofluorescence, or NAAT can confirm the diagnosis, but PCR-based genotyping is the most definitive.
- Due to availability, NAAT testing is usually preferred and recommended for all patients with proctocolitis.
- Finding *Chlamydia trachomatis* in a genital, lymph node, or rectal specimens through culture, direct immunofluorescence, or NAAT is diagnostic and confirmatory.
- Men who have sex with men and have proctocolitis should be tested for all strains of *C. trachomatis.*
- HIV testing is especially recommended in this patient population.

8.3.2.9. Pelvic Inflammatory Disease

- Women: Diagnosis is primarily clinical based on the presence of lower abdominal pain, pelvic discomfort, purulent vaginal discharge, abnormal vaginal bleeding, or dyspareunia.
- Findings suggestive of pelvic inflammatory disease include:
  - Fever higher than 101°F (38.3°C).
  - Cervical friability.
  - Mucopurulent cervical discharge.
  - Saline microscopy of vaginal fluid shows abundant WBCs.
  - Elevated erythrocyte sedimentation rate (ESR) or C-reactive protein.
  - Laboratory confirmation of *N. gonorrhea or C. trachomatis* by NAAT or culture.
  - A diagnosis of pelvic inflammatory disease is unlikely if the cervical discharge is normal and no white blood cells are seen on a wet prep of the vaginal fluid.
- NAAT testing for *N. gonorrhea, C. trachomatis, and M. genitalium* is recommended.
- Serological testing for HIV and *T. pallidum* should also be performed.

- Pregnancy testing should be done, and pelvic ultrasonography should be considered if there is any suspicion of a tubo-ovarian abscess.

8.3.2.10. Mycoplasma genitalium

- Women/Men: Initial diagnosis is primarily clinical based on symptoms and the exclusion of chlamydia and gonorrhea.
- NAAT assays for *M. genitalium* are now available and FDA-approved, with a 96% or higher sensitivity.
- *M. genitalium* should be suspected in all patients with recurrent or persistent gonorrhea or chlamydia infections and intractable urethritis.
- Presumptive treatment can be initiated in suspected cases even without diagnostic confirmation.

8.3.2.11. Syphilis

- Women/Men: The diagnosis is confirmed by a positive finding on serological tests, which include at least one nontreponemal and one treponemal assay.
- No NAAT tests for syphilis are currently available. PCR tests for *T. pallidum* have been developed, but none are FDA-approved.
- Nontreponemal testing, including the Venereal Disease Research Laboratory (VDRL) and rapid plasma reagin (RPR) assays, are non-specific serum antibody tests for syphilis.
    - A negative test would be non-reactive, while a positive test would demonstrate a titer of at least 1:8.
    - If the titer is lower than 1:8, the test should be repeated, and a treponemal assay should also be performed.
    - Nontreponemal tests are simple, inexpensive, and are usually the initial screening tests for syphilis.
    - They will identify roughly 80% of patients with primary syphilis and close to 100% with secondary syphilis.
    - They typically turn positive only after the appearance of the primary chancre.
    - When quantified, they can be used for disease tracking as a four-fold change in activity is generally considered significant.
    - However, they are not specific for syphilis and can often give false-positive results, so they are inadequate for a definitive diagnosis alone without confirmation from a treponemal test.
- Treponemal testing, including the fluorescent treponemal antibody absorption and the *Treponema pallidum* particle agglutination assays, are needed to confirm the diagnosis.
- While specific treponemal antibodies appear early, their level does not correlate well with disease activity or stage.
- They typically remain positive for life even after successful treatment, making them ineffective for disease tracking.
- A positive result on at least 1

nontreponemal and 1 treponemal test is required to confirm a syphilis diagnosis definitively.

- Only quantifiable nontreponemal tests can be used for disease tracking.
- Darkfield microscopy can identify the infecting spirochete in 80% of cases even before serological testing becomes positive but is rarely performed due to technical difficulties.
- Patients who present with possible neurosyphilis will need a cerebral spinal fluid sample to assist with the diagnostic workup.
- VDRL testing of the cerebrospinal fluid is highly specific for neurosyphilis but not very sensitive (opposite of blood testing).
- Treponemal testing of the cerebrospinal fluid is highly sensitive but less specific than the VDRL test for neurosyphilis (the treponemal antibodies often diffuse from the blood into the cerebral spinal fluid, which can also be contaminated by blood cells).
- HIV testing should especially be performed on all patients testing positive for syphilis.
- For further details on the complexities of diagnostic testing, see StatPearls' companion reference on "Syphilis."

8.3.2.12. Trichomoniasis

- Women: Diagnosis using NAAT of the vagina, endocervical swab, urine analysis, or urethral sample.
- Alternatively, a wet mount will show motile flagellated protozoa.
- Patients diagnosed with trichomoniasis should also be tested for chlamydia, gonorrhea, HIV, and syphilis.

8.3.3. Pregnancy—STI Screening Recommendations from the CDC 2021 Guidelines

Serious health consequences for both the mother and the fetus may result from sexually transmitted infections. The CDC now advises the following standard STI screenings during pregnancy as a result.

- First Prenatal Visit
  - All pregnant women should be tested for HIV, hepatitis B, hepatitis C, and syphilis.
  - All pregnant women who are at increased risk for infection should also be tested for chlamydia and gonorrhea.
  - Pregnant women who test positive for chlamydia should be retested 3 to 4 weeks after treatment and again within 3 months.
- **Third Trimester Visit (preferably at or before 36 weeks).**
  - Rescreen women younger than 25 years of age or at continued high risk and all those not previously tested for chlamydia, gonorrhea, and syphilis.
  - Pregnant women with high-risk factors or who were not previously tested should be screened for HIV and hepatitis B.
  - Those patients who tested positive for syphilis at the

prenatal visit should be retested.

High-Risk Factors Include

- New or multiple sex partners;
- Inconsistent use of condoms;
- A sexual partner with concurrent or multiple partners;
- A sexual partner who has a sexually transmitted infection;
- History of illegal drug use or prostitution;
- Living in an area with a high rate of STIs;
- Incarcerated individuals.

8.4. Management and Treatment of Symptomatic Sexually Transmitted Infections

8.4.1. Sexually Transmitted Infection Syndromes and the Syndromic Approach to Patient Management

STIs and RTIs are caused by a wide variety of pathogens, but many of them share a similar or overlapping clinical appearance, which is referred to as a sign or symptom. Signs are what the patient or a healthcare provider sees during an examination; symptoms are what the patient feels, like pain or itching. Healthcare professionals can diagnose patients based on signs and symptoms. For instance, trichomoniasis is characterized by a copious, purulent, and malodorous vaginal discharge. However, infections other than STIs, like bacterial vaginosis and vulvovaginal candidiasis, can also cause vaginal discharge. The infection frequently has multiple etiological causes or microbes involved. Trichomonas and gonorrhea change the discharge. Because of this, an etiological diagnosis cannot always be made based solely on the signs and symptoms.

Laboratory testing is the conventional (and gold standard) approach for STI/RTI diagnosis. However, STI testing is frequently unavailable at district hospitals in low-resource environments and is not offered in first-line medical facilities. Certain laboratory tests used to diagnose STIs are pricy or require sophisticated methods. Because of this, the World Health Organization has advised a syndromic approach to STI diagnosis and management in low- and middle-income countries since the 1990s, and in the majority of these settings, this approach has been the method of choice ever since. The method is predicated on a collection of symptoms and instantly identifiable indicators linked to several distinct etiologies. Many studies have demonstrated the efficacy of syndromic management in treating STIs and reducing their spread. After the implementation of syndromic approach-based control measures, there have been notable reductions in the rates of sexually transmitted infections (STIs) (Vuylsteke, 2004).

Common symptoms and signs (syndromes) are:

- Urethral discharge in men;
- Genital ulcer;
- Inguinal bulbs;
- Scrotal swelling;
- Vaginal discharge;
- Lower abdominal pain in women;
- Neonatal conjunctivitis.

The syndromic approach is one that was developed through science. The antimicrobial regimens are selected to address the principal pathogens accountable for the syndromes within a particular geographic region. As a result, recommendations vary from nation to nation depending on the epidemiological pattern of sexually transmitted infections and antibiotic resistance; for this reason, no single treatment strategy works in every situation. Flow charts are typically promoted to help medical professionals choose the best course of action. The WHO has developed training modules that are available in multiple languages, and many nations have customized them to reflect the STI resistance patterns that are observed locally.

The management of STIs is not dependent on laboratory investigations, which are not available in many first-line health facilities. This is an advantage of employing the signs and symptoms-based approach. Furthermore, nurses and clinicians can treat patients just as well as specialists. Syndromic management is not, however, universally endorsed. It has been reviewed that syndromic management of STIs is generally effective in treating genital ulcer disease and urethral discharge STIs in men (level 1 evidence). Since the syndromes and symptoms are less specific in women, vaginal discharge and PID present the biggest challenges (Vuylsteke, 2004) (Figure 8.1).

The fact that infections are frequently asymptomatic presents another significant obstacle to STI control. For the treatment of asymptomatic infections that need to be screened for, syndromic management is not appropriate. Except for syphilis testing during pregnancy, which presents a significant opportunity not to be missed, screening is sadly unavailable in the majority of primary-level or district healthcare settings in lower-resource countries (see more under Linkages). Additionally, control efforts must be focused on several pillars, including the treatment of symptomatic diseases as one, partner notification, preventing risky sexual relations, screening programs during pregnancy, and integrating prevention and control with other reproductive health services, among others (WHO, 2007).

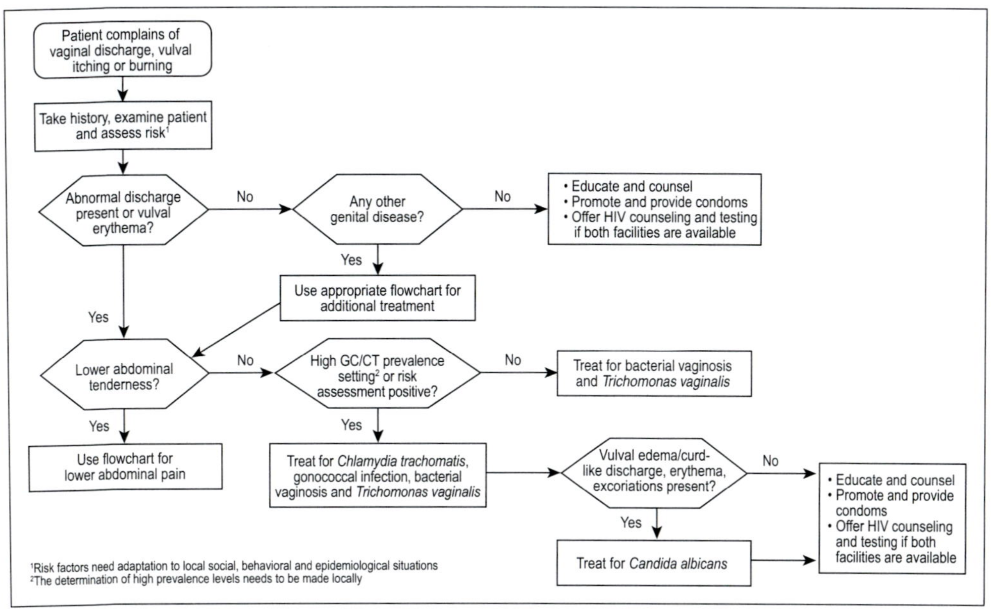

Figure 8.1. *Syndromic approach: vaginal discharge.*

Source: WHO treatment modules, 2007. https://www.glowm.com/pdf/Chap-17_Hanson%20and%20Delvaux.pdf.

The fact that infections are often asymptomatic creates another major challenge for STI control. For treating asymptomatic infections that require screening, syndromic management isn't suitable. With the exception of syphilis testing during pregnancy, which presents a significant opportunity not to be missed, screening is sadly unavailable in the majority of primary level or district healthcare settings in lower-resource countries (see more under Linkages). Additionally, control efforts must be focused on a number of pillars, including the treatment of symptomatic diseases as one, partner notification, preventing risky sexual relations, screening programs during pregnancy, and integrating prevention and control with other reproductive health services (WHO, 2007).

Figure 8.2 illustrates syndromic management: lower abdominal pain.

The syndromic approach was specifically created with primary healthcare in mind. In hospitals, additional testing like gynecological exams, syphilis confirmation tests, and Gram staining can be performed to treat patients who have not responded well to syndromic management. These tests should be used to supplement syndromic management in cases like these. At this level, not only are third-line therapeutic options probably available, but more sophisticated laboratory diagnostics and investigations as well.

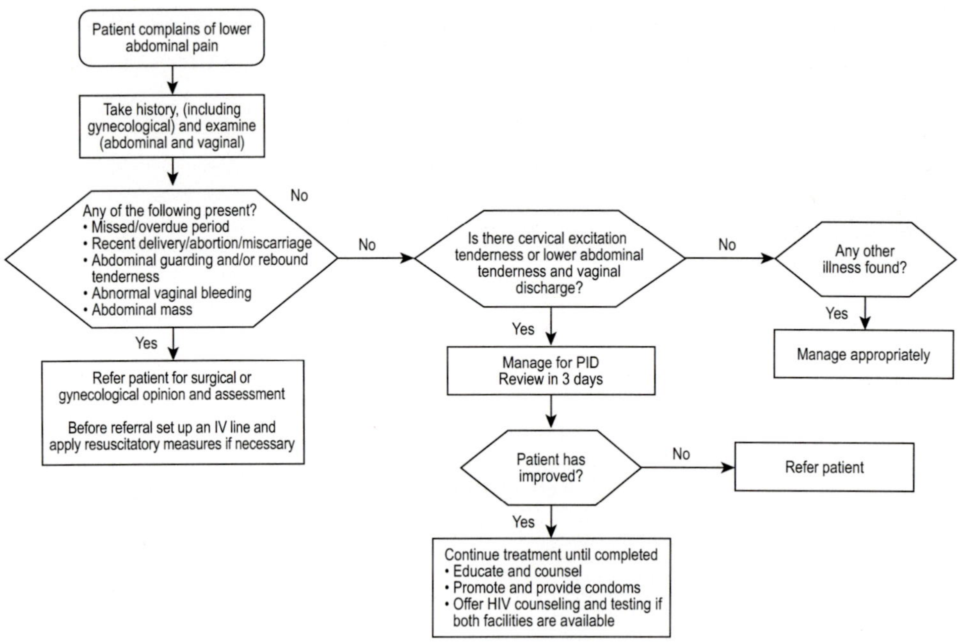

Figure 8.2. *Syndromic management: lower abdominal pain.*

Source: https://www.glowm.com/pdf/Chap-17_Hanson%20and%20Delvaux.pdf.

The recommendations provide the best care possible for patients receiving outpatient services and primary healthcare. However, since the epidemiological patterns of STIs and resistance to antibiotic regimens vary slightly across all countries, we will not offer specific treatment recommendations for syndromic management.

An overview of clinical presentation, symptoms, and potential advanced diagnostics is intended to be provided in the ensuing sections. More sophisticated diagnostic and laboratory facilities are available at district hospitals, and patients who have recurrent STIs or RTIs or who were not cured after the first course of treatment should make use of them.

8.4.2. Clinical and Etiological Diagnostic and Management of Symptomatic Sexually Transmitted Infections

8.4.2.1. The Normal Vaginal Flora

The pH 4.5 vaginal environment is kept slightly acidic by a variety of bacterial species that produce lactobacilli, which make up the normal vaginal flora. This serves as a natural defense against infections, which is important. Hormonal levels affect the type and quantity of natural fluids found in the upper genital tract, cervical mucus, and cells. Therefore, women may experience an increase in vaginal excretion or cervical mucus during the middle of their menstrual cycle, which they may mistake for a vaginal discharge. When oral contraceptives are used, these cyclic variations do not happen.

A vaginal secretion suspended in 0.5 ml of normal saline and placed on a slide for microscopy analysis is known as a wet mount preparation, which allows for the analysis of the normal flora (Figure 8.3). Several superficial epithelial cells, few white blood cells, and few to no clue cells are visible when normal vaginal secretion is examined under a microscope. If a microscope is easily accessible in or close to the consultation room, the same saline preparation can be used to check vaginal secretion in cases of symptomatic STIs/RTIs.

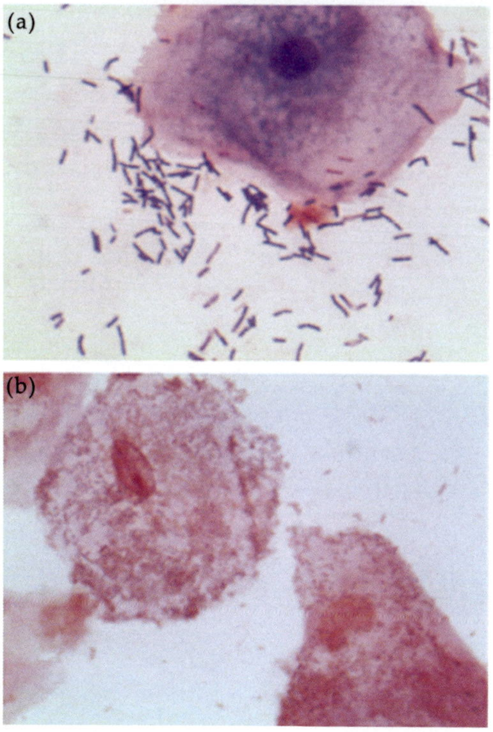

Figure 8.3. *(a) Normal vaginal flora (gram stain); (b) high nugent score, bacterial vaginosis (gram stain).*

Source: https://www.glowm.com/pdf/Chap-17_Hanson%20and%20Delvaux.pdf.

8.4.2.2. Vaginitis

1. **Bacterial vaginosis:** A change in the normal bacterial flora that causes an overgrowth of mostly anaerobic bacteria and the loss of lactobacilli is known as bacterial vaginosis (BV), formerly known as non-specific vaginitis. As a result, the normally 1% concentration of anaerobic bacteria is increased by 100–1000 times. Therefore, vaginal flora imbalance, rather than pathogenic bacterial infection, is what causes BV. This type of vaginitis is the most prevalent. STIs, antibiotic treatment for other conditions, and vaginal douche are risk factors.

Many studies have indicated that women with BV are at increased risk of PID and post-abortal pelvic infection. During pregnancy, BV can cause premature rupture of membranes, preterm labor and delivery.

- Diagnosis: pH is higher that 4.5 (usually 4.7–6); vaginal discharge with fishy odor; vaginal secretions are grey and thinly coat the vaginal walls.
- At the health center or district hospital levels, microscopy (wet mount) shows an increased number of clue cells, typically >20% of epithelial cells are clue cells in advanced infection. 'Whiff test': fishy odor if potassium hydroxide (KOH 10%) is added.
- At provincial or referral laboratory, a 'Nugent score' can be performed: a score of 7–10 is consistent with BV. The assessment uses Gram stain and determines semiquantitatively the presence of large Gram-positive *Lacto bacillus* morphotypes (Table 8.1).
- Treatment: see Table 8.2.

Table 8.1. *Scoring System (0–10) for Gram-Stained Vaginal Smears**

Score†	*Lactobacillus morphotypes*	*Gardnerella and Bacteroides spp. morphotypes*	*Curved Gram-variable rods*
0	4+	0	0
1	3+	1+	1+ or 2+
2	2+	2+	3+ or 4+
3	1+	3+	
4	0	4+	

*Morphotypes are scored as the average number seen per oil immersion field. Note that less weight is given to curved Gram-variable rods. Total score = lactobacilli + G. vaginalis and Bacteroides spp. + curved rods. † 0, no morphotypes present; 1, < 1 morphotype present; 2, 1–4 morphotypes present; 3, 5–30 morphotypes present; 4, >30 morphotypes present.

Source: https://www.glowm.com/pdf/Chap-17_Hanson%20and%20Delvaux.pdf.

2. **Vulvovaginal candidiasis:** Because it affects celibate women and Candida is thought to be a normal component of the vaginal flora, vulvovaginal candidiasis, or VVC, has not historically been regarded as a sexually transmitted infection (STI). Although there is no known etiology or precipitating factor for the majority of women with sporadic and infrequent VVC infections, use of antibiotics, pregnancy, diabetes, or HIV infection may increase the risk of VVC. However, research has demonstrated that both vaginal sex and other types of sexual activity can transmit Candida organisms (Nyirjesy et al., 2003).

Table 8.2. *Overview of Common Infections and Treatment Suggestions*

Infection	*Treatment*
Vaginitis	
Bacterial vaginosis	Metronidazole 2 g orally (single dose) *or*
Trichomoniasis	Metronidazole 500 mg orally twice a day for 7 days
Candidiasis (yeast)	Miconazole 200 mg vaginal suppository, once a day for 3 days *or*
	Clotrimazole 100 mg vaginal tablets, 2 times a day for 3 days *or*
	Fluconazole 150 mg oral tablet (single dose) *or*
	Nystatin 100,000 units, vaginal tablets once a day for 14 days
Cervicitis	
Gonorrhea	Cefixime 400 mg orally (single dose) *or*
	Ceftriaxone 125 mg, by intramuscular injection *or*
	Spectinomycin 2 g by intramuscular injection
Chlamydia	Azithromycin 1 g orally (single dose) *or*
	Doxycycline 100 mg orally twice a day for 7 days
	(*Pregnant women*: azithromycin 1 g orally (single dose) *or* erythromycin 500 mg 4 times a day for 7 days)
Pelvic inflammatory disease (PID)	Treat for gonorrhea and chlamydia (see above) plus for anaerobic infections with
	Metronidazole 500 mg orally twice a day for 7 days *or*
	Ampicillin 2 g by intravenous or intramuscular injection, then 1 g every 6 h *plus*
	Gentamicin 80 mg by intramuscular injection every 8 h *plus*
	Metronidazole 500 mg or 100 ml by intravenous infusion every 8 h
Genital ulcers	
Syphilis	Benzathine penicillin G 2.4 million units intramuscular injection
Genital herpes	Aciclovir 400 mg orally, 3 times a day for 7 days
Chancroids	Ciprofloxacin 500 mg twice a day for 3 days *or*
	Azithromycin, 1 g orally (single dose) *or*
	Erythromycin 500 mg orally 4 times a day for 7 days (also if patient pregnant) *or*
	Ceftriaxone 250 mg intramuscular injection (single dose)
Lymphogranuloma venereum (LGV)	Doxycycline 100 mg orally twice a day for 14 days *or*
	Erythromycin 500 mg 4 times a day for 14 days
Granuloma venereum (donovanosis)	Azithromycin 1 g orally (single dose) *or*
	Doxycycline 100 mg orally twice a day
Infections following miscarriage, induced abortion or delivery	
Septic abortion, post-partum endometritis	Ampicillin 2 g intravenously or intramuscularly, then 1 g every 6 h *plus*
	Gentamycin 80 mg intramuscularly every 8 h *plus*
	Metronidazole 500 mg orally or intravenously every 8 h

Source: https://www.glowm.com/pdf/Chap-17_Hanson%20and%20Delvaux.pdf.

- Diagnosis: vaginal discharge which typically resembles cottage cheese; pruritus, inflammation, vaginal soreness; discharge can vary from watery to thick; pH of the vagina is normal (≤4.5).
- Fungal elements can be confirmed by microscopy (simple saline preparation – wet mount).
- At the referral laboratory a culture on Saboraud medium can be performed.

3. ***Trichomonas vaginalis***: *Trichomonas vaginalis* (Figure 8.4) is a flagellated parasite that causes trichomoniasis and requires an anaerobic environment to thrive. There is a very high transmission rate. The majority of people get the illness from just one encounter

with an infected person. Often, BV coexists with trichomoniasis. Specifically, the infection may result in premature membrane rupture and preterm delivery.

- Diagnosis: profuse, purulent, malodorous vaginal discharge with bubbles; pH is higher than 5.0.
- Microscopy (simple saline–wet–mount preparation) reveals motile (jerky movements) *T. vaginalis* and increased numbers of leukocytes. At the central laboratory, culture and possible DNA amplification (PCR) can also be performed.
- Treatment: see Table 8.2.

Differential Diagnosis of Vaginitis

In cases where a microscopic diagnosis of trichomoniasis, candidiasis, or BV is not possible, the guidelines for the country-specific syndromic approach should be followed.

8.4.2.3. Cervicitis

1. **Gonorrhea:** Neisseria gonorrhoeae, a Gram-negative diplococcus, is the cause of gonorrhea. The majority of women with gonococcal infections are asymptomatic, although the clinical signs of gonococcal urethritis in men include dysuria and urethral discharge, which is frequently profuse.

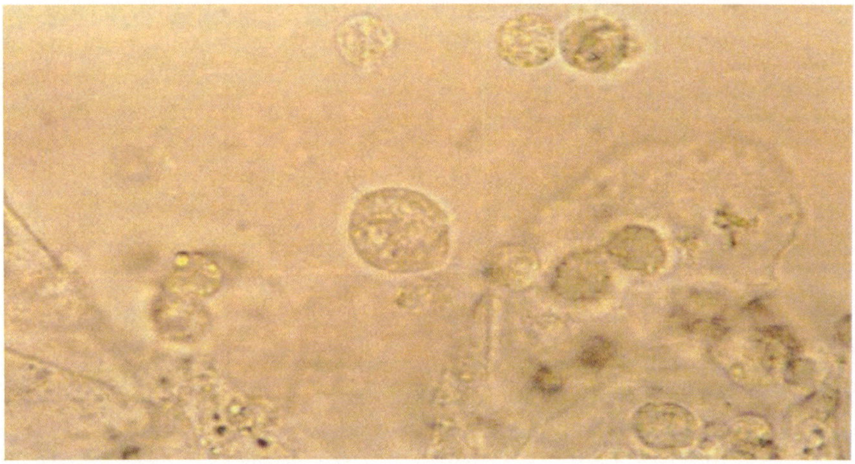

Figure 8.4. *Trichomonas vaginalis (wet mount).*

Source: *https://www.glowm.com/pdf/Chap-17_Hanson%20and%20Delvaux.pdf.*

- **Diagnosis:** No test is available at the first and second levels of care. A reliable and sensitive rapid test is still under development. Gram staining of urethral discharge of men can be done and Gram-negative diplococci are seen inside the leukocytes. Among women, only culture on selective and enriched medium and specific molecular amplification techniques (PCR) can make a definite diagnosis.
- **Treatment:** See Table 8.2.

2. **Chlamydia:** Chlamydia trachomatis is the cause of chlamydial infection. The infection often exhibits mild clinical manifestations and lack of specificity in its symptoms.

- Diagnosis – laboratory: only at the referral or central laboratory with cell culture, antigen detection by direct immunofluorescence or enzyme immunoassay, or molecular amplification. Rapid tests are commercially available but they lack sensitivity; more promising tests are under development.
- Treatment: see Table 8.2. Note: for C. trachomatis infection in pregnancy, erythromycin is recommended (level of evidence 1).

8.4.2.4. Pelvic Inflammatory Disease

Microorganisms that colonize the endocervix and move up to the endometrium and fallopian tubes are the cause of PID. This clinical diagnosis suggests that the patient has inflammation and an upper genital tract infection. Anywhere along a continuum that includes endometritis, salpingitis, and peritonitis, inflammation can be present. Usually, sexually transmitted infections like N are the cause of PID. Gonorrhoeae, or C. trachomatis. An end-stage tuba ovarian abscess is the condition. BV is frequently present in PID.

- **Diagnosis:** A triad of symptoms and signs including pelvic pain, adnexal tenderness, and fever. Many patients present with mild symptoms or no symptoms at all. Genitourinary tract infections may indicate PID.
- **Treatment:** See Table 8.2. Tubo-ovarian abscess normally responds to an antibiotic regimen, but surgical intervention with drainage might become necessary. On ultrasound large masses in the ovaries can be seen and free fluid in Douglas' pouch. If in doubt aspiration of this fluid will distinguish pus from blood. Drainage with a Foley catheter and posterior culdotomy is explained in (HIV-related gynecological problems). If the symptoms persist a laparotomy with drainage might become necessary.

8.4.2.6.1. Differential Diagnosis of PID

PID is particularly challenging to diagnose and treat because it frequently worsens without symptoms being noticed, especially in cases of chlamydial infection. Numerous other conditions, including endometriosis, benign and malignant ovarian cysts, adnexal torsion, and ectopic pregnancy, can also result in lower abdominal pain. Furthermore, individuals experiencing infertility or marital issues may exhibit symptoms of lower abdominal pain, and they frequently receive excessive antibiotic treatment.

8.4.2.5. Ophthalmia Neonatorum

Ophthalmia neonatorum is a condition where newborns can develop swollen eyelids with pus discharge in one or both eyes, typically caused by the bacteria Neisseria gonorrhoeae or Chlamydia trachomatis during childbirth (Figure 8.5).

- **Treatment:** newborns should be treated with ceftriaxone 125 mg intramuscularly as a single dose. Note: the mother and partner should also be treated for gonorrhea and chlamydia inflection.

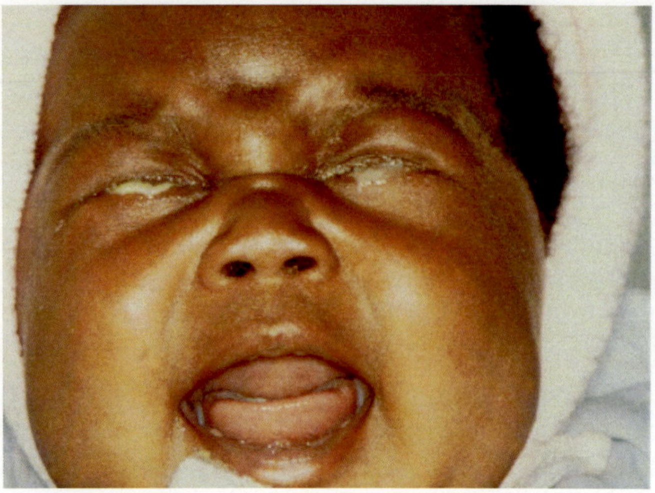

Figure 8.5. *Gonococcal ophthalmia neonatorum.*

Source: https://www.glowm.com/pdf/Chap-17_Hanson%20and%20Delvaux.pdf.

8.4.2.6. Genital Ulcer Diseases

The three main causes of genital ulcer diseases are chancroid, genital herpes, and syphilis (Figure 8.6).

1. Syphilis

- **Diagnosis:** Ulcers caused by syphilis are normally bigger, relatively painless, and have a smooth, indurated border and a smooth base. They are not accompanied by lymphadenopathy. These signs of primary syphilis are seen about 2–10 weeks after infection. The secondary stage of syphilis develops 1–3 months after the primary stage. They appear as a macular–papular rash and/or moist papules (condylomata lata). After this secondary stage, the infection enters a latent phase without any signs and symptoms that can last for years. The tertiary stage is characterized by granulomas of the skin, the bones, and internal organs. Cardiovascular or neurosyphilis may occur.

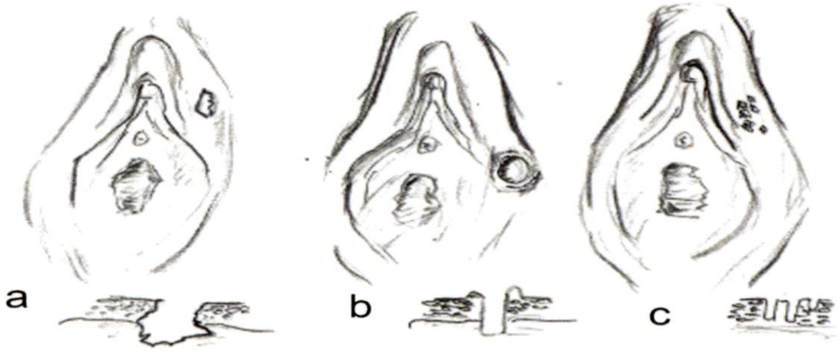

Figure 8.6. *Genital ulcer disease: (a) chancroid; (b) syphilis; and (c) herpes simplex ulcers.*

Source: https://www.glowm.com/pdf/Chap-17_Hanson%20and%20Delvaux.pdf.

- **Laboratory:** Positive non-treponemal rapid plasma reagin (RPR) test or venereal disease research laboratory (VDRL) test, the Treponema – specific TPHA (*Treponema pallidum* hemagglutination assay) test or the new rapid tests can be used (WHO, 2006).

The first option recommended by the WHO for syphilis diagnosis is RPR confirmed by TPHA. Unfortunately, some resource-poor settings have not been able to fully utilize the RPR due to the lengthy shaking procedure and interpretation challenges. Since it has been available for a few years, a novel dipstick-style Treponema specific serological test known as "rapid tests" offers a reliable substitute in situations where RPR testing has proven challenging (Watson-Jones et al., 2005) and is currently advised as a screening examination18. This new rapid test is a treponemal test that is very simple to use, can be kept at room temperature, and can be used with whole blood, serum, or plasma (Table 8.3). The test's inability to differentiate between an active infection and one that has already been treated is a drawback, shared by other treponemal tests. By using the RPR (non-treponemal test), it ought to be verified. The World Health Organization advises against using the RPR test in areas where serum is required and a refrigerator is required. Instead, it is best to use the treponemal rapid test.

- Screening for syphilis should be done on-site, and results and treatment should be made available to the woman before she leaves the clinic. Syphilis screening using the RPR is recommended during antenatal care.

i. ***Congenital syphilis***: In certain countries in sub-Saharan Africa, the prevalence of syphilis among expectant mothers still surpasses 5%. 25% of pregnancies in women with untreated early syphilis may result in abortions or stillbirths, and 14% may result in neonatal deaths. Furthermore, congenital syphilis affects approximately one-third of newborns born to infected mothers. According to WHO estimates, there are 1.5 million cases of congenital syphilis annually. It has been demonstrated that syphilis screening and treatment can reduce stillbirth by 80% (Figure 8.7).

Congenital syphilis might present with hepatosplenomegaly, lymph node swelling, rhinitis, and maculopapular exanthema with moist papules. Late signs of secondary congenital syphilis are teeth deformities, deformities of the skeletal system, and deafness.

Pregnancy-related screening and treatment for the mother can help prevent congenital syphilis. For many years, syphilis screening has been emphasized as a crucial component of prenatal care and as an extremely economical public health intervention. When RPR is unavailable, a new, extremely straightforward rapid point-of-care treponemal test has emerged in recent years that offers a practical, affordable substitute for screening for syphilis in expectant mothers (Rydzak et al., 2008).

Table 8.3. *Interpretation of Serological Tests for Syphilis if the New Rapid Test Is Used as a First-Choice Screening Test*

Treponemal test (rapid test)	*Non-treponemal test (RPR, VDRL)*	*Likely interpretation*
+	+	Syphilis
–	+	False-positive RPR (no syphilis)
+	–	Primary or latent syphilis, previously treated syphilis
–	–	No syphilis

RPR, rapid plasma regain; VDRL, Venereal Disease Research Laboratory.

Source: https://www.glowm.com/pdf/Chap-17_Hanson%20and%20Delvaux.pdf.

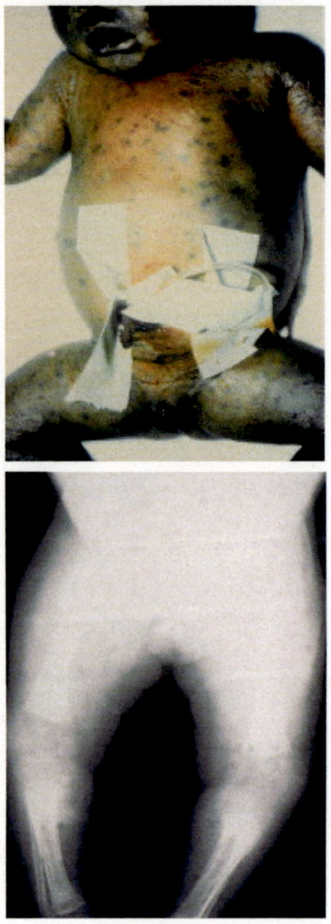

Figure 8.7. *Congenital syphilis.*

Source: https://www.glowm.com/pdf/Chap-17_Hanson%20and%20Delvaux.pdf.

- **Treatment:** children with signs of congenital syphilis and a mother with a positive syphilis test should be treated with aqueous crystalline benzylpenicillin 100,000–150,000 units/kg of body weight intravenously or intramuscularly twice a day for

7 days followed by three times a day for 3 more days or procaine benzylpenicillin 50,000 units/kg of body weight intramuscularly once a day for 10 days. Children born to a syphi lispositive mother should receive 50,000 units/kg of body weight, intramuscularly, in a single dose.

2. **Genital Herpes:** This is the most frequent cause of genital ulcers. The ulcers are often vesicular lesions and look like tiny blisters.

- Diagnosis: grouped vesicles mixed with small ulcers, particularly with a history of such lesions.
- Laboratory: cell culture, serology, DNA amplification.
- Treatment: see Table 8.2. Note: aciclovir may not be available in many countries or only in clinics specialized for the treatment of opportunistic infections of HIV. In this case, the patient has to wait for spontaneous remission which normally occurs in a few days. Treatment may include medication with painkillers. Patients should be advised to abstain from sexual intercourse or to use condoms.

3. **Chancroid:** In 70% of cases, the ulcers caused by Haemophilus ducreyi are accompanied by tender inguinal lymphadenopathy, also known as inguinal bubo, and have deep, uneven margins. They are also exceedingly painful.

- **Laboratory**: culture on specific media, DNA amplification.
- **Treatment:** see Table 8.2. Note: other therapeutic regimens based on erythromycin or cotrimoxazole might be efficient.

4. Lymphogranuloma venereum

- **Diagnosis:** lymphogranuloma venereum is caused by Chlamydia trachomatis, serovar L1, L2 and L3 and is more frequent in men than women. The disease presents with a transient, often painless genital or anorectal ulcer which disappears mostly undiagnosed. Two to three weeks later confluent inguinal nodes develop and might show multiple fistulae. These inguinal bubos are often multiple and have fistulae, which helps to distinguish them from a bubo caused by chancroid.
- **Laboratory:** lesion swabs or bubo aspirate can be tested for C. trachomatis by cell culture, direct immunofluorescence, or molecular amplification. Serovar identification can be performed by various molecular methods. However, diagnosis is mostly done based on clinical appearance.
- **Treatment:** see Table 8.2.

5. **Granuloma Inguinale:** Granuloma inguinale is an uncommon sexually transmitted infection (STI) that is only found in a small number of countries, including parts of South Africa, Brazil, the Caribbean, and parts of Asia (Papua New Guinea and India). The pathogen, which is also known as donovanosis, is brought on by Klebsiella granulomatis.

- **Diagnosis:** clinically, the disease commonly presents with a painless, slowly progressing ulcer. The ulcerations bleed easily on contact.
- **Laboratory:** observation of Donovan bodies within histiocytes

in Giemsa, Leishman, or Wright's-stained tissue smear. An alternative is a histological examination for Donovan's body using Giemsa or silver stain. Amplification methods are not commercially available.

- **Treatment:** see Table 8.2.

6. **Genital Wart and Condylomata Acuminata:** HPV subtypes 6 and 11 are the cause of condylomata acuminata and genital warts. As opposed to subtypes 16 and 18, which cause cervical cancer but not genital warts, these two subtypes of HPV are referred to as low-risk because they have little to no chance of developing a malignant illness. In contrast to the typical condylomata acuminata with verrucous and exophytic lesions, flat papular warts have a different appearance. Treatment for condyloma acuminata may not affect the spread of the virus, and the condition may resolve on its own or stay unchanged. Nonetheless, a lot of women would rather have the lesions removed, and this can be done with electrosurgical or sharp excision. If available, self-treatment with a 0–5% podophyllotoxin solution or a 10–25% podophyllin tincture administered by a healthcare professional is advised.

- **Vaccine:** For a few years, two HPV vaccines have been marketed that help protect against two (Cervarix®) or four (Gardasil®) types of HPV. In girls and young women aged 9–26 years, both vaccines help protect against two types of HPV (16, 18) that cause about 75% of cervical cancer cases, while one of them (Cervarix®) also helps protect against two more types (6, 11) that cause 90% of genital warts cases. The operational issues and effectiveness related to the implementation of this intervention at a wider scale in low-resource countries are being studied. Rwanda is the first country in sub-Saharan Africa to introduce large-scale HPV vaccination[23].

8.4.2.7. Post-Abortion Infections

Any type of abortion, whether induced or spontaneous (miscarriages), can result in infections after the procedure, also known as septic abortions. Even so, it is more prevalent after unfinished and illegal abortions. The spectrum of bacteria that cause infections that arise after an induced abortion is different from that of common STIs/RTIs, and these infections are also referred to as iatrogenic or exogenous infections. As a result, the suggested treatment plan deviates slightly from the standard plan, which focuses mainly on gonococci and chlamydia. The uterus will become infected initially, but it may spread quickly to the lower abdomen and manifest as PID symptoms.

- **Diagnosis:** a triad of symptoms and signs including pelvic pain, adnexal tenderness, and fever, foul-smelling vaginal discharge; history of abortion – speculum examination might show residuals of placenta and/or bleeding.
- **Treatment:** see Table 8.2. Infections not involving deep tissue can be treated with amoxicillin 500 mg orally three times daily for 5 days PLUS metro nidazole 400–500 mg orally three times a day. Severe infection should be treated with intravenous treatment 24. The therapy should be continued for 2 days after the patient is fever-free.

8.4.3. The Consultation for Sexually Transmitted Infections

A good STI/RTI consultation needs a trained provider with sufficient training, experience, and expertise. Elements of a good consultation are:

- Friendly and respectful reception.
- Sufficient history-taking.
- Clinical examination.
- Making a diagnosis.
- Full treatment course based on the diagnosis.
- Providing education and counselling.
- Partner notification.
- Documentation and registration.

A speculum examination is not always part of the initial clinical examination, but it should be done if one is available. To rule out cervical cancer, a speculum examination should be carried out in cases of "recurrent vaginal discharge." Clear instructions on how to take prescribed medications, when to visit the clinic again, and a partner treatment discussion are also crucial. It is advisable to counsel patients to refrain from having sex until they fully recover. A STI consultation must include counselling on STIs, including HIV, as well as recommendations for HIV testing.

Patients of both sexes should receive counselling regarding the risks associated with STIs, such as the possibility of spontaneous abortion, infertility, and premature rupture of the membranes (if pregnant).

8.4.4. Essentials on Diagnosis and Treatment Using the Syndromic Approach

Genital ulcers, lower abdominal pain, and vaginal discharge are the common syndromes that are distinguished in the syndromic management of STIs in women (Table 8.4.).

Flowcharts help the providers to make the diagnosis and treat the patients accordingly. For example, the flowchart on vaginal discharge starts with history taking and examination of signs and symptoms. The provider should verify:

- Whether the patient has abnormal vaginal discharge.
- Whether there is any other sign of another STI/ RTI such as sores or ulcers.
- Whether the patient also has abdominal tenderness.
- How the discharge looks - cord-like discharge indicating Candida albicans - or other types of discharge indicating BV and trichomoniasis.

The flowcharts always remind us about counselling, condom promotion, and counselling and testing for HIV if available.

Table 8.4. *Syndromic Approach Related to STIs/RTIs Among Women: Symptoms, Signs, and Most Common Causes*

Syndrome	*Symptoms*	*Signs*	*Most common causes*
Vaginal discharge	Unusual vaginal discharge; vaginal itching; dysuria (pain of urination); dyspareunia (pain during sexual intercourse)	Abnormal vaginal discharge	*Vaginitis*: • Trichomoniasis • Bacterial vaginosis • Candidiasis *Cervicitis*: • Gonorrhea • Chlamydia
Lower abdominal pain	Lower abdominal pain; dyspareunia	Vaginal discharge; lower abdominal tenderness or palpation; temperature >38°C	Gonorrhea Chlamydia Mixed anaerobes
Genital ulcer	Genital sore	Genital ulcer	Syphilis Chancroid Genital herpes
Neonatal conjunctivitis	Swollen eyelids; discharge; baby cannot open eyes	Edema of the eyelids; purulent discharge	Gonorrhea Chlamydia

Source: https://www.glowm.com/pdf/Chap-17_Hanson%20and%20Delvaux.pdf.

8.4.4.1. Vaginal Discharge

Abdominal tenderness, the type of discharge, and the presence of any additional STI symptoms are typically evaluated during syndromic management. Treatment recommendations frequently include care for cervicitis and vaginitis, which includes care for trichomoniasis, gonococcal or chlamydial infections, and BV. Treatment options are restricted to antifungal therapy only in cases where the discharge is unmistakably caused by Candida albicans (cord-like discharge). Treatment recommendations can be restricted to trichomoniasis and bacterial vaginosis if there are no clear indications of cervicitis and neither chlamydial nor gonococcal infections are very common in the relevant environment.

Vaginal discharge that smells can be a sign of advanced cervical cancer. Patients who experience "vaginal discharge" regularly should undergo a visual inspection using acetic acid (VIA) and a speculum examination.

8.4.4.2. Lower Abdominal Pain

Flowcharts for lower abdominal pain typically attempt to rule out the possibility that the pain is being caused by anything other than an infection (see differential diagnosis of PID). When fever and vaginal discharge are present along with palpable abdominal pain, PID is a fairly obvious diagnosis. Treatment recommendations address chlamydial or gonococcal infections.

8.4.4.3. Genital Ulcer

Treatment recommendations typically address both syphilis and chancroid, despite the differences in their clinical presentations. The current revision of syndromic management guidelines for genital ulcers includes treatment for herpes genitalis, which has emerged as the most common cause of genital ulcer disease in areas where STI programs have effectively decreased the prevalence of syphilis and chancroid in the population. As previously mentioned, the suggested treatment plans for the syndromic approach vary slightly amongst nations due to variations in the epidemiology and resistance patterns of microbes. Due to local resistance to the first-line drugs that were previously recommended, the treatment for gonorrhea in particular has recently been revised. Using the national syndromic approach treatment guidelines is advised for clinicians and nurses, especially those working in first-line health facilities.

8.4.5. Improved Treatment of Sexually Transmitted Infections for HIV Prevention

It has been demonstrated in Tanzania that syndromic management and enhanced STI treatment lower the prevalence of HIV in the population. Nevertheless, the overall impact on HIV incidence at the population level appears to vary depending on the setting and the stage of the epidemic, that is, how far the infection has advanced from being restricted to a subgroup to the majority of infections occurring in the general, typically low-risk population. According to a recent Cochrane review, there is insufficient evidence in the published trials to conclude that improved STI treatment significantly lowers HIV incidence in the population (level of evidence 1). On the other hand, better STI treatment can significantly raise the standard of care given to the patient and significantly lower the prevalence of STIs, especially syphilis infections, in a community.

8.4.6. Linkages between Sexually Transmitted Infections/HIV and Sexual and Reproductive Health Services

Hence, every interaction with the healthcare system should be optimized to deliver care, whether it be information and counselling, screening, or treatment. Prevention and control of STIs/RTIs encompass information, counselling, and testing, as well as the treatment of symptomatic diseases. Therefore, the following slogan should be closely followed in STI/RTI prevention and care:

'Counselling at any visits: don't miss the opportunity.'

It is crucial to address STI/HIV in prenatal care, particularly to guarantee that testing for syphilis and HIV is done during the initial visit (refer to the section on syphilis screening). It has been suggested that family planning and STI services be connected to enhance the standard of care and service uptake. STI clinics should discuss and provide family planning as part of the consultation, or at the very least, refer patients to the appropriate health provider/clinic if the service cannot be provided at the same time. Family planning services should not only provide information but also screening and treatment for symptomatic STIs.

Additionally, the STI/RTI consultation offers a significant window of opportunity for additional preventive services, like acetic acid screening for cervical cancer. Post-abortion care should include HIV/STI counselling as well.

8.4.7. Dual Protection

"Dual protection" refers to defense against STIs and unintended pregnancy. The cornerstone of dual protection is a pair of condoms, which can be used either alone as a backup form of contraception in case of emergencies or conjunction with non-barrier methods such as sterilization. Condom use as a stand-alone strategy for dual protection may be jeopardized because sexually active individuals frequently refuse to use condoms consistently for a variety of reasons, which lowers the effectiveness of the device. As a result, the use of another method of contraception is necessary for dual protection against unwanted pregnancy to be mostly effective.(Vuylsteke et al., 2004; Pettifor et al., 2000).

8.5. Management of Asymptomatic Sexually Transmitted Infections: Screening

A lot of STIs have no symptoms. For this reason, screening programs are especially crucial in preventing the spread of STIs. When gonococcal and/or chlamydial infections occur, up to 70% of women and a sizable portion of men may show no symptoms at all.

Additionally, some people choose not to seek medical attention despite exhibiting symptoms due to stigma or limited access to healthcare facilities. As previously mentioned, accurate diagnosis is frequently a challenge in low-resource environments where laboratory tests are either scarce or nonexistent. Even with an accurate diagnosis, patients may not finish their recommended course of treatment if the prescribed medications are not readily available. It is generally believed that very few persons with STIs or RTIs receive a cure.

As a result, a significant issue with STI treatment is that effective treatment only reaches a small percentage of patients. However, over-treatment is also a known issue with syndromic management; patients may receive treatment for STIs even though other disorders may be the cause of their symptoms. As a result, there are issues with both serious under- and overtreatment of STIs and RTIs. Figure 8.8 illustrates the operational model for STI/RTI control.

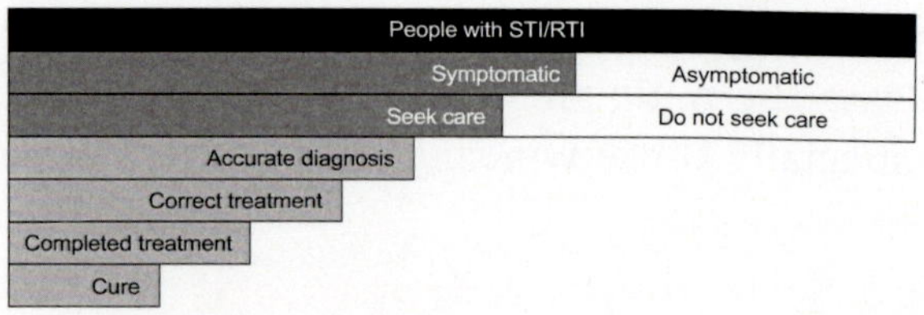

Figure 8.8. *Operational model for STI/RTI control: asymptomatic cases and people who don't seek care.*

Source: https://www.glowm.com/pdf/Chap-17_Hanson%20and%20Delvaux.pdf.

For infections like gonococcal or chlamydial, which are frequently asymptomatic, screening would be the best course of action. Nevertheless, there is currently no straightforward, sensitive, specific, or reasonably priced test for these two agents, although research and development are ongoing.

8.5.1. Syphilis Screening

There are currently only inexpensive, straightforward screening tests available for syphilis. Prenatal care must include the detection of asymptomatic infection to prevent and control syphilis and its side effects, which include stillbirth and spontaneous abortion. For this reason, it has long been advised that syphilis screening and treatment be provided at the initial prenatal care visit as a standard component of prenatal care (WHO, 2007). Given that the procedures require very similar knowledge and interventions, there are opportunities to strengthen syphilis screening through the continued roll-out and support of PMTCT services19. Thus, integrating PMTCT and syphilis screening offers a critical window of opportunity to lessen the prevalence of STIs.

If testing is available, screening for other STIs/RTIs, such as HIV, BV, and cervical infections, should also be provided during prenatal care. Unfortunately, there are currently no accessible, low-cost tests for cervicitis. In most settings, what can and should be done is ask women about STI symptoms in both themselves and their partner during prenatal care, and treat symptomatic women using the syndromic approach. Additionally, it is important to encourage STI prevention during pregnancy to protect the unborn child as well as future fertility.

8.5.2. Periodic Presumptive Treatment

To stop the spread of HIV, Rakai, Uganda, has conducted studies on the use of metronidazole, Cipro, ofloxacin, and azithromycin in large-scale adult treatment. Nonetheless, no discernible distinction was found between the group receiving treatment and a group receiving no treatment for comparison. Currently, mass treatment of the entire population is not advised (Wawer et al., 1999).

However, systematic treatment periodically can be used in high-risk groups, like female sex workers. It is especially advised during the first visit. The following factors will determine whether presumptive treatment should be administered at follow-up appointments: (1) re-infection rate; (2) feasibility; and (3) local resistance patterns. Counselling, screening, and other STI control measures ought to be used in every situation.

8.5.3. Partner Notification

Partner notification is a collection of public health initiatives designed to inform partners of individuals living with sexually transmitted infections (STIs) or HIV, as well as to provide those individuals with relevant services and risk education. Partner notification aims to break the cycle of sexually transmitted infections and prevent re-infection in the patient, while also protecting partners from complications and secondary infections. In cases where a partner exhibits no symptoms, partner treatment may be deemed a "presumptive treatment." Notifying partners should also include educating and counselling them about HIV and STIs.

Offering free care is one strategy, along with the use of referral or notification slips, to promote partner notification and treatment. The most popular strategy is patient referral since it doesn't call for extra resources. It is advised that patients get in touch with their sexual partners on their own. They frequently receive a referral sheet with the patient's diagnosis listed on it or a code that indicates the diagnosis of the patient who came in with symptoms. Another way to guarantee partner treatment is to have medical professionals with specialized training alert sexual partners and make the necessary treatment arrangements. Although far more costly, this is also more efficient. Another option is to combine the two approaches; alternatively, the patient could receive their partner's treatment.

Not every STI or RTI is spread through sex. STI treatment and partner notification ought to guarantee that patients are not stigmatized or given incorrect labels. In cases where index male patients with STIs need to treat their female partners, partner notification should be encouraged due to the limitations of the syndromic approach among women.

8.6. Prevention of Sexually Transmitted Infections

The best way to prevent STIs is to either never have sex or limit your sexual activity to long-term, mutually monogamous relationships with uninfected partners.

8.6.1. Male or Female Condoms

These have been shown to be very successful in preventing infection when used correctly and consistently.

8.6.1.1. Female Condom

Polyurethane was used to make the first female condom, which went by the names Femy, Femidom, and Reality. In 2007, a new version known as the female condom 2, which was made of less expensive nitrile material, was introduced, and mass production of the device started. Findings from qualitative research indicate that when using the female condom as opposed to the male condom or unprotected sex, women living with HIV in particular can feel more in control. At the international level, the female condom has not gotten enough attention thus far.

8.6.2. Adult Male Circumcision

Adult male circumcision is less effective than abstinence, faithfulness, and condom use, but it is promising for reducing the spread of HIV and possibly other STIs. According to multiple reviews, men have a 50–60% lower risk of HIV transmission (level of evidence 1). Male circumcision in adulthood does not appear to negatively affect sexual function, and it may be a very affordable method of HIV prevention. While the evidence is still being gathered, there are some encouraging results suggesting that male circumcision can also prevent other STIs. There are still a lot of operational problems that need to be resolved before this intervention can be widely implemented. Male circumcision cannot be encouraged to lower female infections because there is no proof that it has a direct impact on the transmission of HIV or other STIs from male to female.

8.6.3. Microbicides

Topical microbicides are substances that can be used to treat STIs, such as HIV, inside the rectum or vagina. They can be made into suppositories, films, gels, or creams. The contraceptive effect, or spermicidal activity, of microbicides is uncertain. There isn't currently a microbicide on the market that works well. However, after 30 months, women who used tenofovir (antiretroviral) gel had a 39% lower overall rate of HIV infection. This was the finding of a recent study. Infection was 54% lower in women who took the medication regularly. According to the study, the gel also lowered the risk of genital herpes by 51%.

8.6.4. Prevention of Ophthalmia Neonatorum

Another very successful preventive method is the use of eye ointments containing erythromycin or tetracycline to prevent ophthalmia neonatorum. Credé developed the ocular 2% silver nitrate prophylaxis in 1881, which was subsequently called the Credé prophylaxis in his honor. It has been demonstrated that prophylaxis with silver nitrate, 1% erythromycin, 1% tetracycline solution, or povidone-iodine is effective against the infectious agents that cause ophthalmia neonatorum, primarily gonococci and chlamydia. In the 20th century, prophylactic use significantly decreased blindness and gonococci conjunctivitis in newborns in Western nations. As of right now, preventing ophthalmia neonatorum with a solution of 1% erythromycin or 1% tetracycline is included in the essential care package for newborns. Using eye ointment is simple, affordable, and efficient. Despite the widespread availability of 1% erythromycin or

1% tetracycline solution, the prevention of ophthalmia neonatorum is still not well implemented in many settings. Nurses, midwives, and clinicians must provide reinforcement.

8.6.5. Prevention of Septic Abortion

To prevent unsafe and septic abortions, a health district and district hospital should make a significant effort to provide family planning, safe abortion when permitted, and appropriate post-abortion care. To prevent septic abortion in both spontaneous and induced abortions, good clinical practice should be followed when emptying the uterus following an abortion or miscarriage using medical or surgical procedures (manual vacuum aspiration).

8.6.6. Prevention of Iatrogenic or Exogenous Infection

Finally, following infection control protocols during gynecological procedures and properly decontaminating and sterilizing equipment are important components of preventing iatrogenic or exogenous infections. National guidelines for infection prevention are available in most countries and ought to be adhered to religiously (Watson-Jones et al., 2005; Ishaque et al., 2011).

A Closer Look

Human Papillomavirus

Human papillomavirus (HPV) is a group of more than 200 related viruses, some of which are associated with various cancers and other diseases. HPV is the most common sexually transmitted infection globally, affecting both men and women. The virus is typically spread through intimate skin-to-skin contact, often during vaginal, anal, or oral sex. HPV infections are usually asymptomatic and may resolve on their own, but certain high-risk strains can persist and lead to serious health issues.

There are two main categories of HPV: low-risk and high-risk types. Low-risk HPVs, such as types 6 and 11, can cause benign conditions like genital warts and respiratory papillomatosis. High-risk HPVs, particularly types 16 and 18, are strongly linked to the development of cancers, including cervical, anal, oropharyngeal, penile, vulvar, and vaginal cancers. HPV 16 and 18 are responsible for approximately 70% of cervical cancer cases worldwide.

HPV-related cancers often develop years after the initial infection, underscoring the importance of early detection and prevention. Regular screening for cervical cancer through Pap tests (Pap smears) and HPV tests can detect precancerous changes in the cervix, allowing for timely intervention. Vaccination is a highly effective preventive measure. The HPV vaccine, recommended for preteens (boys and girls) aged 11 or 12, can prevent the majority of HPV-related cancers and genital warts by protecting against the most common high-risk and low-risk types.

Public health efforts focus on increasing vaccine uptake and regular screening to reduce the burden of HPV-associated diseases. Despite the availability of effective vaccines, vaccination rates remain suboptimal in many regions due to factors such as lack of awareness, access issues, and vaccine hesitancy. Education campaigns and healthcare provider recommendations play a crucial role in improving vaccination coverage.

HPV is a prevalent and potentially serious virus with a significant impact on public health. Prevention through vaccination, early detection through screening, and education are key strategies in combating the adverse effects of HPV and reducing the incidence of related cancers and diseases.

Summary

- The prevention of sexually transmitted diseases (STDs) and HIV is a critical public health priority aimed at reducing the incidence and impact of these infections.
- Male circumcision appears to significantly reduce the likelihood of acquiring several STIs, including human papillomavirus, genital herpes, and especially human immunodeficiency virus (HIV), where the infective risk decreases by 50% to 60%.
- Pelvic inflammatory disease (PID) is a sexually transmitted infection that affects the upper female genital tract. It can have serious implications for long-term fertility.
- Ulcerative infections of the genitalia to exclude, which also cause inguinal lymphadenopathy, would be chancroid, herpes, granuloma inguinale, and syphilis.
- The syndromic approach is scientifically derived. The antimicrobial regimens are chosen to cover major pathogens responsible for the syndromes in a specific geographical area.
- The normal vaginal flora is composed of several species of bacteria producing lactobacilli which are maintaining a slightly acid vaginal environment of pH 4.5.
- Partner notification is the set of public health activities that aims at informing the partners of people infected with STI or HIV, and at offering those infected appropriate services and counselling about their risks.
- Prevention of iatrogenic or exogenous infection should include adherence to infection prevention measures when performing any gynecological procedures as well as proper decontamination and sterilization of equipment.

References

1. Abdool Karim, Q., Abdool Karim, S. S., Frohlich, J. A., et al. (2010). Effectiveness and safety of tenofovir gel, an antiretroviral microbicide, for the prevention of HIV infection in women. *Science, 329*(5996), 1168–1174. https://doi.org/10.1126/science.1193748.
2. Andrist, L. C. (1988). Taking a sexual history and educating clients about safe sex. *The Nursing Clinics of North America, 23*(4), 959–973.
3. Anon. (2011). Financing HPV vaccination in developing countries. *The Lancet, 377*(9777), 1544. https://doi.org/10.1016/S0140-6736(11)60611-5.
4. Berer, M. (2003). Integration of sexual and reproductive health services: A health sector priority. *Reproductive Health Matters, 11*(21), 6–15. https://doi.org/10.1016/S0968-8080(03)02152-9.
5. Bray, F., Ferlay, J., Soerjomataram, I., Siegel, R. L., Torre, L. A., & Jemal, A. (2018). Global cancer statistics 2018: GLOBOCAN estimates of incidence and mortality worldwide for 36 cancers in 185 countries. *CA: A Cancer Journal for Clinicians, 68*(6), 394–424. https://doi.org/10.3322/caac.21492.
6. Brocklehurst, P. (2002). Antibiotics for gonorrhea in pregnancy. *Cochrane Database of Systematic Reviews, 2*, CD000098. https://doi.org/10.1002/14651858.CD000098.
7. Brocklehurst, P., & Rooney, G. (1998). Interventions for treating genital *Chlamydia trachomatis* infection in pregnancy. *Cochrane Database of Systematic Reviews, 4*, CD000054. https://doi.org/10.1002/14651858.CD000054.

8. Bugg, C. W., Taira, T., & Zaurova, M. (2016). Pelvic inflammatory disease: Diagnosis and treatment in the emergency department [Digest]. *Emergency Medicine Practice, 18*(12 Suppl Points & Pearls), S1–S2.

9. Capriotti, T. (2018). HIV/AIDS: An update for home healthcare clinicians. *Home Healthcare Now, 36*(6), 348–355. https://doi.org/10.1097/NHH.0000000000000728.

10. Chesson, H. W., Heffelfinger, J. D., Voigt, R. F., & Collins, D. (2005). Estimates of primary and secondary syphilis rates in persons with HIV in the United States, 2002. *Sexually Transmitted Diseases, 32*(5), 265–269. https://doi.org/10.1097/01.olq.0000154505.00898.db.

11. Cook, R. L., Hutchison, S. L., Østergaard, L., Braithwaite, R. S., & Ness, R. B. (2005). Systematic review: Noninvasive testing for *Chlamydia trachomatis* and *Neisseria gonorrhoeae*. *Annals of Internal Medicine, 142*(11), 914–925. https://doi.org/10.7326/0003-4819-142-11-200506070-00011.

12. De Schryver, A., & Meheus, A. (1990). Epidemiology of sexually transmitted diseases: The global picture. *Bulletin of the World Health Organization, 68*(5), 639–654.

13. Doyle, S. M., Kahn, J. G., Hosang, N., & Carroll, P. R. (2010). The impact of male circumcision on HIV transmission. *Journal of Urology, 183*(1), 21–26. https://doi.org/10.1016/j.juro.2009.09.098.

14. Falagas, M. E., Betsi, G. I., & Athanasiou, S. (2007). Probiotics for the treatment of women with bacterial vaginosis. *Clinical Microbiology and Infection, 13*(7), 657–664. https://doi.org/10.1111/j.1469-0691.2007.01722.x.

15. Farley, T. M., Samuelson, J., Grabowski, M. K., et al. (2020). Impact of male circumcision on risk of HIV infection in men in a changing epidemic context: Systematic review and meta-analysis. *Journal of the International AIDS Society, 23*(6), e25490. https://doi.org/10.1002/jia2.25490.

16. Fleming, D., & Wasserheit, J. (1999). From epidemiological synergy to public health policy and practice: The contribution of other sexually transmitted diseases to sexual transmission of HIV infection. *Sexually Transmitted Infections, 75*(1), 3–17. https://doi.org/10.1136/sti.75.1.3.

17. Glatz, M., Juricevic, N., Altwegg, M., Bruisten, S., Komericki, P., Lautenschlager, S., Weber, R., & Bosshard, P. P. (2014). A multicenter prospective trial to assess a new real-time polymerase chain reaction for detection of *Treponema pallidum*, herpes simplex-1/2, and *Haemophilus ducreyi* in genital, anal, and oropharyngeal ulcers. *Clinical Microbiology and Infection, 20*(12), O1020–O1027. https://doi.org/10.1111/1469-0691.12616.

18. Gray, R. H., Kigozi, G., Kong, X., et al. (2012). The effectiveness of male circumcision for HIV prevention and effects on risk behaviors in a posttrial follow-up study. *AIDS, 26*(5), 609–615. https://doi.org/10.1097/QAD.0b013e3283504a3f.

19. Grosskurth, H., Todd, J., Mwijarubi, E., et al. (1995). Impact of improved treatment of sexually transmitted diseases on HIV infection in rural Tanzania: Randomized controlled trial. *The Lancet, 346*(8974), 530–536. https://doi.org/10.1016/S0140-6736(95)91380-7.

20. Guaschino, S. (2000). [Complications of sexually transmitted diseases: Clinical course and treatment]. *Annali dell'Istituto Superiore di Sanità, 36*(4), 431–435.

21. Hayes, R., Schulz, K., & Plummer, F. (1995). The cofactor effect of genital ulcers on the per-exposure risk of HIV transmission in sub-Saharan Africa. *Journal of Tropical Medicine and*

Hygiene, 98(1), 1–8.

22. Hook, E. W. (2017). Syphilis. *The Lancet, 389*(10078), 1550–1557. https://doi.org/10.1016/S0140-6736(16)32411-4.
23. Hussain, S. A., & Vaidya, R. (2023). Congenital syphilis. In *StatPearls [Internet]*. StatPearls Publishing. Retrieved from: https://www.ncbi.nlm.nih.gov/books/NBK556046/ (accessed on 3 September 2024).
24. Huynh, K., & Kahwaji, C. I. (2023). HIV testing. In *StatPearls [Internet]*. StatPearls Publishing. Retrieved from: https://www.ncbi.nlm.nih.gov/books/NBK441872/ (accessed on 3 September 2024).
25. Irizarry, L., Velasquez, J., & Wray, A. A. (2023). Chancroid. In *StatPearls [Internet]*. StatPearls Publishing. Retrieved from: https://www.ncbi.nlm.nih.gov/books/NBK555904/ (accessed on 3 September 2024).
26. Ishaque, S., Yakoob, M., Imdad, A., et al. (2011). Effectiveness of interventions to screen and manage infections during pregnancy on reducing stillbirths: A review. *BMC Public Health, 11*(Suppl. 3), S3. https://doi.org/10.1186/1471-2458-11-S3-S3.
27. Jain, B. (2017). The key role of differential diagnosis in diagnosis. *Diagnosis, 4*(4), 239–240. https://doi.org/10.1515/dx-2017-0027.
28. James, C., Harfouche, M., Welton, N. J., Turner, K. M., Abu-Raddad, L. J., Gottlieb, S. L., & Looker, K. J. (2020). Herpes simplex virus: Global infection prevalence and incidence estimates, 2016. *Bulletin of the World Health Organization, 98*(5), 315–329. https://doi.org/10.2471/BLT.19.237149.
29. Jennings, L. K., & Krywko, D. M. (2023). Pelvic inflammatory disease. In *StatPearls [Internet]*. StatPearls Publishing. Retrieved from: https://www.ncbi.nlm.nih.gov/books/NBK448185/ (accessed on 3 September 2024).
30. Justiz Vaillant, A. A., & Gulick, P. G. (2022). HIV and AIDS syndrome. In *StatPearls [Internet]*. StatPearls Publishing. Retrieved from: https://www.ncbi.nlm.nih.gov/books/NBK513295/ (accessed on 3 September 2024).
31. Kissinger, P. (2015). Epidemiology and treatment of trichomoniasis. *Current Infectious Disease Reports, 17*(6), 484. https://doi.org/10.1007/s11908-015-0484-x.
32. Lanao, A. E., Chakraborty, R. K., & Pearson-Shaver, A. L. (2023). Mycoplasma infections. In *StatPearls [Internet]*. StatPearls Publishing. Retrieved from: https://www.ncbi.nlm.nih.gov/books/NBK556046/ (accessed on 3 September 2024).
33. Lawrence, H. C., & Ness, D. L. (2017). Planned Parenthood provides essential services that improve women's health. *Annals of Internal Medicine, 166*(6), 443–444. https://doi.org/10.7326/M17-0192.
34. Lo Oker, J., Garnett, G., & Schmid, G. (2008). An estimate of the global prevalence and incidence of herpes simplex virus type 2 infection. *Bulletin of the World Health Organization, 86*, 805–812. https://doi.org/10.2471/BLT.07.046128.
35. Luria, L., & Cardoza-Favarato, G. (2023). Human papillomavirus. In *StatPearls [Internet]*. StatPearls Publishing. Retrieved from: https://www.ncbi.nlm.nih.gov/books/NBK526098/ (accessed on 3 September 2024).

36. Martín-Sánchez, M., Ong, J. J., Fairley, C. K., Chen, M. Y., Williamson, D. A., Maddaford, K., Aung, E. T., Carter, G., Bradshaw, C. S., & Chow, E. P. F. (2020). Clinical presentation of asymptomatic and symptomatic heterosexual men who tested positive for urethral gonorrhoea at a sexual health clinic in Melbourne, Australia. *BMC Infectious Diseases, 20*(1), 486. https://doi.org/10.1186/s12879-020-05218-3.

37. Mathew, J., Jr., & Sapra, A. (2023). Herpes simplex type 2. In *StatPearls [Internet]*. StatPearls Publishing. Retrieved from: https://www.ncbi.nlm.nih.gov/books/NBK538263/ (accessed on 3 September 2024).

38. Mayaud, P., & Mabey, D. (2004). Approaches to the control of sexually transmitted infections in developing countries: Old problems and modern challenges. *Sexually Transmitted Infections, 80*(3), 174–182. https://doi.org/10.1136/sti.2002.004101.

39. Mayhew, S. H. (1996). Integrating MCH/FP and STD/HIV services: Current debates and future directions. *Health Policy and Planning, 11*(4), 339–353. https://doi.org/10.1093/heapol/11.4.339.

40. Mohseni, M., Sung, S., & Takov, V. (2023). Chlamydia. In *StatPearls [Internet]*. StatPearls Publishing. Retrieved from: https://www.ncbi.nlm.nih.gov/books/NBK459171/ (accessed on 3 September 2024).

41. Ng, B., Butler, L., Horvath, T., & Rutherford, G. (2011). Population-based biomedical sexually transmitted infection control interventions for reducing HIV infection. *Cochrane Database of Systematic Reviews, 2011*(3), CD001220. https://doi.org/10.1002/14651858.CD001220.pub3.

42. Nyirjesy, P., & Sobel, J. D. (2003). Vulvovaginal candidiasis. *Obstetrics and Gynecology Clinics of North America, 30*(4), 671–684. https://doi.org/10.1016/S0889-8545(03)00095-8.

43. Peters, A., Jansen, W., & van Driel, F. (2010). The female condom: The international denial of a strong potential. *Reproductive Health Matters, 18*(35), 119–128. https://doi.org/10.1016/S0968-8080(10)35498-4.

44. Pettifor, A., Walsh, J., Wilkins, V., & Raghunathan, P. (2000). How effective is syndromic management of STDs? A review of current studies. *Sexually Transmitted Diseases, 27*(7), 371–385. https://doi.org/10.1097/00007435-200007000-00008.

45. Rawla, P., Thandra, K. C., & Limaiem, F. (2023). Lymphogranuloma venereum. In *StatPearls [Internet]*. StatPearls Publishing. Retrieved from: https://www.ncbi.nlm.nih.gov/books/NBK559267/ (accessed on 3 September 2024).

46. Rupp, T. J., & Leslie, S. W. (2023). Epididymitis. In *StatPearls [Internet]*. StatPearls Publishing. Retrieved from: https://www.ncbi.nlm.nih.gov/books/NBK459317/ (accessed on 3 September 2024).

47. Rydzak, C. E., & Goldie, S. J. (2008). Cost-effectiveness of rapid point-of-care prenatal syphilis screening in sub-Saharan Africa. *Sexually Transmitted Diseases, 35*(9), 775–784. https://doi.org/10.1097/OLQ.0b013e3181761967.

48. Saleh, D., Yarrarapu, S. N. S., & Sharma, S. (2023). Herpes simplex type 1. In *StatPearls [Internet]*. StatPearls Publishing. Retrieved from: https://www.ncbi.nlm.nih.gov/books/NBK525776/ (accessed on 3 September 2024).

49. Santiago-Wickey, J. N., & Crosby, B. (2023). Granuloma inguinale. In *StatPearls [Internet]*.

StatPearls Publishing. Retrieved from: https://www.ncbi.nlm.nih.gov/books/NBK470548/ (accessed on 3 September 2024).

50. Schumann, J. A., & Plasner, S. (2023). Trichomoniasis. In *StatPearls [Internet]*. StatPearls Publishing. Retrieved from: https://www.ncbi.nlm.nih.gov/books/NBK441851/ (accessed on 3 September 2024).

51. Smith, L., & Angarone, M. P. (2015). Sexually transmitted infections. *Urologic Clinics of North America, 42*(4), 507–518. https://doi.org/10.1016/j.ucl.2015.07.009.

52. Springer, C., & Salen, P. (2023). Gonorrhea. In *StatPearls [Internet]*. StatPearls Publishing. Retrieved from: https://www.ncbi.nlm.nih.gov/books/NBK532932/ (accessed on 3 September 2024).

53. Tobian, A. A. R., Serwadda, D., Quinn, T. C., et al. (2009). Male circumcision for the prevention of HSV-2 and HPV infections and syphilis. *The New England Journal of Medicine, 360*(13), 1298–1309. https://doi.org/10.1056/NEJMoa0802556.

54. Tudor, M. E., Al Aboud, A. M., Leslie, S. W., & Gossman, W. (2023). Syphilis. In *StatPearls [Internet]*. StatPearls Publishing. Retrieved from: https://www.ncbi.nlm.nih.gov/books/NBK441912/ (accessed on 3 September 2024).

55. Vuylsteke, B. (2004). Current status of syndromic management of sexually transmitted infections in developing countries. *Sexually Transmitted Infections, 80*(5), 333–334. https://doi.org/10.1136/sti.2004.010249.

56. Wagenlehner, F. M., Brockmeyer, N. H., Discher, T., Friese, K., & Wichelhaus, T. A. (2016). The presentation, diagnosis, and treatment of sexually transmitted infections. *Deutsches Ärzteblatt International, 113*(1–2), 11–22. https://doi.org/10.3238/arztebl.2016.0011.

57. Wald, A., & Link, K. (2002). Risk of human immunodeficiency virus infection in herpes simplex virus type 2-seropositive persons: A meta-analysis. *Journal of Infectious Diseases, 185*(1), 45–52. https://doi.org/10.1086/338115.

58. Watson-Jones, D., Oliff, M., Terris-Prestholt, F., et al. (2005). Antenatal syphilis screening in sub-Saharan Africa: Lessons learned from Tanzania. *Tropical Medicine & International Health, 10*(9), 934–943. https://doi.org/10.1111/j.1365-3156.2005.01477.x.

59. Wawer, M. J., Sewankambo, N. K., Serwadda, D., et al. (1999). Control of sexually transmitted diseases for AIDS prevention in Uganda: A randomized community trial. *The Lancet, 353*(9152), 525–535. https://doi.org/10.1016/S0140-6736(98)06439-3.

60. Waymack, J. R., & Sundareshan, V. (2023). Acquired immune deficiency syndrome. In *StatPearls [Internet]*. StatPearls Publishing. Retrieved from: https://www.ncbi.nlm.nih.gov/books/NBK538460/ (accessed on 3 September 2024).

61. Welbourn, A. (2006). Sex, life, and the female condom: Some views of HIV-positive women. *Reproductive Health Matters, 14*(28), 32–40. https://doi.org/10.1016/S0968-8080(06)28256-4.

62. Wiysonge, C. S., Kongnyuy, E. J., Shey, M., et al. (2011). Male circumcision for prevention of homosexual acquisition of HIV in men. *Cochrane Database of Systematic Reviews, 2011*(4), CD007496. https://doi.org/10.1002/14651858.CD007496.pub2.

63. Workowski, K. A., & Bolan, G. A. (2015). Sexually transmitted diseases treatment guidelines, 2015. *MMWR Recommendations and Reports, 64*(RR-03), 1–137. https://www.cdc.gov/std/tg2015/default.htm (accessed on 3 September 2024).

64. World Health Organization, ICM. (2008). *Managing Incomplete Abortion*. Geneva: WHO.

65. World Health Organization, TDR. (2006). *Rapid Syphilis Test*. Geneva: WHO.

66. World Health Organization. (2000). *Joint WHO/UNAIDS/UNFPA Policy Statement: Dual Protection Against Unwanted Pregnancy and Sexually Transmitted Infections, Including HIV*. Geneva: WHO.

67. World Health Organization. (2005). *Sexually Transmitted and Other Reproductive Tract Infections: A Guide to Essential Practice*. Geneva: WHO. Retrieved from: http://whqlibdoc.who.int/publications/2005/9241592656.pdf (accessed on 3 September 2024).

68. World Health Organization. (2007). *Global Strategy for the Prevention and Control of Sexually Transmitted Infections: 2006–2015. Breaking the Chain of Transmission*. Geneva: WHO.

69. World Health Organization. (2007). *The Global Elimination of Congenital Syphilis: Rationale and Strategy for Action*. Geneva: WHO.

70. World Health Organization. (2011). *Prevalence and Incidence of Selected Sexually Transmitted Infections: Methods and Results Used by WHO to Generate 2005 Estimates*. Geneva: WHO. Retrieved from: http://whqlibdoc.who.int/publications/2011/9789241502450_eng.pdf (accessed on 3 September 2024).

71. Xu, F., Sternberg, M. R., Kottiri, B. J., McQuillan, G. M., Lee, F. K., Nahmias, A. J., Berman, S. M., & Markowitz, L. E. (2006). Trends in herpes simplex virus type 1 and type 2 seroprevalence in the United States. *JAMA, 296*(8), 964–973. https://doi.org/10.1001/jama.296.8.964.

72. Ye, X., Liu, J., & Yi, Z. (2019). Trends in the epidemiology of sexually transmitted disease, acquired immune deficiency syndrome (AIDS), gonorrhea, and syphilis, in the 31 provinces of Mainland China. *Medical Science Monitor, 25*, 5657–5665. https://doi.org/10.12659/MSM.916645.

73. Zuppa, A. A., D'Andrea, V., Catenazzi, P., et al. (2011). Ophthalmia neonatorum: What kind of prophylaxis? *Journal of Maternal-Fetal & Neonatal Medicine, 24*(6), 769–773. https://doi.org/10.3109/14767058.2010.514921.

Chapter 9

WOMEN'S AND ADOLESCENT HEALTH

Contents

Introduction

Women and adolescent health is a critical time for young women to develop good health habits that will help them in their future lives.

The broad category of women's health includes conditions like diabetes and heart disease that may affect women differently from men as well as conditions that are specific to women, like menstruation and pregnancy.

As a transitional period from childhood to adulthood, adolescence is a crucial and significant time in life that ushers in a period of physical, psychological, and social change (Dick and Ferguson, 2015). Those between the ages of 10 and 19 are considered adolescents (Melaku et al., 2015). More than 25% of people on the planet are adolescents (Taghizadeh Moghaddam et al., 2016). Since they make up a sizable portion of the population in our country, their health should be given careful thought (Panjalipour et al., 2018). The importance of female adolescent health is further reinforced by the features of female puberty, the physical and psychological difficulties of adolescence, and the crucial role of female infertility. Women's adolescence shapes their later years and has a significant influence on their ability to start and raise families (Jaskiewicz, 2009). Assembling and organizing care strategies begins with determining what the target groups' needs are. The distinction between the needs of adults and adolescents was highlighted at the International Conference on Population and Development. It was requested of the participating countries to determine and attend to these needs (Chandra-Mouli et al., 2015). There are inherent differences among adolescent populations, but not much research has been done to evaluate their particular health needs.

Orientation and Directional Terms

Term	Definition	Illustration
Anemia	Anemia is a blood disorder that occurs when the body doesn't produce enough healthy red blood cells, which means the body doesn't get enough oxygen-rich blood.	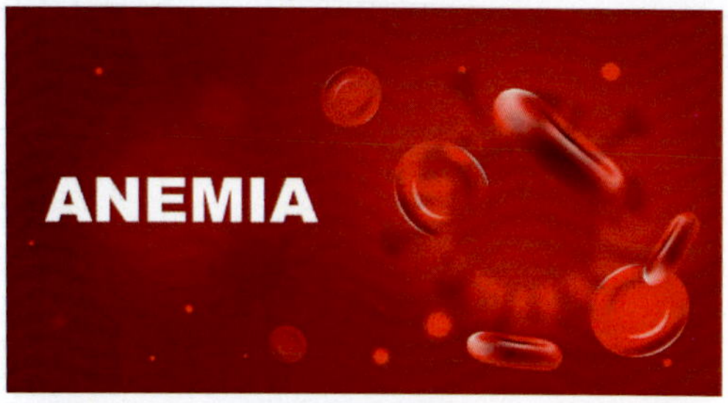
Cancer	Cancer is a group of diseases involving abnormal cell growth with the potential to invade or spread to other parts of the body.	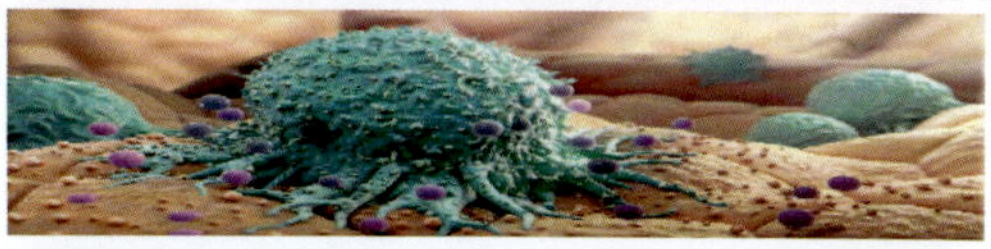
Cardiovascular disease	Cardiovascular disease is caused by narrowing or blockages in the arteries (i.e., blood vessels carrying oxygen to the heart).	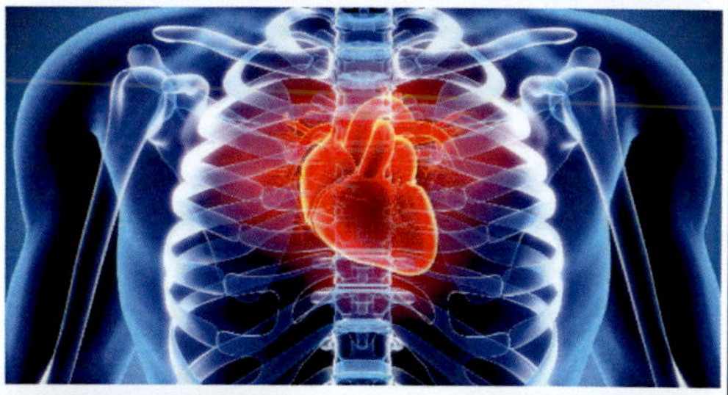
,Depression	Depression is a mental disorder that can affect a person's thoughts, feelings, behavior, and sense of well-being. It can cause a persistent feeling of sadness and loss of interest in activities, and can make it difficult to do normal day-to-day activities.	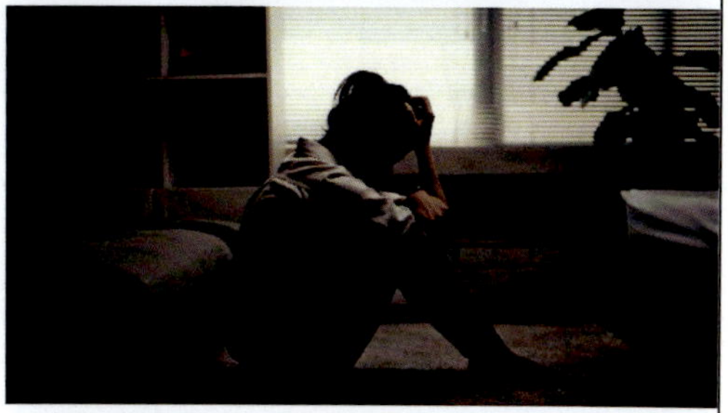
Lung disease	Lung disease is any condition that prevents the lungs from functioning properly, affecting respiratory function and pulmonary function.	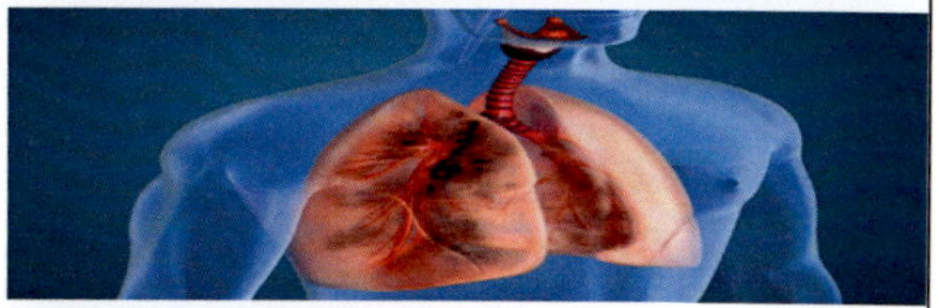
Osteoporosis	Osteoporosis is a bone disease that occurs when the body loses too much bone, makes too little bone, or both.	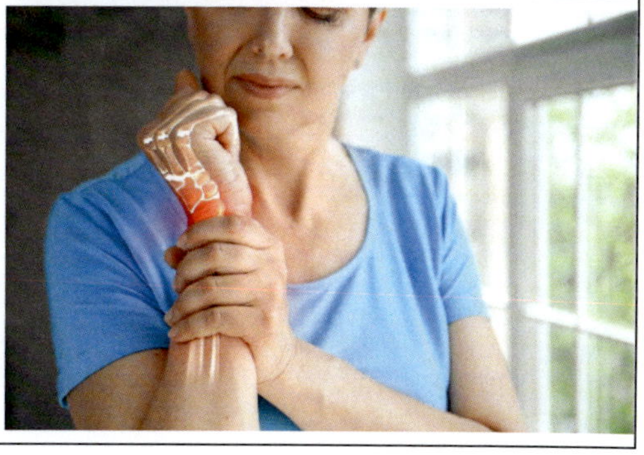

9.1. Women's Health

There are numerous distinct ways in which the health of women and men is different. The World Health Organization (WHO) defines health as "a state of complete physical, mental and social well-being and not merely the absence of disease or infirmity." Women's health is an example of population health. Many groups argue for a broader definition pertaining to women's overall health, better expressed as "The health of women." Women's reproductive health is often treated as a monolithic concept. These disparities are made worse in developing nations where women face additional disadvantages and whose health encompasses both risks and experiences.

Although women and men experience the major causes of death—heart disease, cancer, and lung disease—at similar rates, women's experiences are distinct. The primary cause of cancer-related mortality in women is now lung cancer, surpassing all other cancer subtypes. Breast cancer, colorectal, ovarian, uterine, and cervical cancers follow lung cancer in terms of importance. Although smoking is the primary cause of lung cancer, women who do not smoke have a three times higher risk of developing the disease than men who do not smoke. Despite this, cervical cancer continues to be one of the most common cancers in developing countries and is linked to the human papilloma virus (HPV), a sexually transmitted infection. Breast cancer, on the other hand, is still the most common cancer in women in developed countries and is one of the major chronic diseases affecting women. The HPV vaccine and screening together hold the key to preventing and treating these illnesses. Osteoporosis, anemia, depression, dementia, and cardiovascular disease are other significant health concerns for women.

In 176 of the 178 countries where life expectancy data is available, women's life expectancy is higher than men's. This has been the case in Western Europe since at least 1750. Gender continues to be a significant social determinant of health because conditions like poverty, work, and family responsibilities affect women's health in addition to their biology. Women have historically experienced disadvantage in a variety of areas, including social and economic power, which limits their access to basic needs like health care. The more disadvantage a woman faces, such as in developing nations, the more detrimental effects this disadvantage has on her health.

The reproductive and sexual health of women differs significantly from that of men. Maternal mortality accounts for over a quarter of a million deaths annually, with significant differences between developed and developing nations. Pregnancy and childbirth are associated with significant risks to women even in developed nations. Preeclampsia is one of the pregnancy's morbidities and mortality rates that are influenced by comorbidity from other non-reproductive diseases like cardiovascular disease. Sexually transmitted infections can have fatal effects on women and babies. For example, transmission from mother to child can result in stillbirths and neonatal deaths, and pelvic inflammatory disease can cause infertility. Women are also burdened by rape, unintended pregnancies, birth control, infertility from a variety of other causes, and the fight to obtain access to abortions.

9.1.1. Definitions and Scope of Women's Health

Women's experiences with health and illness are different from men's because of their own biological, social, and behavioral characteristics. Biological variations show distinct risks for the emergence of illness and range from phenotypes to cellular biology. WHO defines health as "a state of complete physical, mental and social well-being and not merely the absence of disease or infirmity." One example of population health, or the health of a particular, defined population, is the condition of women.

Women's health has been described as "a patchwork quilt with gaps." A broader understanding of women's health to include all aspects of women's health has been urged, replacing "Women's Health" with "The Health of Women," despite the fact that many issues surrounding women's health are related to their reproductive health, including maternal and child health, genital health and breast health, and endocrine (hormonal) health, including menstruation, birth control, and menopause. According to WHO, one of the main obstacles to guaranteeing that all women have access to high-quality healthcare is the overemphasis placed on reproductive health. Osteoporosis and cardiovascular disease are two conditions that affect both men and women, but they present differently in women. Women's health issues also include medical conditions where women deal with issues unrelated to their biology, such as socioeconomic status and unequal access to healthcare. Because women are disadvantaged by pervasive discrimination worldwide, women's health is especially important.

Several proponents of health and medical research, including the Society for Women's Health Research in the US, are in favor of this more inclusive definition, which goes beyond problems unique to human female anatomy to encompass regions where biological sex differences exist between men and women. In addition, women use the healthcare system and have greater needs for care than do men. Their need for reproductive and sexual health plays a role in this, but they also experience a higher prevalence of chronic non-reproductive health conditions like diabetes, cancer, heart disease, and osteoporosis. Understanding that events affect women's growth, development, and health throughout their entire life cycle, or life-course, from infancy to old age, is another crucial viewpoint. One of the World Health Organization's primary tactics is the life course perspective.

9.1.1.1. Global Perspective

When considering many aspects of health, gender disparities in disease susceptibility, symptoms, and response to treatment are especially evident when considering these factors globally. Although developed countries provide the majority of the information available, there are notable differences between developed and developing nations when it comes to women's roles and health. The global viewpoint is defined as the "area for study, research and practice that places a priority on improving health and achieving health equity for all people worldwide." The World Health Organization listed the following ten conditions as the top ten threats to women's health in 2015: cancer, HIV, STIs, maternal health, sexually transmitted infections, violence, mental health, non-communicable diseases, youth, and aging.

9.1.2. Women's Life Expectancy

Regardless of ethnicity or location, women have longer life expectancies than men and experience fewer deaths overall. However, historically, the mortality rate for women was higher, mostly due to maternal deaths (death during childbirth). After the industrial revolution, the gender gap decreased and eventually reversed in industrialized nations, especially the most developed. Despite these variations, women suffer worse outcomes and more severe illnesses at an earlier age in many health-related domains.

Notwithstanding these distinctions, heart disease—which accounts for 25% of all deaths in the US—is the leading cause of death for both men and women. Cancer, lung disease, and stroke follow in order of prevalence. Women are more likely than men to die from dementia, but they are less likely to die from suicide or unintentional injuries.

The childbearing years account for the majority of the differences in women's life expectancy between developed and developing nations. If a woman makes it through this time, the differences between the two regions become less noticeable because, in later life, non-communicable diseases (NCDs) become the leading causes of death for women worldwide. In older women, cardiovascular disease accounts for 45% of deaths, followed by lung disease (10%) and cancer (15%). The resources of developing nations are further burdened by these. A growing number of women in these countries are suffering from obesity and diabetes, and their chances of developing cardiovascular disease and other non-communicable diseases (NCDs) are rising as a result of changing lifestyles that include food, physical activity, and cultural norms that support larger body sizes in women.

Compared to women who are not socially marginalized, women who are have a higher risk of dying young. The life expectancy of women with substance abuse disorders, homelessness, sex work, and/or incarceration is considerably lower than that of other women. Women in these overlapping, stigmatized groups have a 10–13 times higher death rate than average women their age at any given time.

9.2. Women's Health Issues

The average lifespan of a woman increased from 48.3 years in 1900 to 79.4 years in 1997. Making those extra years of life healthy and productive is our current challenge. Women make up 51% of the US population overall, 59% of those over 65, and 71% of those over 85, the group with the quickest rate of population growth. Additionally, 46% of the workforce in the country is made up of women. They comprise 52% of the population of voting age, and compared to men, they vote more frequently in national elections. 52.8% of men and 55.5% of women cast ballots in the 1996 election.

A woman's unique biology and her social, cultural, and environmental contexts all influence her health. These elements have an impact on her life's duration as well as quality. For instance, a woman's average life expectancy varies significantly based on her race. Compared to African American women, white women had an average life expectancy of 80 years versus 75 years in 1997, a difference of 5 years. Women who are impoverished or whose education level is below that of a high school graduate have shorter life expectancies, greater rates of disease, injury, disability, and death, and more restricted access to high-quality medical care.

In the past, women have also served as their families' primary healthcare providers and decision-makers. In a recent nationwide survey, nearly two-thirds of women said they were the only ones in their family who made decisions about health care, and 83% said they were in charge of making decisions about family finances related to health care alone or jointly. In addition, women tend to sick or disabled family members' needs more often than men do. An estimated 72% of the estimated 15% of Americans who provide informal care are women, many of whom are juggling taking care of their own children and an ailing relative.

9.2.1. Barriers to Women's Health Care

9.2.1.1. Medical Research

Women have long been underrepresented in clinical trials and many health issues important to women have been largely ignored by medical research until recently. In the past, many studies on other diseases concentrated on men, while research on women's health primarily addressed conditions that impact fertility and reproduction. Nowadays, the majority of women get diagnoses and treatments based on what has been successful for men. Nonetheless, a broader research agenda has resulted from the work of advocates for women's health and the discovery of disparities in medical research. Men and women differ and are similar in terms of their health, and this research is starting to shed light on these differences.

9.2.1.2. Health Care Practices

Women frequently encounter systemic fragmentation when attempting to access other health care services and reproductive health care. In addition, women visit the doctor more frequently than men do. Women have a keen interest in and knowledge of health-related topics. On the other hand, trustworthy information regarding medical care has not been widely accessible. According to national studies, women might not be as happy as men are with the information they get from their healthcare providers or the degree of communication they have with them.

Moreover, a number of studies have shown that medical professionals treat women and men differently. Health care providers may treat women less thoroughly than they treat men for similar complaints, downplay their symptoms, perform fewer interventions for the same diagnoses, prescribe certain medications more frequently, or give less information when asked questions.

9.2.1.3. Access to Health Insurance

Despite the fact that the US economy is doing better than it has ever been, more women than ever do not have health insurance. Between 1993 and 1998, the percentage of women under 65 without health insurance increased from 14% to 18%. Even more striking, the 1998 Commonwealth Fund Survey of Women's Health revealed that a startling 26% of women under 65 did not have health insurance for all or part of 1998.

Women of color, those with health issues, and those with low to moderate incomes are the groups most likely to lack health insurance. Over 80% of women without health insurance either work or are married to someone who does. Medical care becomes much less accessible and of lower quality when one is uninsured.

In 1997, 12% of women under 65 had Medicaid coverage, and 70% of women under 65 had private health insurance. The Medicare program covers almost all Americans 65 and older, including 92% of those who also have private insurance.

9.2.2. Types of Women's Health Issues

Women must exercise greater caution and awareness of the issues related to their health. Let's examine some of the major health issues that women today face.

9.2.2.1. Heart Disease

The leading cause of death for American women is heart disease. Heart disease kills more women than men each year, despite the common perception that it only affects men. Heart disease typically strikes women later in life than it does men. Furthermore, compared to men, women are more likely to have other chronic coexisting conditions that could mask their heart disease symptoms. Women may experience different heart attack symptoms than men do, which can result in a misdiagnosis of the condition in these patients. Compared to men, women who survive a heart attack are more likely to have a stroke or experience another heart attack. In actuality, compared to 24% of men, 42% of women pass away a year after having a heart attack.

9.2.2.2. Cancer

The second most common cause of death for American women is cancer. With an estimated 66,000 deaths from the disease in 1999, lung cancer has been the primary cause of cancer-related deaths among women in the US since 1987. Men's lung cancer death rates have decreased over the last ten years, while women's rates have increased. Women are underrecognized for these concerning trends, which are almost entirely attributable to rising rates of female cigarette smoking. With 43,300 women lost to breast cancer in 1999, breast cancer is currently the second most common cause of cancer-related deaths among American women. Between 1940 and 1990, the incidence of breast cancer increased gradually before stabilizing at about 0 cases per 100,000 women. The increased use of mammography screening has led to a rise in the early detection of breast cancers, when they are more treatable. The number of deaths from breast cancer has decreased as a result of early detection and better treatment. The death rate from breast cancer fell by 5.6% between 1990 and 1994. Compared to African American women, whose mortality rate decreased by just 1%, white women experienced a more marked decline in mortality—dropping 6.1%.

In American women, colorectal cancer ranks as the third most common cause of cancer-related deaths. A diet high in fruits, vegetables, and whole grains, low in fat, and regular exercise can all help prevent many cases. However, it is anticipated that 28,800 women will lose their lives to colorectal cancer in 1999.

Cervical cancer early detection and prevention have significantly improved since the introduction of the Pap smear. Since the early 1970s, there has been a 40% decrease in the disease's incidence and death rates. However, because they are not getting regular Pap tests, a large number of elderly, low-income, and rural women continue to be at high risk for this illness. Cigarette smoking and infection with specific strains of the human papillomavirus (HPV) are two other significant risk factors. In 1999, it is anticipated that 12,800 new cases of cervical cancer will be diagnosed. Additionally, 4,800 people are predicted to pass away from the illness in that year.

The detection of endometrial (uterine lining) cancer, which claimed an estimated 37,400 new cases and 6,400 deaths in 1999, is only partially achieved by the Pap smear and pelvic examination. Of all the cancers of the female reproductive system, ovarian cancer is the most deadly, despite having a lower incidence. Frequently, symptoms don't show up until the disease is in its most advanced stages. Over 14,500 people died from ovarian cancer in 1999, out of approximately 25,200 cases.

The most dangerous type of skin cancer, melanoma, is most common in women 25 to 29 years old and second most common (after breast cancer) in women 30 to 34 years old. Although women are less likely than men to get skin cancer overall, the fastest-growing group of skin cancer patients is women under 40. In addition, the number of newly diagnosed cases of melanoma is rising. From 6 cases per 100,000 people in 1973 to 13 cases per 100,000 people in 1995, it has doubled.

9.2.2.3. Stroke

A clot that obstructs blood flow to a portion of the brain is typically the cause of a stroke. A stroke can result in memory loss, paralysis, and speech impairment. More than twice as many women die from stroke each year as from breast cancer, making it the third most common cause of death for American women. In this nation, it is the most frequent cause of adult disability.

Women make up 43% (or 240,000) of the annual 550,000 stroke cases as well as 61% (97,227 of 159,791 annual deaths) of stroke deaths. Compared to white women, African American and Hispanic women experience strokes at higher rates.

When combined, heart disease and stroke kill almost twice as many American women as all cancers combined. In this nation, over one in five women suffers from a serious heart or blood vessel condition known as cardiovascular disease. But according to a 1997 nationwide survey, only 8% of American women said that heart disease and stroke were the main causes of death for women.

9.2.2.4. Chronic Obstructive Pulmonary Disease (COPD)

Emphyzema, asthmatic bronchitis, and chronic bronchitis are all conditions that impair lung airflow and are categorized under COPD. 53,045 women died from COPD in 1997, making it the fourth most common cause of death in this age group. In 1997, there were 17.7 deaths per 100,000 people due to this disease. Men die from COPD at a far higher rate than women do, but since 1979, the rate for women has almost doubled. Women 75 years of age and older have experienced the fastest increases.

9.2.2.5. HIV/AIDS

HIV/AIDS, once thought to be a sickness exclusive to men, is now a public health concern for women. It is the third most common cause of death for African American women in this age range and the fifth most common cause of death for women ages 25 to 44. 10,841 new cases of AIDS among adult and adolescent women were reported between July 1998 and June 1999. The percentage of documented cases of AIDS among women rose from 7% to 23% between 1985 and 1999. Girls made up half of all AIDS cases reported in 1998 among those aged 13 to 19. A total of 114,621 women were reported to have AIDS by June 1999, with African Americans and Latinas accounting for 77% of those diagnoses.

Thankfully, there has been a noticeable decrease in the transmission of HIV during pregnancy thanks to improved treatment and expanded HIV screening among women of reproductive age. Their contribution has been instrumental in the 75% reduction in the percentage of infants diagnosed with perinatally acquired AIDS since 1993. Intravenous drug use is the second most common method of HIV infection among adult and adolescent women, after heterosexual contact. Both in the mode of infection and over the course of the illness, there are notable gender differences. These variations highlight the necessity of gender-sensitive care and preventative measures in the fight against AIDS.

9.2.2.6. Autoimmune Diseases

The onset of autoimmune diseases occurs when the body launches an inexplicable offensive against itself, attacking healthy tissue with antibodies. Rheumatoid arthritis, scleroderma, diabetes Type I, multiple sclerosis, Sjogren's syndrome, autoimmune thyroid disease, and systemic lupus erythematosus (SLE) affect women about 75% of the time. As distinct medical conditions, autoimmune diseases are relatively uncommon. Altogether, though, they account for the fourth most common cause of disability among American women. These illnesses are still misdiagnosed and misunderstood.

9.2.2.7. Mental Illness

Every year, one in ten Americans goes through a depressive episode. About twice as many women as men suffer from major depression and dysthymia, a milder, more chronic form of depression. In the United States, women are estimated to experience a major depression at a rate of 12% versus 7% for men; additionally, 42% of women experience dysthymia. Certain anxiety disorders, such as panic, anxiety, and phobic disorders, are two to three times more common in women. Women account for at least 90% of all eating disorder cases. Furthermore, there seems to be a strong link between eating disorders and substance abuse as well as between eating disorders and depression.

Mental illness can be lethal if left untreated. In 1994, suicide ranked as the fourth most common cause of death for young women between the ages of 15 and 24 and the fifth most common among women between the ages of 25 and 44. Compared to men, women are more likely to attempt suicide. But because men are more likely to use a firearm, women are much less likely to die in their attempt or attempts.

9.2.2.8. Substance Abuse

Alcohol and other legal and illicit drug abuse is a major and persistent issue among women in the United States. An estimated 120,000 fatalities annually are linked to drug and alcohol abuse. The estimated costs of alcohol and drug abuse to society and health in 1998 were $238 billion. Currently, over 1.2 million women in this nation abuse prescription medications for purposes other than those prescribed to them, and nearly 4.1 million women use illegal drugs. 4.5 million Women between the ages of 15 and 44 reported using illicit drugs in 1997 and 1998; 1.6 million of these women also had children living with them. Merely 3.2% of expectant mothers were present drug users. But among women who were not pregnant and who had a child under the age of two, the rate rose to 6.2%. An estimated 37% of people using illegal drugs in this nation are women.

Compared to men, women are less likely to abuse or use alcohol. However, the death rate for female alcoholics is 50–100% higher than that of male alcoholics. In 1998, 2.1% of American women reported heavy drinking, 8.6% reported binge drinking (consuming more than five drinks at once), and 45.1% reported having consumed at least one alcoholic beverage within the previous month. In 1997, among teenage girls, 29% reported binge drinking and 40% reported consuming alcohol at least once in the previous month.

Significant birth defects, such as mental retardation, nervous system problems, aberrant facial and head features, and slowed growth, have been directly linked to heavy drinking during pregnancy. There is no proven safe amount of drinking during pregnancy; abstinence is the only recommended course of action due to the unknown effects of moderate drinking (one to two drinks per day). 1.3% of pregnant women reported binge drinking, 0.5% reported heavy drinking (five drinks or more per day), and 16.1% reported never drinking alcohol in 1996.

A large number of women who abuse alcohol or drugs have a history of mental illness. More than 80% of respondents say they have a family member who is addicted to drugs or alcohol, and 70% report having experienced sexual abuse before the age of 16. Planning their course of treatment and their illness are made more difficult by these factors. In addition, women who abuse drugs or alcohol are more vulnerable to injuries, pharyngeal and oral cancers, HIV/AIDS, tuberculosis, and sexually transmitted diseases (STDs).

9.2.2.9. Smoking

In this nation, smoking cigarettes is the biggest preventable cause of death, accounting for a significant portion of deaths from heart disease, stroke, lung disease, cancer, and other illnesses. Since 1965, when smoking rates peaked, women's smoking rates have dropped by 35%. However, in 1997, 22.3 million adult women, or 22.1% of this population, were still smokers. In contrast to their adult counterparts, teenage girls have been smoking at a higher rate—from 27% in 1991 to 37% in 1997. 70% of girls in high school had tried smoking cigarettes in 1997. Smoking during pregnancy significantly raises the developing fetus's health risks. It is the primary cause of preterm births and significantly raises the risk of low birth weight, mental retardation, miscarriage, and other serious health issues in newborns.

According to the 1997 National Household Survey on Drug Abuse, 19.9% of pregnant women smoked, with the highest rates among those who were in their first trimester and the lowest among those who were in their third. Women with children under the age of two had a smoking rate of 26.6%. According to this statistic, some women may decide not to smoke while they are pregnant but pick back up after the baby is born.

Children who have been around secondhand smoke are more vulnerable to serious respiratory conditions like bronchitis, pneumonia, and asthma; they are also more likely to experience recurrent ear infections and Sudden Infant Death Syndrome (SIDS).

9.2.2.10. Violence

One of the biggest public health issues facing American women is violence. Every year, more than 4.5 million women fall victim to violence. Almost two out of every three of these women report having been attacked by a family member or acquaintance. Women are ten times more likely than men to experience sexual assault, and they are six times more likely to experience abuse at the hands of a known individual. 10–20%, or one or two young women out of ten, are thought to have experienced sexual abuse.

Homicide was the sixth most common cause of death for women aged 25 to 44 in 1997, and the second most common cause of death for women aged 15 to 24. It is the primary reason why women die at work.

Concern among researchers is growing that one significant contributing factor to maternal mortality may be violence. According to reports, between 4 and 8% of pregnancies involve violence. It can be concluded that between 152,000 and 325,000 pregnant women in the US experienced violence, based on the application of these percentages to the 3.9 million women who gave birth to live babies in 1995. So, rather than preeclampsia, gestational diabetes, or placenta previa, violence may be a more common issue for expectant mothers.

9.2.2.11. Reproductive Health

Women's lives and experiences with health are significantly shaped by their ability to procreate. By the time they are 45, more than 80% of American women have given birth, and the average woman has 2.2 children.

While many women view becoming a mother as a defining aspect of adulthood, the majority of them attempt to avoid becoming pregnant for the majority of their reproductive years. The percentage of women who use contraception, aged 15 to 44, has increased to 64% from 56% in 1982 and 60% in 1988. The percentage of women using contraception during their first sexual encounters increased from 64% in the late 1980s to 76% in 1995.

The percentage of unplanned pregnancies fell by 16% between 1987 and 1994. The use of contraceptives has increased, and their effectiveness has improved, which is most likely the cause of this decline. Still, 49% of pregnancies in 1994 were not planned. When an unplanned pregnancy occurred in 1994, almost half of the women had used contraception.

Male sterilization (4.2 million), birth control pills (10.4 million), male condoms (7.9 million), and female sterilization (10.7 million women) are the most often used forms of contraception. Less than 1% of women used female condoms as a form of contraception in 1995, while 2% of women used injectable hormones and 1% used hormonal implants.

Women's gynecological health plays a significant role in their overall health, not just when they are reproductively active. A third of a woman's life is spent after menopause on average. Although many older women wrongly think that they no longer need to have regular gynecological exams, this is the exact time in life when they are more vulnerable to reproductive system cancers and other gynecological issues like uterine prolapse.

The risk of reproductive health issues linked to sexually transmitted diseases (STDs) is higher in younger women. One in four teenagers get an STD annually, and two thirds of all STD cases affect people under the age of 25. Biologically speaking, women are more likely than men to contract STDs, and because of variations in cervical anatomy, younger women are more vulnerable than older ones.

Compared to men, women are less likely to exhibit STD infection symptoms. For instance, only 25% of women experience symptoms from chlamydia, the most common infectious disease in the country that is curable. In contrast, 50% of men experience these symptoms. Untreated gonorrhea infections cause 10–40% of women infected with chlamydia infections to develop pelvic inflammatory disease (PID). PID then causes ectopic pregnancy in 9% of cases, chronic pelvic pain in 18% of cases, and infertility in 20% of cases. High rates of STD infection among adolescent women not only increase a person's vulnerability to HIV, but they also cause direct health problems. In 1998, American women were reported to have had 501,128 new cases of chlamydia. 179,651 new cases of gonorrhea were reported in the same year. (The highest rates of gonorrhea infection were seen in young women, ages 15 to 19. Furthermore, 18,179 syphilis cases were documented. About one in four women (or 25% of this population) and one in five men (or 20% of men) are infected with herpes simplex virus type 2 (HSV-2).

Women who are of reproductive age frequently experience gynecological issues. Every year, over 4.5 million women between the ages of 18 and 50 report having at least one chronic gynecological condition. 10% of women who menstruate experience dysmenorrhea, a severe form of pain that disrupts their daily routine, and half of all women experience some pain during their menstrual cycle. Premenstrual syndrome (PMS) affects nearly two out of every five women between the ages of 14 and 50. Of these, 10% have symptoms severe enough to interfere with daily activities.

Endometriosis, which can result in infertility and chronic pain, affects up to 10% of American women. 10–20% of women have fibroids, which are non-cancerous growths in the uterus. Half of the more than 580,000 hysterectomies carried out annually in the United States are linked to endometriosis and fibroids combined. Uterine prolapse, excessive bleeding or pain, and cancer are additional causes. Hysterectomy is the second most common surgical procedure in the country, with one in three women over 60 having had one.

9.2.2.12. Fertility and Infertility

In the United States, 3,880,894 live births occurred in 1997. The birth rate fell from 24 live births per 1,000 people in 1950 to 14.5 live births per 1,000 people in 1997. The majority of American women who give birth are in the 20–29 age range. Nonetheless, over the course of this decade, there has been a rise in the percentage of pregnant women in their thirties and forties. In 1997, there were 483,220 births to teenage girls, a 16% decrease from 1991.

6.1 million Women suffered from infertility in 1997, compared to 4.6 million in 1988. This increase was partly caused by older baby boomers and postponed childbearing. Conditions affecting the male partner, the female partner, and both partners equally make up the causes of infertility. The American Society for Reproductive Medicine estimates that approximately one in four infertile couples are unable to conceive due to STDs.

Prenatal care that is provided on time and to a sufficient standard increases the likelihood of a successful pregnancy outcome, according to numerous studies. Over 82.5% of all expectant mothers received prenatal care during their first trimester in 1997—a continuous improvement since 1970. Nevertheless, 3.9% of expectant mothers either received no prenatal care at all or only in the third trimester.

In 1997, there were 7.2 infant deaths for every 1,000 live births, a record low. A 15% estimated decline in Sudden Infant Death Syndrome (SIDS) between 1995 and 1996 is linked to about one-third of that reduction. The infant mortality rate in the United States continues to be among the highest in the industrialized world despite these advancements.

Since 1950, the rate of maternal mortality has dropped by more than ten times. 7.6 maternal deaths occurred for every 100,000 live births in 1997. The rate of maternal mortality linked to heart conditions, embolism, bleeding, high blood pressure, domestic abuse, and infection, however, may be greater than current estimates suggest due to new and improved data collection techniques.

9.2.2.13. Environmental Health

A large number of diseases that affect women are caused by environmental factors. Unfavorable environmental circumstances include workplace contamination as well as pollution of the air, water, and soil. Exposure to lead, chemicals, pesticides, tobacco smoke, and constant noise are examples of occupational hazards. Women's health is impacted by environmental factors both at home and in the community, such as lead-based paints, radon, electromagnetic fields, food, and cosmetics, as well as heatstroke, hypothermia, and violence. We still don't fully understand how environmental factors can interfere with a woman's endocrine, reproductive, central nervous, and immune systems, leading to particular diseases like cancer, autoimmune disorders, endometriosis, and osteoporosis.

9.2.2.14. Chronic Disabling Conditions

Women are more likely than men to experience chronic disabling conditions like diabetes, osteoporosis, osteoarthritis, obesity, urinary incontinence, Alzheimer's disease, fibromyalgia, and chronic fatigue syndrome. This is partly because women typically live longer than men. These ailments not only impair function but also carry the potential to be fatal in the long run. A protracted trajectory of increasing impairment is a defining feature of each of these disorders.

Family members and other caregivers suffer negative consequences from chronic illnesses in addition to the patient. To ascertain whether particular gender-related factors are involved in the higher incidence of these illnesses in women, more research is required.

1. **Diabetes Mellitus:** 16 million Americans are thought to have diabetes. Only 10.3 million cases are diagnosed, with 8.1 million of those being in women. Compared to white women, Black, Hispanic, American Indian, and Asian Pacific Islander women have a 2–4 times higher prevalence of diabetes.

Diabetes can be managed with medication, exercise, weight loss, and a healthy diet. Diabetes can cause serious vision loss, heart problems, strokes, kidney problems, lower limb amputations, and even death if left untreated. Diabetes is the sixth most common cause of death for Asian American women, the seventh most common cause for white women, and the fourth most common cause of death for African American, Native American, and Hispanic women.

2. **Osteoporosis:** Bone fractures can result from osteoporosis, a disorder marked by the thinning and increasing brittleness of bones. Over 25 million Americans suffer from it; 80% of them are women. This condition affects more than half of all women over the age of 65. 1.5 million Fractures of the hip, wrist, vertebrae, and other bones occur as a result of osteoporosis each year. It is responsible for 70% of all fractures that occur in adults over 45 in a given year. Within a year after suffering a hip fracture, 20% of women pass away.

Osteoporosis is a major cause of admission to nursing homes and is estimated to cost over $10 billion annually. Osteoporosis prevention is a lifelong endeavor, despite the fact that the condition is commonly associated with advanced age. By the age of 18, a woman has gained about 60% of her final bone mass, and by the age of 35, her bone density has reached its peak. Girls and women of all ages should avoid tobacco use, excessive alcohol or caffeine consumption, and consume foods high in calcium in addition to getting regular exercise and building and maintaining healthy bones. Supplementing with calcium and vitamin D, receiving estrogen replacement therapy during menopause, and using non-hormonal medication to prevent bone loss are additional treatment approaches.

3. **Alzheimer's Disease:** Alzheimer's disease affects an estimated 4 million people in the US. More than 13,600 women lost their lives to the illness in 1995. For people over 65, it is the most typical cause of dementia. The annual cost of Alzheimer's disease is estimated to be between $80 and $100 billion, placing a significant burden on society. It also has a severe negative impact on those who care for those with Alzheimer's, mostly women.
4. **Urinary Incontinence:** Thirteen million Americans—eleven millions of whom are women—are affected by urinary incontinence, or the inadvertent loss of urine. While incontinence affects half of the elderly population, it is not a condition that only affects the elderly. Urinary incontinence affects one in four women between the ages of thirty and fifty-nine. Due to weakening pelvic muscles or pelvic trauma, women are more likely to experience this issue during pregnancy, childbirth, physical activity, or after menopause. In eight out of ten cases, incontinence can be treated. Less than half of those who encounter this issue, nevertheless, talk to a medical professional about it.
5. **Obesity:** The percentage of obese females has risen to 36% since the 1970s, an increase of more than one-fourth. Mexican-American women (50.1%) and African-American women (52.3%) have particularly high rates. A significant portion of this rising rate is linked to overeating and a growing lack of physical activity. Women who are overweight are more susceptible to high blood pressure, diabetes, heart disease, arthritis, and some types of cancer. Of the 42.7 million Americans who suffer from arthritis, nearly 26.4 million are female. It is the most prevalent chronic illness that disables people that women report having. An estimated 4.6 million American women, or 4.6% of the total population, claim that their daily activities are restricted by arthritis. African American women (6.5%) and Native American women (6.9%) report higher rates than do white women (4.2%).

A collection of more than 100 conditions affecting the muscles, tendons, joints, bones, or nerves are collectively referred to as arthritis. These ailments can be minor or severe. The hands, feet, knees, and hips are the joints where arthritis most frequently causes pain or stiffness. Risk factors include advancing years, trauma, obesity, and inherited susceptibility. Despite the fact that arthritis is more prevalent in older people, half of all Americans with the condition are under 65. Medication, physical activity, applying heat or cold to the afflicted area, weight management, and surgery are all part of the treatment for arthritis.

6. **Fibromyalgia:** Three to six million Americans suffer from fibromyalgia, according to the American College of Rheumatology. Women make up the majority of those affected—an estimated 80% of them are of childbearing age. Fibromyalgia is a common disorder that manifests as multiple tender points in the neck, spine, shoulders, and hips, as well as widespread musculoskeletal pain and fatigue. In addition to these symptoms, fibromyalgia patients may also have anxiety, irritable bowel syndrome, insomnia, and morning stiffness.
7. **Chronic Fatigue:** The hallmarks of Chronic Fatigue and Immune Dysfunction Syndrome (CFIDS) include debilitating, persistent fatigue as well as nonspecific symptoms like headaches, sore throats, sore muscles, joint pain, trouble thinking, and short-term memory loss. According to estimates, up to 500,000 Americans may be affected by CFIDS. Women make up about 80% of those with the syndrome diagnoses.

9.2.2.15. Disease Prevention/Health Promotion

Over half of all chronic illnesses in the United States are related to behavioral and lifestyle factors, accounting for the majority of the country's health care burden. It is estimated that changing lifestyle behaviors (such as diet, physical activity, use of helmets and seatbelts, sexual behavior, alcohol and drug abuse, and tobacco use) could prevent 47% of premature deaths in the United States. Mitigating environmental risks has the potential to prevent an estimated 20% of these preventable deaths. Improving the quality and length of life requires the development of successful behavior modification techniques as well as programs targeted specifically at women that support health.

9.2.3. Special Populations

9.2.3.1. Minority Women

Premature death, disease, and disability continue to disproportionately affect a large number of women of color. For white women in 1997, the life expectancy was 79.4, for African American women it was 74.9, and for women from other minorities it was 75.7. In addition, chronic conditions like diabetes, lupus, some forms of cancer, cardiovascular disease, and some infectious diseases like AIDS, tuberculosis, and hepatitis are more common in women of color. Maternal mortality is more common among African American, Hispanic, and American Indian/Alaskan Native women than it is among white women, and infant mortality is highest among African American and Puerto Rican women. In addition, compared to white women, African American and Hispanic women are more likely to experience homicide and HIV/AIDS.

Compared to white women, women of color are more likely to be poor, which is strongly associated with higher rates of illness and early death. Women of color are more likely than White women to have limited access to healthcare and lower utilization rates for many preventive health services. The systemic, cultural, social, and financial barriers that minority women face in accessing health care, the scarcity of minority health care providers, and the historical legacies of discrimination are all contributing factors to these disparities.

9.2.3.2. Adolescent Girls

The adolescent years are a vibrant, formative time in life. Young women make crucial decisions about their lifestyles, such as what to eat, how active they are, whether to have sex, and whether to use drugs, alcohol, or tobacco. All of these choices will have an impact on their health and happiness as adults.

Unintentional injury ranks first among the leading causes of death for teenage girls. More than one in five high school-age girls report having experienced physical or sexual abuse, and one in four of these girls exhibit depressive symptoms. According to surveys, 8% of high school girls regularly binge and purge, 60% report trying to lose weight, and 28% believe they are overweight. According to estimates, 37% of teenage girls reported smoking in the previous month, 48% admit to regular drinking, and 15% say they use a seat belt infrequently or never.

The age group in this country that receives the least medical care is youth and young adults under the age of 24. Approximately 27% of teenagers between the ages of 10 and 18 and 27% of those between the ages of 19 and 24 do not have health insurance. Many more do not have access to services that are comprehensive, cost-effective, private, and tailored to their individual needs.

9.2.3.3. Older Women

On average, women outlive men by seven years. It is projected that life expectancy will rise for the next century, with women expected to benefit more than men. There were 14.3 million men and 20.3 million women over 65 in 1998. It is projected that by 2030, the percentage of Americans over 65 will have doubled, and the number of Americans over 85 will have tripled. Seven out of ten baby-boom wives are expected to outlive their husbands, typically by 15 to 20 years.

Women are more likely than men to experience chronic illnesses and disabilities that worsen with age, including cancer, obesity, osteoporosis, arthritis, and heart disease. This is because women tend to live longer than men do.

In comparison to older men, older women are also more likely to be impoverished. Women make up nearly 75% of the elderly impoverished in the country. Furthermore, compared to men, women spend up to 25% more of their disposable income on out-of-pocket medical expenses. Because of the expense of these tests, their perception that they are unnecessary, or the lack of a recommendation from their doctor, two thirds of older women do not use preventive screening services like mammography.

Positive developments are taking place for the growing number of senior women. The percentage of people with disabilities is rapidly declining, and women are becoming more educated and financially independent. Women will live longer and actually healthier lives in the twenty-first century if they actively adopt healthy habits.

9.2.3.4. Incarcerated Women

Women make up the fastest growing segment of the prison population in the United States, despite making up only 6.5% of all inmates nationwide. For the third year in a row, the number of women under the control of state or federal prison authorities surpassed the increase in the male population, totaling 84,427. Furthermore, at the middle of 1998, 737,958 female juvenile arrests had occurred, and 63,791 women were being held in jails every day.

The healthcare needs of female inmates differ from those of male inmates. These disparities are caused by a number of things, including the comparatively complicated reproductive systems of women, their status as mothers and pregnant women, their role as caregivers for minor children, their increasingly risky illicit drug use, their higher rates of HIV positivity, and their pasts of sexual and physical abuse.(Chandra-Mouli et al., 2015; Clawson et al., 1996).

9.3. School Age and Adolescent Health

For some ethnic and religious groups, reaching the age of seven marks an important developmental turning point. This age is designated as the First Holy Communion age by the Catholic Church because it believes that children have reached the capacity for reason at this point. At this age, a person begins formal schooling, develops a conscience and morality, and gains the ability to live independently of their family.

Twenty years of age is another important developmental milestone. Childhood and adolescence are drawing to an end, and the person must now be psychologically and physically ready to take on the responsibilities and benefits of adulthood.

9.3.1. School Age: 7 to 11 Years

The school-age years of 7 to 11 are a comparatively carefree time for children when compared to earlier and later ages. Psychosexual issues are dormant, and a great deal of challenging physical and psychological tasks have been mastered. Now that she is an independent adult, the child can develop her cognitive, social, and motor abilities as well as explore the outside world with peers and novel experiences. Erikson defined this stage as "industry versus inferiority" and stated that acquiring these abilities through diligence (i.e., industry) can foster a sense of competence that lasts a lifetime. In contrast, a persistent sense of low self-esteem may arise from not achieving these goals.

9.3.1.1. School and Learning

In the United States, formal education starts at around age seven, similar to most other modern societies. Children begin to develop the ability to reason logically at this age. Piaget labeled this developmental stage the stage of concrete operations and observed that it was essential to possess this ability in order to reason and learn mathematical concepts.

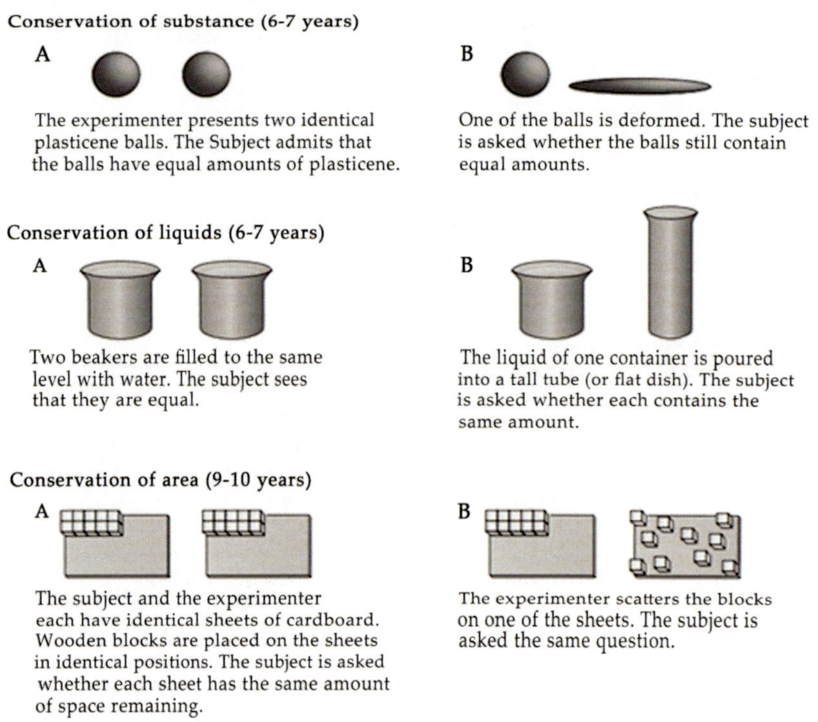

Figure 9.1. *Tests evaluating the concept of conservation.*

Source: Barbara Fadem. Behavioral Science in Medicine. Lippincott Williams & Wilkins. ISBN 978-1-60913-664-2.

A child possessing concrete operational skills, for instance, can comprehend that an object can have multiple properties, such as being both red and metal, and that the amount of a substance stays constant regardless of the size of the container it is in.

The latter idea was dubbed the concept of conservation by Piaget. For instance, even though one container is a tall, thin tube and the other is a short, wide bowl, the 7-year-old child can understand that both contain the same amount of water, but not the 4-year-old child (Figure 9.1). Due to the rapidity with which these skills must be acquired, learning issues that were previously undetected frequently surface at the onset of formal education.

9.3.1.2. Play and Peer Relationships

For children of school age, school is the center of their social life, along with extracurricular activities like sports. Through these activities, kids develop a feeling of competence and self-worth and start interacting socially with adults who aren't their primary caretakers. The child grows to value the approval and support of teachers, sports coaches, and scout leaders as additional role models. By pursuing hobbies, kids can also gain a sense of competence. Here, they can catalog and manage collections of items, like stamps, coins, dolls, or trading cards, using their newly developed organizing skills.

During the school-age years, peer relationships—especially those involving children of the same sex—also become more significant. Youngsters of this age usually have a small circle of friends with whom they interact, frequently discussing the differences between other kids in the group and their shared attitudes and beliefs. Children who are popular usually have good social skills and abide by the rules. Youngsters who are rejected by the group and don't "fit in" typically fall into one of two categories: those who are extremely aggressive or "bossy," or those who are melancholy, anxious, and low on self-esteem. Children who aren't popular can benefit from social skills exercises because they can develop new friendships. Additionally, since these kids usually have negative attitudes toward school, these interventions also have the added advantage of raising academic achievement.

9.3.1.3. Sexuality

Freud named this developmental period "latency" because the 7–11 year old age group exhibits a quiescent sexuality, a precursor to the sexual and romantic feelings of adolescence. When a child reaches latency, they usually associate themselves with a parent or caregiver of the same sex and aspire to be just like them when they grow up. Additionally, at this age, children show little social interest in people of the other sex. Boys like to play with other boys, girls with other girls. They might even say that kids of the other sex are goofy or gross. In a few years, this attitude will have drastically changed.

9.3.1.4. The Development of Morality

6- to 7-year-old children have started to acquire the capacity to empathize with others and to internalize a sense of right and wrong, in contrast to younger children who are almost entirely self-absorbed. These moral and empathetic sentiments continue to develop during the academic years.

Like a convert to a new religion, the child is in the early stages of moving from self-involvement to understanding others and is more rule-conscious and aware of right and wrong than an older child or adult. The 7-year-old is adamant about the Monopoly board game being played by the exact rules; he says that no player can leave jail until he forfeits three turns. Later on, when the child starts to comprehend the perspective of others, he exhibits greater acceptance and adaptability in social situations. After just one missed turn, the 12-year-old can break the rules and let losing players get out of jail and continue playing.

The nervous system of a child at latency can become mature enough for them to perform intricate motor tasks. This, along with the child's developing moral compass, leads to her interest in and proficiency with the frequently intricate regulations of team sports.

9.3.1.5. Illness

Children of school age handle illness and hospitalization better than younger or older kids do. Therefore, if given the option, this is the ideal age for elective surgery. Some school-age children (and adolescents) who are unwell or have an unwell sibling or parent may react by misbehaving at home or school, even though the majority cope well. Some might experience anxiety, depression, or withdrawal.

Understanding that death is final is another significant turning point at this age. The six-year-old starts to realize that death is inevitable and starts to worry that his parents will pass away and leave him. Around the age of nine, the child starts to realize that other people can die, and he or she may start to worry about dying. It can be challenging for parents and doctors to decide whether, when, and how to inform a child who is truly seriously or even terminally ill about his prognosis.

9.3.2. Adolescence: 11 to 20 Years

Adolescence can be conveniently categorized into three phases: early (ages 11 to 14), middle (ages 15 to 17), and late (ages 18 to 20). The increasing development of independence and autonomy as well as the additional demands of individual decision-making define all three phases.

Adolescent-related alterations in the brain include the persistence of myelination that started earlier in development, which results in an increase in the volume of white matter to gray matter. The adolescent's enhanced cognitive abilities are positively correlated with this increase, which is especially evident in the frontal and parietal lobes. Along with a reduction in the metabolism of glucose and oxygen, the brain also undergoes pruning of up to 50% of the wildly formed synaptic connections during childhood.

9.3.2.1. Early Adolescence (11 to 14 years)

The outward sign of the onset of adolescence is puberty. Increased skeletal growth and the emergence of primary and secondary sex traits indicate this milestone. Girls go through puberty before boys do. The average age at which pubertal development begins in the United States is 10.5 years for girls (normal range: 8.0 to 13.5 years) and 11.5 years for boys (normal range: 9.5 to 13.5 years). The first ejaculation, a sign of male puberty, happens between the ages of 12 and 15 years, while the first menstrual cycle, or menarche, typically happens between the ages of 11 and 14. With typical ranges of 10.5 to 17.0 and 13.5 to 17.0 for girls and boys, respectively, the physical process of puberty is typically finished by the average age of 13.5 years for girls and 15.0 years for boys. Tanner staging divides puberty into five stages based on the emergence of traits associated with secondary sex: immature, Stage 1, mature, Stage 5 (Table 9.1).

Table 9.1. *Tanner Stages of Sexual Development*

	CHARACTERISTICS		
TANNER STAGE	**FEMALE**	**MALE**	**BOTH**
Stage 1	Preadolescent	Preadolescent	Preadolescent
Stage 2	• Nipples (papillae) slightly elevated • Areola enlarges • Breast tissue slightly elevated	• Testes enlarge • Penis enlarges • Scrotum enlarges and develops some texture	• Scant, straight pubic hair
Stage 3	• Breast and areola enlarge but no separation in contour	• Testes enlarge further • Penis increases further in length	• Pubic hair increases over the pubis and becomes curly
Stage 4	• Areola rises above the rest of the breast	• Penis increases in width • Glans develops • Scrotal skin darkens	• Pubic hair resembles adult type but less in quantity
Stage 5	• Breast and pubic hair like adult	• Male sex organs and pubic hair like adult	• Pubic hair also on medial surface of thighs

Source: Barbara Fadem. Behavioral Science in Medicine. Lippincott Williams & Wilkins. ISBN 978-1-60913-664-2.

Teenagers' heightened self-consciousness about their appearance combined with the remarkable physical changes of puberty can make any deviation from the typical developmental pattern—like acne, obesity, or delayed breast development—extremely distressing. Unlike older teens, early adolescents are typically obedient and unlikely to seriously challenge parental authority, even though they are sensitive to the opinions of their peers.

9.3.2.2. Middle Adolescence

The adolescent becomes very interested in body image and popularity among peers of the same and opposite sexes by the time they are 15 years old. The middle adolescent adopts current styles in music and clothes to blend in with their peers, and they would rather hang out with friends than their family. Although this conduct is expected and typical, it may cause problems with parents.

The middle adolescent is also more likely than younger or older adolescents to take risks due in part to a willingness to break the rules and feelings of invulnerability. This conduct, which can include abstaining from birth control, using drugs, and smoking cigarettes, can have detrimental effects on one's health. It is not always effective to warn an adolescent about the long-term effects of her risk-taking behavior. Education about apparent short-term benefits is more likely to reduce an adolescent's undesired behavior, especially when it comes to physical appearance or popularity. For instance, a teenager's smoking behavior is more likely to be influenced by being told that smoking will result in bad breath or discolored teeth than it is by being informed that smoking increases her long-term risk of developing lung cancer.

Medically ill middle adolescents may be reluctant to follow medical advice because it may mean temporarily losing their valued, recently acquired autonomy and need for privacy. Even the most committed physician may find it difficult to tolerate this response.

9.3.2.3. Late Adolescence (18 to 20 years)

An identity crisis is linked to late adolescence, during which the teen must clarify and enhance his position in the world. When this crisis is resolved, morality, ethics, and self-control are typically strengthened along with the capacity to evaluate oneself honestly. This age group, which is primarily college students, starts protest movements for social change and speaks out about global issues and humanitarian concerns in most countries. According to Erikson, role confusion is a common trait among teenagers who struggle to define their identities and find their places in the world. Adolescents experiencing role confusion may exhibit aberrant behaviors like drug addiction, criminal activity, or cult membership.

In terms of education, some late adolescents—but not all—acquire the formal, hypothetical, or abstract reasoning skills necessary for calculus. This phase of cognitive development was dubbed formal operations by Piaget.

9.3.2.4. Teenage Sexuality and Pregnancy

Adolescence is characterized by intense sexual feelings in addition to personality development and cognitive maturation. Masturbating and engaging in physical activity are two ways that these emotions are expressed. During adolescence (and beyond), daily masturbation is a common occurrence, and feelings of love for an unattainable person, like a rock star, are known as heterosexual or homosexual crushes. Adolescents may have homosexual experiences, which may or may not be the first indications of a homosexual orientation. Additionally, this kind of practice is typical development, despite the fact that parents may become alarmed.

The average age of first sexual encounters in the US is roughly 16 years old. Most men and women have had sex by the time they are 19 years of age. In this society, having sex before marriage is commonplace due to the average age of first marriage being roughly 23.

Less than half of teenagers who are sexually active take contraception on a regular basis. Teenagers are frequently of the belief that they are unique and different, and as a result, they will not become pregnant or contract an STD. There are several reasons for this. This belief is not supported by evidence. Age-specific gonorrhea rates in 2000 were highest in women (716 cases per 100,000) and third highest in men (328 cases per 100,000) in the 15–19 age group. One of the most prevalent STDs, chlamydia, affects teenage girls more frequently than it does older women. Teens' inability to use contraceptives can also be attributed to a lack of access or ignorance of the most effective methods.

Teenage pregnancy is predisposed by emotional and social factors such as depression, low academic achievement, and divorced parents. Approximately one-third of American girls become pregnant before turning 20 years old, despite the fact that the country's teen pregnancy rate is currently declining. On the other hand, older women are becoming more pregnant, especially those who are over 40 (Figure 9.2). Teenagers who are pregnant can be difficult for doctors to treat because they are more likely than older patients to experience obstetric complications. This is partly because teenagers are physically immature and less likely than older patients to seek prenatal care.

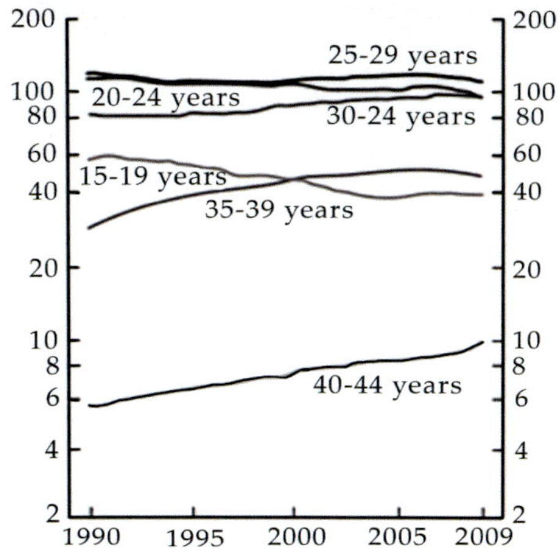

Figure 9.2. *Birth rates in the United States by age of mother: 1990 to 2008 and preliminary 2009.*

Source: Barbara Fadem. Behavioral Science in Medicine. Lippincott Williams & Wilkins. ISBN 978–1-60913–664–2.

The majority of medical care for minors, or those under the age of 18, needs parental approval. Nonetheless, it is typically morally and legally acceptable for medical professionals to treat STDs, pregnancy-related issues, drug and alcohol abuse, and provide minors with sexual counselling and contraception without parental knowledge or consent.

First-trimester abortion became legal in every state in 1973 after the Supreme Court's Roe versus Wade ruling. Only a few states allow abortions during the second trimester. A half a million teenage girls have abortions every year, but in at least half of the states, they have to tell their parents or get their consent.

9.3.3. Problems Affecting Development

While the majority of kids breeze through latency and adolescence, some encounter challenges that impede their ability to learn and interact with others. For instance, attention deficit/hyperactivity disorder (ADHD) and Tourette's syndrome can both lead to behavioral issues, and intellectual disability can result in developmental delays.

Children can experience the same psychiatric disorders as adults, such as anxiety disorders like generalized anxiety disorder, mood disorders like depression, and psychotic disorders like schizophrenia, with the exception of personality disorders, which are not diagnosed in children. Childhood disorders are covered in this section, including selective mutism, ADHD, disruptive behavior disorders, intellectual disability, and separation anxiety disorder. A list of neurodevelopmental and related disorders that are typically first diagnosed in infancy, childhood, or adolescence can be found in Table 9.2.

Table 9.2. *Neurodevelopmental and Related Disorders*

CLASSIFICATIONS	DISORDERS
Intellectual disability	Mild, moderate, severe, profound, or severity unspecified
Specific learning disorders	With impairment in reading, mathematics, or written expression
Motor disorders	Developmental coordination disorder (not because of a general medical condition), stereotyped movement disorder, tic disorders
Communication disorders	Language disorder, speech-sound disorder, childhood-onset fluency disorder (stuttering), social (pragmatic), communication disorder, unspecified communication disorder
Autism spectrum disorder (ASD)	Autism spectrum disorder, level 1 ("requiring support"), level 2 ("requiring substantial support"), or level 3 ("requiring very substantial support")
Feeding and eating disorders	Pica (eating non-food items), rumination disorder (regurgitating and rechewing food), avoidant/restrictive food intake disorder
Tic disorders	Tourette's disorder, persistent (chronic) motor or vocal tic disorder, provisional tic disorder
Elimination disorders	Encopresis: with or without constipation and overflow incontinence Enuresis (not caused by a general medical condition)
Other specified and unspecified neurodevelopmental disorders	Symptoms that impair social or other important areas of function but do not meet the criteria for any of the disorders in the neurodevelopmental disorders class

Source: Barbara Fadem. Behavioral Science in Medicine. Lippincott Williams & Wilkins. ISBN 978-1-60913-664-2.

9.3.3.1. *Intellectual Disability*

Not every child reaches their cognitive development milestones by the anticipated age. A child may be diagnosed with an intellectual disability, formerly known as mental retardation, if her intellectual functioning is noticeably below what is expected for her age and interferes with her ability to function.

Environmental and biological factors can contribute to intellectual disability. The two most prevalent genetic causes are fragile X syndrome (FXS) and Down syndrome. Meiotic nondisjunction-related trisomy of chromosome 21 accounts for about 95% of Down syndrome cases, while translocation and fusion of chromosomes 21 and 13, 14, or 15 account for about 4% of cases. The cause of the remaining 1% of cases is mosaicism brought on by mitotic nondisjunction. People who have this uncommon kind of Down syndrome may exhibit fewer symptoms of the illness and contain a mixture of normal and aberrant cells. A single palmar transverse crease, a protruding tongue, a flat facial profile, hypotonia, epicanthal folds, small ears, and a thick neck are among the physical traits of Down syndrome. Additionally, a higher risk of Alzheimer's disease and premature aging has been connected to Down syndrome. Both sexes are roughly equally affected by Down syndrome.

A single gene on the long arm of the X chromosome at the Xq27 site (the fragile site) has abnormalities in FXS. Although it affects both sexes equally, men are typically more severely affected. Boys diagnosed with frontotemporal syndrome (FXS) commonly exhibit delayed cognitive function, hyperkinetic behavior, and stereotypical hand-flapping gestures. Hyperextensible joints, big ears, an elongated face, and postpubertal testicular enlargement are examples of physical abnormalities. Prenatal and postnatal infections such as rubella and toxoplasmosis, maternal substance abuse, and metabolic factors affecting the mother or fetus are other biological causes of intellectual disability. The cause of intellectual disability is often unknown in many cases. Along with neurological dysfunctions like seizures, hearing issues, vision issues, and developmental disorders like autism, intellectual disability can also occur.

Children and teenagers with mild (IQ of 50 to 69) and moderate (IQ of 35 to 49) intellectual disabilities deal with a variety of social issues. As they get older, they realize how unique they are and frequently give up on trying to blend in and look like everyone else. The ensuing low self-esteem may worsen social disengagement and make it harder to interact with peers. After puberty, avoiding pregnancy can become problematic for people with intellectual disabilities, especially in residential social settings like summer camp or school. Long-acting, reversible contraceptive techniques (like subcutaneous hormone implants) and supervision are especially helpful for these people.

9.3.3.2. Learning and Communication Disorders

When a child does not learn or communicate at a level commensurate with his age and intellectual development, but instead is not intellectually disabled, learning and communication disorders are diagnosed. Reading, math, and written expression disorders are examples of learning disorders. Receptive, expressive, and mixed language disorders are examples of communication disorders. A child with communication disorders is unable to appropriately understand language (receptive), use language (expressive), or both. For instance, a 9-year-old child with expressive language disorder might refer to a bicycle as something to ride on or struggle to explain events from a beach excursion. Additional communication disorders include speech sound disorder, where a child has articulation issues and cannot make the necessary motor movements for accurate speech production, such as lisping, such as saying yeth for the word yes, or leaves out or misplaces speech sounds, such as saying top for stop or ca for cat.

9.3.3.3. Disruptive Behavior Disorders of Childhood

The typical toddler is unyielding and indifferent to other people's emotions. But by the time they are 7 years old, most kids follow their parents' instructions and have empathy for other people. However, some school-age children exhibit difficult, defiant behavior patterns that are persistent and ultimately disruptive.

The inappropriate behavior that ruins relationships with others and impairs academic performance is the hallmark of disruptive behavior disorders, which include conduct disorder and oppositional defiant disorder. When a child exhibits conduct disorder, they seriously transgress social norms (e.g., stealing, truancy, mistreating or torturing animals or small children, and starting fires) are examples of the inattentive behaviors associated with this illness. The diagnosis of ADHD requires evidence of the disorder before the age of twelve and persistence of the symptoms for at least six months, even though the disorder may not be identified until the symptoms interfere with learning and social interactions in the classroom. It must also happen in a minimum of two contexts, i.e., both at home and at school. If a child struggles in one environment but not another, behavioral problems are more likely to be explained by problems in the child's relationship with the teacher or parents. The combined type, predominantly inattentive type, and predominantly hyperactive type are the three specifiers for ADHD (Table 9.3). The primary inattentive type needs to be distinguished from inattention due to absence of epileptic seizures since the child may gaze blankly into space for a brief period of time in both conditions.

Table 9.3. *Symptoms of ADHD and Specifiers*

SYMPTOMS OF HYPERACTIVITY-IMPULSIVITY (H-I)	SYMPTOMS OF INATTENTION
• Shows restlessness and fidgeting, squirms in seat • Shows inappropriate or excessive running and climbing • Shows excessive talking • Cannot remain seated • Cannot play quietly • Acts as if motor-driven • Answers before questions are completed • Cannot await turn • Interrupts or intrudes on conversations of others	• Makes careless mistakes as a result of inattention • Has limited attention span • Does not listen to direct speech • Does not finish work or chores • Cannot organize tasks and activities • Avoids sustained mental effort • Loses necessary objects like books or pencils • Is easily distracted • Is forgetful
ADHD, COMBINED PRESENTATION	
Symptoms of H-I	Symptoms of inattention
ADHD, PREDOMINATELY INATTENTIVE PRESENTATION	
Few symptoms of H-I	Symptoms of inattention
ADHD, PREDOMINATELY HYPERACTIVE PRESENTATION	
Symptoms of H-I	Few symptoms of inattention

Source: Barbara Fadem. Behavioral Science in Medicine. Lippincott Williams & Wilkins. ISBN 978-1-60913-664-2.

Most of the etiology of ADHD is unknown. There may be some mild brain dysfunction, but there isn't any strong proof of a pronounced intellectual disability or significant structural neurological issues. Although there are anecdotal reports, scientific research has not found a link between ADHD and poor eating habits, a high sugar intake, or a sensitivity to food additives like artificial flavors or colors. Due to their problematic behavior, children with ADHD are more likely to experience physical abuse from their parents, even though the etiology of the disorder is unrelated to parenting styles such as excessive punishment or leniency. Additionally, there's a higher chance of disruptive behavior disorders in them.

In addition to pharmacological treatments, psychosocial and educational interventions are part of the management of ADHD. The latter group comprises mainly stimulants of the central nervous system (CNS), like methylphenidate (Ritalin) and dextroamphetamine sulfate (Dexedrine), that act by raising the level of dopamine in the brain. Conversely, more recent medications like guanfacine (Intuniv) and atomoxetine (Strattera) function by controlling norepinephrine levels in the brain. While the exact mechanism of these CNS agents' action on ADHD remains unclear, it appears that they aid in decreasing activity levels and lengthening attention spans, which enhances the child's concentration. Children using stimulant drugs may exhibit stunted growth and inability to gain weight because these medications also reduce appetite. However, after the child stops taking the medication, their weight and growth typically return to normal. Use of the agents only, when necessary, like on school days, can lessen these adverse effects. Anxiety and depression, two characteristics of ADHD that are linked to other medications.

Adolescence often brings some improvement in symptoms for many children with ADHD, especially a decrease in activity level. By adulthood, the majority of adolescents with ADHD continue to improve in all symptom areas. There is disagreement over the diagnosis and management of ADHD. Some contend that some children who are diagnosed with ADHD may actually just be too active for their parents or teachers to handle. This could result in needless medication and all of its side effects, as well as a higher chance of drug abuse in the future. The potential issues associated with misdiagnosis can be minimized by improving the diagnostic criteria for ADHD and increasing the use of social and psychological interventions for parents and children who are very active. Recent research indicates that children who take stimulants for ADHD are not more likely to abuse drugs as adults, even if the child does require medication (Wilens et al., 2003).

9.3.3.4. Separation Anxiety Disorder

Separation anxiety disorder, often known as school phobia or school refusal because the primary symptom is a refusal to attend school, is defined by an intense fear of losing a significant attachment figure, especially the mother. The child avoids leaving the mother and going to school because of this fear, blaming physical symptoms like headaches or stomachaches for their absence.

Up to 4% of school-age children suffer from separation anxiety disorder. While 7 to 8 years old is the most common age of onset, the disorder can manifest at any later age. The prognosis is worse for separation anxiety disorder that manifests later in life. The genesis of separation anxiety disorder involves both family and social factors. For instance, a stressful life event like moving or the loss of a pet or family member may trigger the disorder. Parents of children affected by this disorder frequently exhibit excessive concern for their child's welfare and are more likely to suffer from anxiety disorders themselves. The kids themselves have a higher chance of developing anxiety disorders as adults, especially agoraphobia. The best course of action for children with this disorder is gradual reintroduction to school in conjunction with family therapy. Antidepressants are among the medications that are helpful for treating the related symptoms.

9.3.3.5. Selective Mutism

Rarely, children (usually girls) with selective mutism speak in specific social contexts (e.g., home) but not in other contexts (e.g., in the classroom). Occasionally, the child uses hand gestures or whispers to communicate. Apart from the speech issue, the child behaves in a socially appropriate manner. Selective mutism is therefore more than just being shy. Selective mutism typically manifests at the age of six, and it can linger for months or even years. If the disorder continues after the age of ten, the prognosis is worse. Similar to separation anxiety disorder, selective mutism is frequently brought on by a traumatic life event, and behavioral and family therapy are the most successful forms of treatment (Dunn et al., 1992; Faust et al., 1977).

A Closer Look

Maternal Health

Pregnancy presents substantial health risks, even in developed countries, despite advances in obstetrical science and practice. Maternal mortality remains a major problem in global health and is considered a sentinel event in judging the quality of healthcare systems. Adolescent pregnancy represents a particular problem, whether intended or unintended, and whether within marriage or a union or not. Pregnancy results in major changes in a girl's life, physically, emotionally, socially, and economically and jeopardizes her transition into adulthood. Adolescent pregnancy, more often than not, stems from a girl's lack of choices. or abuse. Child marriage is a major contributor worldwide since 90% of births to girls aged 15–19 occur within marriage.

Maternal Death

In 2013 about 289,000 women (800 per day) in the world died due to pregnancy-related causes, with large differences between developed and developing countries. In developed nations maternal mortality has been steadily falling and on average means 16 deaths per 100,000 live births, as measured by the maternal mortality ratio (MMR). By contrast rates as high as 1,000 deaths per 100,000 live births are reported in the rest of the world, with the highest rates in Sub-Saharan Africa and South Asia, which account for 86% of such deaths. These deaths are rarely investigated, yet the World Health Organization considers that 99% of these deaths, the majority of which occur within 24 hours of childbirth, are preventable if the appropriate infrastructure, training, and facilities are in place. In these resource-poor countries, maternal health is further eroded by poverty and adverse economic factors that impact the roads, health care facilities, equipment, and supplies in addition to limited skilled personnel. Other problems include cultural attitudes towards sexuality, contraception, child marriage, home birth, and the ability to recognize medical emergencies. The direct causes of these maternal deaths are hemorrhage, eclampsia, obstructed labor, sepsis, and unskilled abortion. In addition, malaria and AIDS can also endanger pregnancy. In the period 2003–2009, hemorrhage was the leading cause of death, accounting for 27% of deaths in developing countries and 16% in developed countries.

Non-reproductive health remains an important predictor of maternal health. In the United States, the leading causes of maternal death are cardiovascular disease (15% of deaths), endocrine, respiratory and gastrointestinal disorders, infection, hemorrhage, and hypertensive disorders of pregnancy.

In 2000, the United Nations created Millennium Development Goal (MDG) 5 to improve maternal health. Target 5A sought to reduce maternal mortality by three quarters from 1990 to 2015, using two indicators, 5.1 the MMR and 5.2 the proportion of deliveries attended by skilled health personnel (physician, nurse, or midwife). Early reports indicated that MDG 5 had made the least progress of all MDGs. By the target date of 2015, the MMR had only declined by 45%, from 380 to 210, most of which occurred after 2000. However, this improvement occurred across all regions, but the highest MMRs were still in Africa and Asia, although South Asia witnessed the largest fall, from 530 to 190 (64%). The smallest decline was seen in the developed countries, from 26 to 16 (37%). In terms of assisted births, this proportion had risen globally from 59 to 71%. Although the numbers were similar for both developed and developing regions, there were wide variations in the latter from 52% in South Asia to 100% in East Asia. The risk of dying in pregnancy in developing countries remains fourteen times higher than in developed countries, but in Sub-Saharan Africa, where the MMR is highest, the risk is 175 times higher. In setting the MDG targets, skilled assisted birth was considered a key strategy, but also an indicator of access to care and closely reflects mortality rates. There are also marked differences within regions with a 31% lower rate in rural areas of developing countries (56 vs. 87%), yet there is no difference in East Asia but a 52% difference in Central Africa (32 vs. 84%). With the completion of the MDG campaign in 2015, new targets are being set for 2030 under the Sustainable Development Goals campaign. Maternal health is placed under Goal 3, Health, with the target being to reduce the global maternal mortality ratio to less than 70. Amongst tools being developed to meet these targets is the WHO Safe Childbirth Checklist.

Improvements in maternal health, in addition to professional assistance at delivery, will require routine antenatal care, and basic emergency obstetric care, including the availability of antibiotics, oxytocics, anticonvulsants, the ability to manually remove a retained placenta, perform instrumented deliveries, and postpartum care that is financially accessible, such as through insurance. Research has shown the most effective programs are those focusing on patient and community education, prenatal care, emergency obstetrics (including access to cesarean sections) and transportation. As with women's health in general, solutions to maternal health require a broad view encompassing many of the other MDG goals, such as poverty and status, and given that most deaths occur in the immediate intrapartum period, it has been recommended that intrapartum care (delivery) be a core strategy. New guidelines on antenatal care were issued by WHO in November 2016.

Complications of Pregnancy

In addition to death occurring in pregnancy and childbirth, pregnancy can result in many non-fatal health problems including obstetrical fistulae, ectopic pregnancy, preterm labor, gestational diabetes, hyperemesis gravidarum, hypertensive states including preeclampsia, and anemia. Globally, complications of pregnancy vastly outway maternal deaths, with an estimated 9.5 million cases of pregnancy-related illness and 1.4 million near-misses (survival from severe life-threatening complications). Complications of pregnancy may be physical, mental, economic, and social. It is estimated that 10–20 million women will develop physical or mental disability every year, resulting from complications of pregnancy or inadequate care. Consequently, international agencies have developed standards for obstetric care.

Obstetrical Fistula

Of near-miss events, obstetrical fistulae (OF), including vesicovaginal and rectovaginal fistulae, remain one of the most serious and tragic. Although corrective surgery is possible it is often not available and OF is considered completely preventable. If repaired, subsequent pregnancies will require a cesarean section. While unusual in developed countries, it is estimated that up to 100,000 cases occur every year in the world and that about 2 million women are currently living with this condition, with the highest incidence occurring in Africa and parts of Asia. OF results from prolonged obstructed labor without intervention, when continued pressure from the fetus in the birth canal restricts blood supply to the surrounding tissues, with eventual fetal death, necrosis, and expulsion. The damaged pelvic organs then develop a connection (fistula) allowing urine or feces, or both, to be discharged through the vagina with associated urinary and fecal incontinence, vaginal stenosis, nerve damage, and infertility. Severe social and mental consequences are also likely to follow, with the shunning of the women. Apart from lack of access to care, causes include young age and malnourishment. The UNFPA has made prevention a priority and is the lead agency in the Campaign to End Fistula, which issues annual reports and the United Nations observes May 23 as the International Day to End Obstetric Fistula every year. Prevention includes discouraging teenage pregnancy and child marriage, adequate nutrition, and access to skilled care, including cesarean section.

Summary

- Women's health is a broad category that includes health issues that are unique to women, such as menstruation and pregnancy, as well as conditions that affect both men and women, but that may affect women differently, such as heart disease and diabetes.
- Adolescence is a vital and very important stage of life, a passage from childhood to adulthood that marks the beginning of physical, psychological, and social transformation. Adolescence includes individuals aged 10–19 years.
- Women's experience of health and disease differ from those of men, due to unique biological, social and behavioral conditions. Biological differences vary from phenotypes to cellular biology and manifest unique risks for the development of ill health.
- Women's life expectancy is greater than that of men, and they have lower death rates throughout life, regardless of race and geographic region. Historically though, women had higher rates of mortality, primarily from maternal deaths (death in childbirth).
- Heart disease is the number one killer of American women. Although it is typically viewed as a man's disease, more women die of heart disease each year than do men. On average, women develop heart disease later in life than men.
- Cigarette smoking is the leading preventable cause of death in this country, contributing substantially to deaths from cancer, lung disease, heart disease, stroke, and other causes. Smoking rates among women have decreased by 35% since their peak in 1965.
- Violence is a major public health problem for American women. More than 4.5 million women are victims of violence each year. Of these women, nearly two of every three are attacked by a relative or someone they know. Women are 6 times more likely to be abused by someone they know than men and 10 times more likely to be victims of sexual assault. It is estimated that 10 to 20% (or one to two young women in 10) are the victims of sexual abuse.
- The age of 20 years is another significant development milestone. Childhood is over, adolescence is coming to an end, and the individual must now be physically and socially prepared to face the challenges and enjoy the privileges of adult life.
- Puberty is the physical indicator of the start of adolescence. This milestone is marked by increased skeletal growth and the development of primary and secondary sex characteristics. Girls reach puberty earlier than boys.
- By about age 15 years, the adolescent has a great interest in body image and popularity with same- and opposite-sex peers. To fit in with peers, the middle adolescent embraces current fashions in clothing and music and prefers to spend time with friends rather than family. This behavior is expected and normal, but it can lead to conflict with parents.
- Late adolescence is associated with an identity crisis, in which the teen must define and refine his place in the world. Resolution of this crisis usually results in the further development of morals, ethics, and self-control, as well as the ability to realistically appraise one's own abilities.

- Adolescence is marked not only by cognitive maturation and personality formation, but also by strong sexual feelings. These feelings are expressed through physical activity and masturbation.

References

1. Centers for Disease Control. (2000). *STDs in Adolescents and Young Adults: National STD Surveillance Report*. Centers for Disease Control and Prevention.
2. Chandra-Mouli, V., Svanemyr, J., Amin, A., Fogstad, H., Say, L., Girard, F., & Temmerman, M. (2015). Twenty years after the International Conference on Population and Development: Where are we with adolescent sexual and reproductive health and rights? *Journal of Adolescent Health, 56*(S1–S6). https://doi.org/10.1016/j.jadohealth.2014.09.015.
3. Clawson, J. A. (1996). A child with chronic illness and the process of family adaptation. *Journal of Pediatric Nursing, 11*, 52–61.
4. Dick, B., & Ferguson, B. J. (2015). Health for the world's adolescents: A second chance in the second decade. *Journal of Adolescent Health, 56*, 3–6. https://doi.org/10.1016/j.jadohealth.2014.10.260.
5. Dunn, J., & McGuire, S. (1992). Sibling and peer relationships in childhood. *Journal of Child Psychology and Psychiatry, 33*, 67–105.
6. Faust, M. S. (1977). Somatic development of adolescent girls. *Monographs of the Society for Research in Child Development, 42*, 75–82.
7. Jaskiewicz, M. G. (2009). An integrative review of the health care needs of female adolescents. *Journal of the Nurse Practitioner, 5*, 274–283. https://doi.org/10.1016/j.nurpra.2008.05.016.
8. Kurian, R. (2010). Tourette's syndrome. *New England Journal of Medicine, 363*, 2332–2338.
9. Lightbody, A. A., & Reiss, A. L. (2009). Gene, brain, and behavior relationships in Fragile X syndrome: Evidence from neuroimaging studies. *Developmental Disabilities Research Reviews, 15*(4), 343–352.
10. Melaku, Y. A., Zello, G. A., Gill, T. K., Adams, R. J., & Shi, Z. (2015). Prevalence and factors associated with stunting and thinness among adolescent students in Northern Ethiopia: A comparison to World Health Organization standards. *Archives of Public Health, 73*, 44. https://doi.org/10.1186/s13690-015-0093-9.
11. Panjalipour, S., Bostani Khalesi, Z., & Mirhaghjoo, S. N. (2018). Iranian female adolescents' reproductive health needs: A systematic review. *International Journal of Women's Health and Reproductive Sciences, 6*, 226–232. https://doi.org/10.15296/ijwhr.2018.39.
12. Piaget, J., & Inhelder, B. (1969). *The Psychology of the Child*. Basic Books.
13. Sadler, T. W. (2000). *Langman's Medical Embryology* (8th ed.). Lippincott Williams & Wilkins.
14. Shapiro, T., & Hertzig, M. (1988). Normal child and adolescent development. In J. A. Talbott, R. E. Hales, & S. C. Yudofsky (Eds.), *American Psychiatric Press Textbook of Psychiatry*. American Psychiatric Press.
15. Shapiro, T., & Perry, R. (1976). Latency revisited: The age 7 plus or minus 1. *Psychoanalytic Study of the Child, 31*, 79–105.

16. Taghizadeh Moghaddam, H., Bahreini, A., Ajilian Abbasi, M., Fazli, F., & Saeidi, M. (2016). Adolescence health: The needs, problems, and attention. *International Journal of Pediatrics, 4*, 1423–1438.

17. Tanner, J. M. (1970). Physical growth. In P. H. Mussen (Ed.), *Camichel's Manual of Child Development* (3rd ed., pp. 77–155). Wiley.

18. Wilens, T. E., Faraone, S. V., Biederman, J., & Gunawardene, S. (2003). Does stimulant therapy for attention-deficit/hyperactivity disorder beget later substance abuse? A meta-analytic review of the literature. *Pediatrics, 111*, 179–185.

Chapter 10

OBESITY AND NUTRITION

Contents

Introduction

Obesity and nutrition are intrinsically linked aspects of public health that significantly impact individuals and communities worldwide. Obesity is defined as an excessive accumulation of body fat that presents a health risk, commonly measured by the Body Mass Index (BMI), where a BMI of 30 or above indicates obesity. The prevalence of obesity has reached epidemic proportions globally, affecting both developed and developing countries. This surge is primarily attributed to changes in dietary patterns and lifestyles, characterized by increased consumption of high-calorie, nutrient-poor foods and a decrease in physical activity.

Poor nutrition is a leading contributor to obesity. Diets high in processed foods, sugars, and unhealthy fats, coupled with low intake of fruits, vegetables, and whole grains, contribute to excessive caloric intake and weight gain. These dietary habits are often influenced by factors such as food availability, marketing, socioeconomic status, and cultural preferences. In many communities, especially in urban areas, the easy availability of fast food and sugary beverages, coupled with busy lifestyles, makes it challenging to maintain a healthy diet.

The health consequences of obesity are severe and multifaceted. It increases the risk of various chronic diseases, including type 2 diabetes, cardiovascular diseases, certain cancers, and musculoskeletal disorders. Obesity also has psychological impacts, often contributing to low self-esteem, depression, and social stigmatization. These health issues lead to increased healthcare costs and a significant burden on healthcare systems.

Addressing obesity requires a comprehensive approach that includes promoting healthy nutrition and active lifestyles. Public health initiatives focus on education and awareness campaigns that inform individuals about the benefits of a balanced diet and regular physical activity. Schools play a crucial role by incorporating nutrition education into their curricula and providing healthy meal options. Community programs that offer cooking classes, nutrition counselling, and exercise groups also support individuals in making healthier choices.

Policy interventions are critical in creating environments that promote healthy behaviors. Governments can implement regulations to limit the marketing of unhealthy foods, particularly to children, and provide incentives for the production and consumption of healthier food options. Policies that ensure food labeling transparency help consumers make informed dietary choices. Additionally, urban planning that encourages physical activity through the development of parks, bike paths, and pedestrian-friendly infrastructure can help combat sedentary lifestyles.

Addressing socioeconomic barriers is also essential, as lower-income populations often have limited access to healthy foods and safe spaces for physical activity. Initiatives such as subsidized healthy food programs, farmers' markets in underserved areas, and community gardens can improve access to nutritious foods. Healthcare providers play a vital role by routinely screening for obesity, offering nutritional counselling, and supporting weight management programs.

Overall, tackling obesity and improving nutrition require a multi-faceted strategy that involves individuals, communities, healthcare providers, policymakers, and the food industry. By promoting healthy eating habits, increasing physical activity, and implementing supportive policies, societies can reduce the prevalence of obesity and its associated health risks, leading to improved overall public health and quality of life.

Orientation and Directional Terms

Term	Definition	Illustration
Obesity	Obesity is a chronic complex disease defined by excessive fat deposits that can impair health. Obesity can lead to an increased risk of type 2 diabetes and heart disease, it can affect bone health and reproduction, it increases the risk of certain cancers.	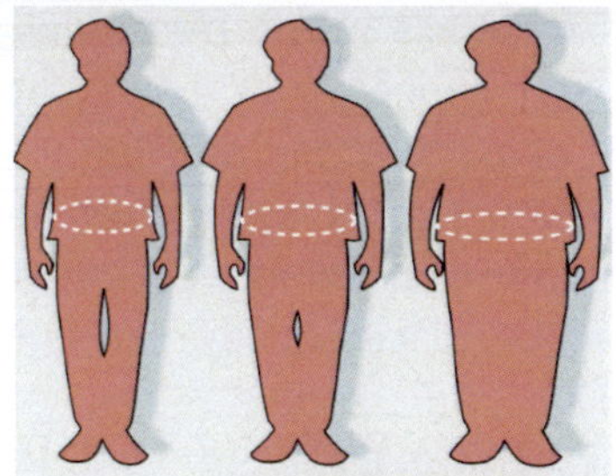
Amniotic fluid	Amniotic fluid is a clear, slightly yellowish liquid that surrounds the unborn baby (fetus) during pregnancy. It is contained in the amniotic sac. Polyhydramnios may occur when a fetus cannot swallow a normal amount of amniotic fluid due to a gastrointestinal, neurological, or other problem.	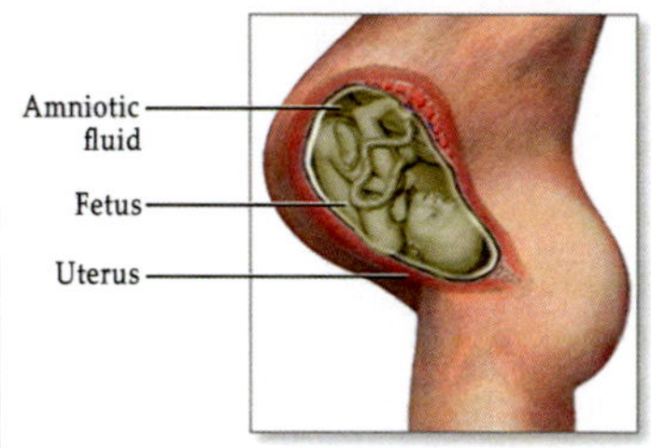
Diabetes mellitus	Diabetes mellitus (DM) is a metabolic disease, involving inappropriately elevated blood glucose levels. DM has several categories, including type 1, type 2, maturity-onset diabetes of the young (MODY), gestational diabetes, neonatal diabetes, and secondary causes due to endocrinopathies, steroid use, etc.	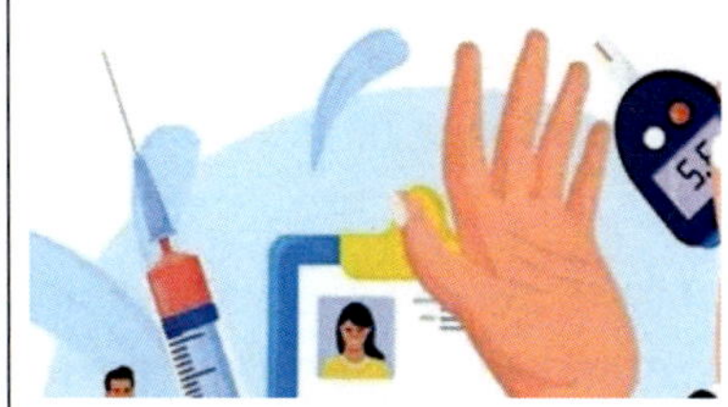
Weight-loss	Weight loss, in the context of medicine, health, or physical fitness, refers to a reduction of the total body mass, by a mean loss of fluid, body fat (adipose tissue), or lean mass (namely bone mineral deposits, muscle, tendon, and other connective tissue).	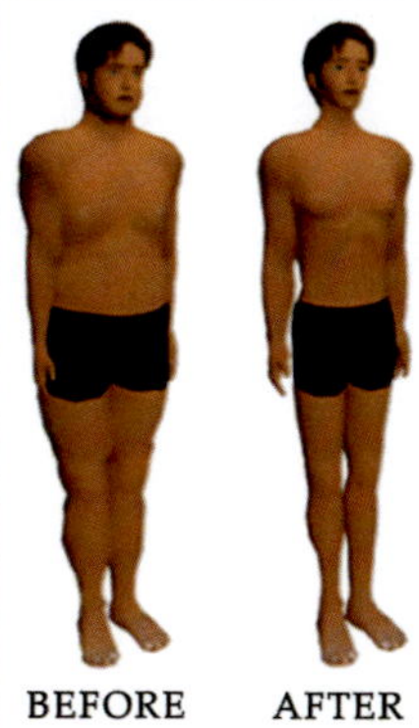
Balanced Diet	A balanced diet contains all of the essential elements that the human body needs. Carbohydrates, lipids, vitamins, minerals, proteins, fiber, and water are all essential components in a well-balanced diet. A nutritious, well-balanced diet lowers the risk of disease and enhances general health.	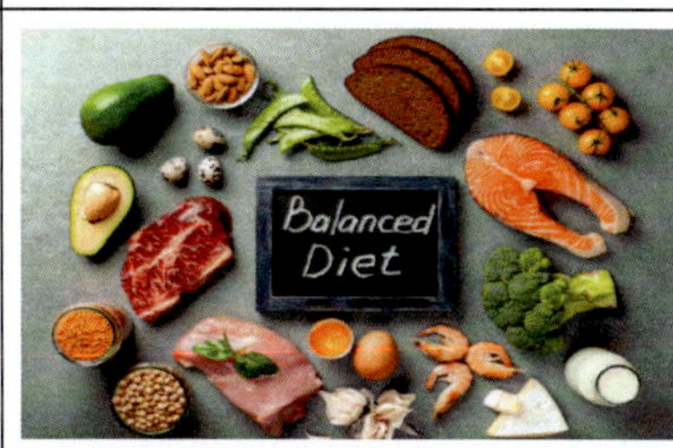

10.1. Definition of Obesity

The condition known as obesity is characterized by an excessive increase in body fat mass relative to non-fat mass and a body weight size that is larger than expected for a given height. The WHO defines obesity as the buildup of fatty tissue that adversely affects an individual's health. It is well known that obesity is a condition in which the body accumulates fat due to overeating.

The Latin term for obesity means "due to eating." In the past, obesity was seen as a sign of good health and was associated with material wealth and high status. Along with the Industrial Revolution, attitudes started to change to refer to negative concepts like lumpishness, trouble, being slow, and being unhealthy. Previously, obesity was sometimes associated with positive concepts like strength, power, sovereignty, imposing presence, fertility, and abundance. These days, a lot of systemic diseases are thought to be preceded by obesity.

Based on conducted research, it has been determined that obesity poses a significant risk for various medical conditions, including but not limited to coronary heart disease, hypertension, stroke, type 2 diabetes, ovarian, breast, prostate, and colon cancer, osteoarthritis, varicose veins, sleep apnea syndrome, difficult childbirth, ovarian cysts, and depression.

10.1.1. Causes of Obesity

Numerous factors contribute to the development of obesity, including genetic predisposition, environmental factors, dietary habits, psychological factors, and demographic factors. Figure 10.1 shows a schematic representation of the factors that contribute to the development of obesity.

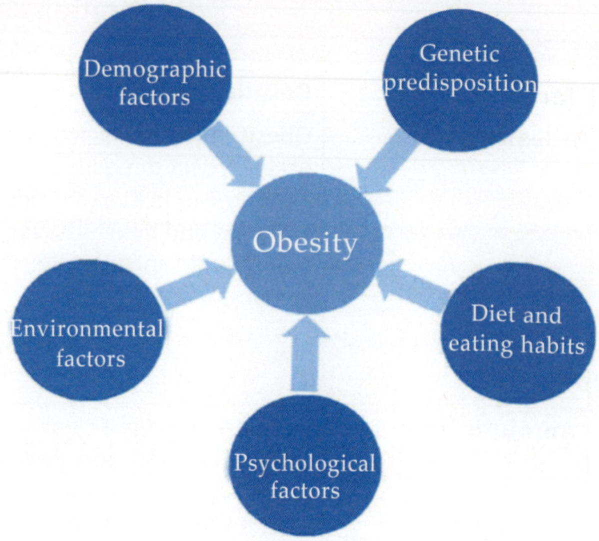

Figure 10.1. *Factors that influence the formation of obesity.*

Source: https://www.researchgate.net/publication/319085839_Obesity_and_nutrition.

10.1.1.1. Demographic Factors

1. **Age:** Every age group is affected by obesity, but in recent years, it has seemed to rise with advancing years. As we age, our body's fat rate rises. Not only do adult males and females exhibit obesity, but small children also exhibit it. It indicates a rise in both males and females with age, at least until the ages of 50 and 60. Childhood obesity may persist into adulthood if preventative measures are not taken. The National Health and Nutrition Examination Survey (NHANES) has been used to study the lowest and highest weight rates in the United States since 1999. The most recent study was carried out in 2012. Obesity prevalence in children under the age of two was found to be 8.1%, while it was found to be 16.9% in children aged two to nineteen. More than 20% of children and adolescents in the European Region

are overweight, and one-third of them are obese, according to data from the World Health Organization's (WHO) Regional Office for Europe. Compared to children of normal weight, obese children have a twice greater chance of becoming obese adults. In the United Kingdom in 1989, there were 15% of overweight children and 5% of obese children; by 1998, these rates had risen to 24% and 9%, respectively. Throughout all of Europe, 8–25% of adolescents between the ages of 12 and 17 are obese. Obesity rates in some countries are as follows: Latin America (4.4%), Africa (3.9%), and Asia (2.9%). With a 10% rate, Russia had the lowest, and with a 36% rate, Italy had the highest obesity rate among the countries reported.

2. **Gender:** When a young person reaches puberty, their body produces more fat due to an increase in estrogen. Because girls' estrogen levels are higher than boys' during adolescence, fat starts to accumulate in the body during this time and is manifested as increased weight in girls. As a result, during puberty, girls are more likely than boys to be obese. Akıs (2003) conducted a study in Bursa-Orhangazi with 5795 children in the 6–14 age group and found that the prevalence of obesity was more in girls than it was in boys. Suzek (2005) conducted a study in Mugla with 6480 students who were between the ages of 6–15 and found that obesity prevalence was 7.6% for girls and 9.1% for boys. The results additionally revealed a high rate of obesity among those aged 10. It is well known that pregnancy and childbirth are the main factors contributing to weight gain in women. Furthermore, a variety of biological conditions that women encounter during menopause may be the cause of their weight issues.

10.1.1.2. Genetic Predisposition

Genetic predisposition to obesity and environmental factors that have an impact later in life are two of the factors contributing to obesity. 40–70% of adult obesity is linked to genetic factors, despite the paucity of research on genetics in children. In genetic studies, a single gene defect linked to obesity has been identified. The Ob gene, which is involved in the production of leptin and regulates cocaine through leptin and transcript (CART) protein regulated by amphetamine, has garnered interest recently. Research is also being done on genes that activate mechanisms other than leptin.

Children's birth weight, eating habits, and weight in three to five years were noted to have similar features throughout the three generations in a cohort study that looked at the genetic components of childhood obesity. A systematic analysis looking at the connection between parents' BMI values and childhood obesity has revealed that there is still a lack of research on this topic, but it has been suggested that pre-pregnancy weight in mothers in particular may have an impact on childhood obesity. However, despite the possibility that some genes increase the susceptibility to obesity in exogenous obesity, family history and way of life continue to be more significant. According to surveys done on families who are at risk, the probability of obesity in children whose parents are normal weight is 7%; however, this probability rises to 40% in cases where one parent is obese and to 80% in cases where both parents are obese.

10.1.1.3. Environmental Factors

Environmental factors have led to a common problem for both developed and developing countries: eating foods high in fat and calories, leading sedentary lives, and having easy access to these foods. The imbalance of energy intake and expenditure—that is, not using as much energy as is taken in—is one of the most significant contributing factors to obesity. Lifestyle modifications have been connected to the sharp rise in obesity prevalence that has occurred recently everywhere in the world. A shift in eating habits toward lower-quality foods and drinks with more energy but fewer nutrients results in an increase in caloric intake. In addition, the scarcity of spaces for kids to play and participate in sports reduces the amount of energy they expend outside and forces them to spend more time inside watching TV or using the computer, which uses less energy. It is well known that prolonged television viewing affects autonomic eating patterns and the preference for unhealthy foods.

Eating high-fat, high-sugar, and high-salt foods and snacks while watching television also contributes to an imbalance between energy expenditure and intake. Obesity is linked to inactivity, and obesity itself causes immobility, creating a vicious cycle. Sedentary behaviors like watching television and using the computer have been linked to the development of obesity, according to a study done in the United States that included 25% of overweight or obese children. Research on the connection between computer use and obesity is lacking, but studies on the effects of excessive television watching—five hours or more a day on average—on childhood obesity have been found. According to reports, children who spend more time on computers—in addition to watching television—are at a higher risk of becoming obese. Children can spend up to 55 hours a week on screens, and the average American home has a television on for eight hours every day. A systematic analysis looking at the connection between obesity and sleep duration found that getting little sleep is primarily associated with an independent risk factor for childhood obesity.

10.1.1.4. Diet and Eating Habits

The mother's diet during pregnancy can have a significant impact on the baby's eating habits afterwards. The main stage of taste development is in utero. Fetal exposure teaches the fetus to accept and even prefer the foods that the mother eats. An amniotic sac regenerates every three hours. A fetus swallows one liter of amniotic fluid on average during the last trimester. Research has shown that the mother's diet during the final few hours of pregnancy affects the flavor of the amniotic fluid. Moreover, during the final months of pregnancy, a fetus swallows and smells the amniotic fluid. Since nutrients from the mother's diet are present in both amniotic fluid and breast milk, a fetus's education regarding food taste begins in utero and during the early stages of development.

The most significant determinants of children's eating habits are the variety, regularity, amount, and composition of the diet that is fed to them starting at birth. Feeding a child high-energy foods from an early age and consuming them for extended periods are behaviors that lead to obesity and expand the child's stomach. It is commonly known that breastfeeding can prevent the development of obesity. Adverse dietary changes can also result from eating more out of doors and drinking sugar-sweetened beverages; portion sizes growing; a lack of variety in nutrients; and consuming fast food and high-energy, high-fat snacks that are readily available, quick to prepare, and seem to be everywhere.

Excessive eating habits are the decisive factor in obesity. Early in life, the rate at which new fat cells are formed is especially rapid. The quantity of fat cells rises along with the rate of fat accumulation. Approximately three times as many fat cells are present in obese children as in normal children. These days, eating fast food that is high in sugar and calories, skipping breakfast, restricting physical activity, and following a diet that is excessively high in calories can all contribute to obesity.

10.1.1.5. Psychological Factors

The etiology of obesity is complex and involves numerous biological, psychological, social, and environmental factors. As a result, managing obese people requires a multifaceted strategy along with psychological support. Research from both domestic and foreign sources indicates that patients seeking obesity treatment require psychosocial support. Obese people are more likely to experience mental and social issues like low self-esteem, a negative body image, depression, suicide, smoking, drinking, and using drugs, as well as unemployment, loneliness, social exclusion, and discrimination. Body image is an important consideration in managing obesity.

In obese people, perceived body weight—rather than actual body weight—is linked to body dissatisfaction. According to a study, people who are overweight or obese have lower self-esteem than people who are normal weight, and there is a correlation between the two variables (self-esteem decreases as BMI rises). BMI and body dissatisfaction are found to be strongly correlated in another study. Furthermore, there is a significant impact of body image on psychosocial health. Obese patients have been found to have a higher prevalence of psychopathological conditions, such as depression and personality disorders. According to reports, most people's eating habits change in response to different emotional states, such as happiness, sadness, stress, etc. Some children exhibit extreme anorexia in response to psychological issues, while others may react by overeating. A person's spiritual structure can be impacted and malnourished by their relationship with their parents, their children, issues in the home, rejection from friends, and academic failure.

10.1.2. Health Problems That Lead to Obesity

Over the world, obesity is a serious public health issue. One of the main health issues facing the globe today is obesity. A person's health is impacted by obesity in several ways; a heavy body is difficult to move. Problems with different organs can shorten life expectancy. Studies have shown that obesity has detrimental effects on human health. Research reveals that individuals aged 40–44 and 20% overweight have a mortality rate that is 30–40% higher than that of people with a normal weight. However, the rate rises to 80–100% in 40% of individuals of the same age who are overweight.

10.1.2.1. Diabetes Mellitus

Diabetes mellitus is a chronic metabolic disorder characterized by elevated blood glucose levels due to the body's inability to produce or effectively use insulin. There are three main types of diabetes: type 1, type 2, and gestational diabetes. Type 1 diabetes, an autoimmune condition, occurs when the body's immune system attacks and destroys insulin-producing beta cells in the pancreas. It typically manifests in childhood or adolescence, requiring lifelong insulin therapy. Type 2 diabetes, the most common form, results from insulin resistance combined with an eventual decline in insulin production. It is closely linked to obesity, sedentary lifestyles, and poor dietary habits and is more prevalent in adults, though its incidence is rising among younger populations. Gestational diabetes develops during pregnancy and usually resolves after childbirth, but it increases the risk of type 2 diabetes for both the mother and child later in life.

The global prevalence of diabetes is rising alarmingly, with the International Diabetes Federation (IDF) reporting that approximately 537 million adults were living with diabetes in 2021. This figure is projected to reach 643 million by 2030 and 783 million by 2045. Diabetes is a significant public health concern due to its association with severe complications such as cardiovascular diseases, kidney failure, nerve damage, and vision impairment, leading to increased morbidity and mortality rates.

Effective management of diabetes involves a combination of lifestyle modifications, medication, and regular monitoring of blood glucose levels. Lifestyle interventions, including a balanced diet, regular physical activity, and weight management, are fundamental in managing and preventing type 2 diabetes. Dietary recommendations focus on consuming whole grains, lean proteins, healthy fats, and plenty of fruits and vegetables while limiting refined sugars and processed foods. Physical activity helps improve insulin sensitivity and aids in maintaining a healthy weight.

Pharmacological treatments for diabetes include oral medications, such as metformin and sulfonylureas, and injectable therapies like insulin and GLP-1 receptor agonists. These treatments aim to lower blood glucose levels, enhance insulin sensitivity, and manage co-existing conditions such as hypertension and hyperlipidemia. Advances in diabetes care have introduced new medications and technologies, such as continuous glucose monitors (CGMs) and insulin pumps, which help patients manage their condition more effectively.

Preventing diabetes, particularly type 2, involves addressing modifiable risk factors through public health initiatives and community programs. Education campaigns that promote healthy eating, regular exercise, and weight control are essential. Screening programs for early detection and intervention in high-risk populations can prevent or delay the onset of diabetes.

Healthcare systems must provide accessible and comprehensive care to manage diabetes effectively, including regular check-ups, education on self-management, and support for lifestyle changes. Multidisciplinary care teams, including endocrinologists, dietitians, and diabetes educators, play a crucial role in delivering personalized care and improving patient outcomes.

10.1.2.2. Hypertension

Hypertension, or high blood pressure, is a chronic medical condition where the force of the blood against the artery walls is consistently too high, leading to health problems such as heart disease and stroke. It is often termed a "silent killer" because it frequently presents without noticeable symptoms, yet significantly increases the risk of cardiovascular events, kidney disease, and other serious health issues. Blood pressure is measured in millimeters of mercury (mm Hg) and is expressed with two numbers: systolic pressure (the pressure when the heart beats) over diastolic pressure (the pressure when the heart is at rest). Hypertension is typically diagnosed when these readings are consistently 130/80 mm Hg or higher. Globally, hypertension is a major public health issue, affecting an estimated 1.13 billion people, with a significant number of cases found in low- and middle-income countries. The prevalence of hypertension increases with age, and it is more common in men than women before age 65, after which the trend reverses. Risk factors for developing hypertension include genetics, age, being overweight or obese, physical inactivity, a diet high in salt and low in potassium, excessive alcohol consumption, smoking, and stress. Chronic conditions such as diabetes and high cholesterol also contribute to the risk.

Managing hypertension involves lifestyle modifications and, when necessary, medication. Lifestyle changes are the first line of defense and include adopting a healthy diet, such as the DASH (Dietary Approaches to Stop Hypertension) diet, which emphasizes fruits, vegetables, whole grains, and low-fat dairy products while reducing salt, red meat, and added sugars. Regular physical activity, maintaining a healthy weight, limiting alcohol intake, and quitting smoking are crucial steps in preventing and controlling hypertension.

Pharmacological treatment includes various classes of antihypertensive medications, such as diuretics, ACE inhibitors, angiotensin II receptor blockers, calcium channel blockers, and beta-blockers. These medications work through different mechanisms to lower blood pressure and reduce the strain on the cardiovascular system. Often, a combination of two or more drugs may be necessary to achieve optimal blood pressure control.

Monitoring blood pressure regularly is essential for managing hypertension. Home blood pressure monitors allow individuals to track their readings and share them with healthcare providers, facilitating better management of the condition. Regular check-ups with healthcare providers help adjust treatment plans and monitor for potential complications.

Public health initiatives play a crucial role in addressing hypertension at a population level. These initiatives include promoting awareness of hypertension and its risks, encouraging healthy lifestyles through community programs, and implementing policies to reduce salt and unhealthy fats in processed foods. Screening programs for early detection and intervention can help identify individuals at risk and provide them with the necessary support and resources to manage their blood pressure.

10.1.2.3. Cancer Types

In recent times, there has been a commensurate rise in the incidence of obesity and the types of cancer. Obesity is now known to play a significant role in the development of many cancer types, particularly in the West. Obesity is said to raise the risk of developing certain cancers, including endometrial, colon, rectum, esophageal, pancreatic, and breast cancers. In the US, two-thirds of adults are becoming more and more overweight or obese. It has been discovered that in about 3.2% of men and 8.8% of women, newly diagnosed cancer is linked to higher BMI.

10.1.2.4. Respiratory (Pulmonary) System Disorders

One major respiratory system-affecting side effect of sleep apnea syndrome is obesity. Excess fat storage in the chest wall and abdomen can impede the chest's ability to breathe. The amount of oxygen needed for breathing processes in people who are morbidly obese is three times greater than in people who are not obese. In between 70 and 80% of cases of sleep apnea, obesity is present. According to studies, there is a 6% increase in the risk of sleep apnea for every 10% increase in body mass index.

10.1.3. Evaluation Procedures for Obesity

Evaluation procedures for obesity involve a comprehensive assessment of an individual's health status, lifestyle, and risk factors to determine the extent of obesity and its potential impact on overall health. These procedures are crucial for developing effective management and treatment plans. The key components of obesity evaluation include:

10.1.3.1. Anthropometric Measurements

- **Body Mass Index (BMI):** BMI is calculated using weight in kilograms divided by height in meters squared (kg/m^2). A BMI of 30 or above indicates obesity.
- **Waist Circumference:** Measuring waist circumference helps assess abdominal fat, which is a significant risk factor for metabolic and cardiovascular diseases. A waist circumference greater than 102 cm (40 inches) in men and 88 cm (35 inches) in women is associated with higher health risks.
- **Waist-to-Hip Ratio (WHR):** This ratio is calculated by dividing waist circumference by hip circumference. A WHR above 0.90 in men and 0.85 in women indicates a higher risk of obesity-related complications.
- **Skinfold Thickness:** Using calipers to measure skinfold thickness at various body sites can estimate body fat percentage.

10.1.3.2. Clinical Assessment

- **Medical History:** A detailed medical history includes assessing family history of obesity-related diseases, previous weight loss attempts, eating and activity habits, and psychological factors such as stress or depression.
- **Physical Examination:** A comprehensive physical exam can identify obesity-related complications, such as high blood pressure, signs of insulin resistance, or orthopedic issues.

10.1.3.3. Laboratory Tests

- **Blood Glucose Levels:** Fasting blood glucose and HbA1c levels help assess for diabetes or prediabetes.
- **Lipid Profile:** Measuring cholesterol levels, including LDL, HDL, and triglycerides, can identify dyslipidemia.
- **Liver Function Tests:** These tests can detect nonalcoholic fatty liver disease (NAFLD), which is common in obese individuals.
- **Thyroid Function Tests:** Assessing thyroid function can rule out hypothyroidism, which can contribute to weight gain.

10.1.3.4. Dietary Assessment

- **24-Hour Dietary Recall:** Patients provide a detailed account of all foods and beverages consumed in the past 24 hours.

- **Food Frequency Questionnaire (FFQ):** This tool assesses habitual intake over a longer period, identifying patterns and frequency of consumption of various food groups.
- **Dietary Logs:** Patients maintain a food diary over several days to provide a more comprehensive view of their eating habits.

10.1.3.5. Physical Activity Assessment

- **Activity Logs:** Patients record their physical activities, including type, duration, and intensity.
- **Questionnaires:** Tools like the International Physical Activity Questionnaire (IPAQ) assess physical activity levels and sedentary behavior.
- **Wearable Devices:** Devices such as pedometers and fitness trackers provide objective data on physical activity and energy expenditure.

10.1.3.6. Psychosocial Assessment

- **Mental Health Screening:** Identifying depression, anxiety, or other psychological issues that may affect eating and physical activity behaviors.
- *Behavioral Assessments*: Evaluating eating behaviors, such as binge eating or emotional eating, and readiness for behavior change.

10.1.3.7. Evaluation of Comorbidities

- Assessing for obesity-related conditions such as hypertension, cardiovascular diseases, sleep apnea, osteoarthritis, and reproductive issues, which can influence the management plan.

10.1.3.8. Assessment of Weight-Related Quality of Life

- Tools such as the Impact of Weight on Quality of Life (IWQOL) questionnaire help understand how obesity affects the patient's daily life and well-being.

10.1.4. Diagnosis of Obesity

Body mass index (BMI) is used to diagnose obesity. BMI does have some restrictions, though. The BMI only slightly modifies results based on ethnic group and ignores factors such as age and sex. The BMI that qualifies as overweight is somewhat lower for individuals of Asian and other ethnic backgrounds. Furthermore, the BMI does not differentiate between fat and lean tissue. Consequently, physicians might not know if a high BMI results from too much fat or muscle (like in bodybuilders). In these situations, they calculate body composition, or the proportion of muscle and fat in the body. Measurement of waist circumference is done. Visceral obesity, or fat that builds up in the abdomen and around the waist, is identified and measured with the use of this measurement. Subcutaneous fat, which is fat beneath the skin that is distributed throughout the body, is not nearly as harmful as abdominal obesity. More accurate than BMI in determining a patient's risk of certain complications (like heart problems) are the patient's waist circumference and the presence of metabolic syndrome.

Body composition (the percentage of body fat and muscle) can be determined using the following:

- Measurement of skinfold thickness and the circumference of the upper arm.

- Bioelectric impedance, which can be done in a doctor's office.
- Underwater (hydrostatic) weighing.

Typically, the skinfold thickness is measured behind the upper arm, over the triceps. Pinching the skin yields the skinfold, which is the measurement of the skin and the layer of fat beneath it. By using bioelectrical impedance analysis, the percentage of body fat is indirectly calculated and the percentage of total body water is estimated directly. People in good health and those with a limited number of chronic conditions, like moderate obesity or diabetes mellitus, are the ones who respond to it the best.

The most accurate technique for calculating body fat percentage is underwater weighing. It takes a lot of money and effort, though. As a result, research uses it more frequently than clinical care. When a man's body fat percentage is more than 25%, he is deemed obese. The percentage is higher than 32% in women. Usually, blood tests are conducted. Measurements of blood sugar (glucose) are used to screen for prediabetes and diabetes, and measurements of cholesterol and other fat levels are used to screen for abnormally high cholesterol and other fat levels. To detect high blood pressure, doctors also take blood pressure readings. By using these tests, physicians can diagnose patients with metabolic syndrome, which is a diagnosis that encompasses all three disorders. In addition, doctors look for other conditions like depression, fatty liver, and obstructive sleep apnea that are frequently seen in obese patients.

10.1.5. Treatment of Obesity

Initially, dietary adjustments, heightened physical activity, and behavioral modifications are all part of the lifestyle modifications used to treat obesity. Both weight-loss (bariatric) surgery and medications are crucial for long-term weight loss, but they are frequently underutilized because of access issues, insurance company reimbursement issues, or personal preferences of the patient or physician. Reducing body weight by even 5 to 10% can have a positive impact on lowering blood pressure, cholesterol, and the risk or severity of weight-related health issues like diabetes. Motivation and preparedness are essential for successful weight loss. The most prosperous people set realistic goals and understand that long-term lifestyle adjustments are necessary for healthy weight loss, not quick fixes or temporary diets. It can be helpful to ask medical professionals for assistance, such as dieticians or physicians. Family support is also very important. Regular contact programs—like WW, formerly known as Weight Watchers—increase accountability and can boost the chances of success. Counselors usually lead weekly meetings, which are enhanced by educational and guidance resources. Like any other chronic illness, obesity requires a lifelong management program because most patients gain weight back after treatment.

10.1.5.1. Changes in Diet

Reducing calories and selecting a variety of nutrient-dense foods are essential components of a healthy, balanced diet for weight loss. A healthy rate of weight loss could be achieved by cutting back on daily caloric intake by 500 to 1,000 calories. Typically, this strategy calls for 1,200–1,500 calories per day. Nonetheless, the body might adapt to the reduction in calories by lowering the metabolic rate, for instance. Weight loss might therefore be less than anticipated. Nevertheless, the most effective way to lose weight and keep it off seems to be a high-fiber diet combined with a calorie restriction of roughly 600 per day and some protein replacement in the form of carbohydrates. Extremely low-calorie diets help people lose weight more quickly, but they should be monitored by a doctor.

The following changes in diet are recommended:

- Eating small meals and avoiding or carefully choosing snacks.
- Eating breakfast (skipping breakfast can lead to consuming too many calories later in the day).
- Eating 5 or more servings of fruits and vegetables a day.
- Substituting fresh fruits and vegetables and salads for refined carbohydrates and processed food.
- Eating lean protein—for example, fish or chicken breast or vegetable protein, such as soy.
- Switching from full-fat to no-fat or low-fat dairy products.
- Eliminating high-calorie beverages, such as soda, juice, or alcohol, and drinking water instead.
- Limiting consumption of restaurant and fast food.
- Limiting alcohol consumption.
- Switching from harmful fats (such as saturated and trans fats) to good fats, such as monounsaturated fats (in olive and canola oils) and polyunsaturated fats (in deep-sea fish and vegetable oils), and limiting the amount of fat consumed.

Consuming foods high in monounsaturated fats from plants, like olive oil, or foods high in fish oils, such as those from deep-sea fish like salmon and tuna, may lower the risk of diabetes and heart problems. Dairy products that are fat-free or low-fat should be consumed to help prevent vitamin D deficiency. Some people find that using meal replacements on a regular or occasional basis helps help them lose weight and keep it off.

10.1.5.2. Physical Activity

Increasing physical activity can aid in healthy weight loss and weight maintenance. Exercise, or organized physical activity, is one type of physical activity. Other types of physical activity include gardening, taking the stairs rather than the elevator, and walking whenever possible rather than driving. Engaging in lifestyle activities can burn a significant amount of calories. It is more likely for someone on a diet to gain back the weight they lose if they do not exercise. Exercises that burn more calories than less active ones include jogging, biking, cross-country skiing, skating, walking quickly (3 to 4 miles [5 to 6 km] per hour), and tennis. One hour of brisk walking per day can burn approximately 240 calories, as an example, as vigorous walking can burn about 4 calories per minute. Approximately 6 to 8 calories are burned per minute when running, or 360 to 480 calories per hour. In general, walking for at least 150 minutes a week is necessary to promote health. People must engage in moderate physical activity for 300–360 minutes per week or vigorous aerobic exercise for 150 minutes per week (such as running or using an elliptical machine) to lose weight and keep it off. In addition to improving endurance, intense aerobic exercise lowers the risk of coronary artery disease.

People should engage in strength training—using weights or another type of resistance—three days a week to reap the greatest benefits from exercise. The body burns more calories when at rest because strength training increases the amount of muscle tissue, which raises the metabolic rate.

10.1.5.3. Changes in Behavior

In the end, behavior modification is required for weight loss to be successful and sustainable. The most successful weight-loss programs support behavioral changes in their participants. To change behavior, people need certain skills, such as:

- Problem-solving;
- Stress management;
- Self-monitoring;
- Contingency management;
- Stimulus control.

Problem solving involves identifying and planning ahead for situations that make unhealthy eating more likely (such as going out to dinner or traveling) or that reduce the opportunity for physical activity (such as driving cross country).

To manage stress, people can learn to identify stressful situations and develop ways to manage the stress that do not involve eating—for example, by going for a walk, meditating, or taking deep breaths.

To monitor themselves, people may keep a food log, including the number of calories in the foods, and weigh themselves regularly. They may record where and when they eat, what their mood is when they eat, and who is with them. With this information, they can observe and record patterns of behavior and eating and may be able to avoid situations that lead to weight gain or unhealthy eating.

Contingency management involves providing rewards (other than food) for behavior that contributes to weight loss or maintenance. For example, if people walk more or eat less of certain foods, they may reward themselves by getting new clothes or going to a movie. Rewards may also come from other people—for example, praise from family members or members of a support group. People can get support by using social media to connect and health care professionals.

To control stimuli that can trigger unhealthy eating, people can learn to identify obstacles to healthy eating and an active lifestyle. Then they can develop strategies to overcome them. For example, people may avoid going by a fast food restaurant on their way to work or not keep sweets in the house. To develop an active lifestyle, they may take up an active hobby (such as gardening), walk more, make a habit of taking the stairs instead of elevators, or park at the far end of parking lots (resulting in a longer walk).

Internet resources, applications for mobile devices, and other technological devices may also help people develop an active lifestyle and maintain weight loss. Applications can help people set a weight-loss goal, monitor their progress, track food consumption, and record physical activity.

10.1.5.4. Medications

Weight-loss drugs, also known as anti-obesity drugs, may be helpful for persons who have obesity or overweight conditions as well as weight-related problems. The best results from medications come from dietary adjustments, increased physical activity, and planned behavior modification programs. Certain drugs used to lose weight are meant to be used temporarily. Some are meant to be used indefinitely. If a patient's weight does not decrease after 12 weeks of treatment, weight-loss medications should be discontinued or modified.

Anti-obesity medications that are currently available include

- Orlistat.
- Phentermine.
- A combination of phentermine and topiramate.
- Lorcaserin (not available in the United States).
- A combination of naltrexone and bupropion.
- Liraglutide.
- Semaglutide.
- Tirzepatide.

These drugs are prescribed to patients with a body mass index (BMI) of 30 or higher, or to those with a BMI of 27 or higher who also have diabetes or high blood pressure.

Orlistat limits the breakdown and absorption of fats in the intestine, producing, in effect, a low-fat diet. Orlistat is available with a prescription or over-the-counter. Fat that has not been absorbed ends up in the digestive system. Bloating, gas, and loose stools are some of the side effects of this fat that usually go away with time. Meals high in fat are the ideal times to take orlistat. The fat-soluble vitamins A, D, E, and K may be more difficult to absorb when taking orlistat. Some people get osteoporosis, which increases the risk of fractures if insufficient vitamin D is absorbed. A vitamin supplement containing these nutrients should be taken by orlistat users. Take the supplement at least two hours before or after taking orlistat.

Phentermine reduces appetite by affecting chemical messengers in the part of the brain that controls appetite. It is available by prescription only. It is taken only for a short time. It can increase blood pressure and heart rate and cause insomnia, anxiety, and constipation.

Phentermine plus topiramate (used to treat seizures and migraines) is available by prescription only. Up to two years of weight loss are achieved with this combination. Women of childbearing age should only take it if they are using birth control and getting monthly pregnancy tests because it can cause birth defects. These drugs may raise heart rate and interfere with sleep and concentration.

Lorcaserin is given by prescription only. Due to worries about a potential elevated risk of cancer, it is not available in the United States. It works by blocking specific brain receptors to reduce appetite. Constipation, dry mouth, headache, nausea, fatigue, and dizziness are some of the side effects that sometimes go away. Taking locarserin while pregnant is not advised. Monoamine oxidase inhibitors, selective serotonin reuptake inhibitors, and serotonin-norepinephrine reuptake inhibitors are among the antidepressants that people taking lorcaserin should avoid taking.

Naltrexone plus bupropion is available by prescription only. In conjunction with diet and exercise, it can aid in weight loss. When used alone, naltrexone can help alcoholics stop drinking and block the effects of opioids. Moreover, naltrexone might lessen appetite. Protripon is prescribed on its own to treat depression and assist smokers in quitting. Additionally, bupropion can reduce appetite. Increased blood pressure, nausea, vomiting, and headaches are among the side effects of the combination medication. This medication should not be taken by anyone with uncontrolled hypertension, a seizure disorder, or a history of seizures.

Liraglutide is used to treat type 2 diabetes and obesity. Liraglutide functions by reducing the rate at which food exits the stomach. Injection delivery is required. Headache, diarrhea, nausea, vomiting, pancreatitis (inflammation of the pancreas), and hypoglycemia (low blood sugar) are among its side effects. Liraglutide should not be administered to patients with medullary thyroid carcinoma, a type of thyroid cancer.

Semaglutide is an injectable medication used to treat type 2 diabetes and obesity. Semaglutide suppresses appetite and aids in the pancreas releasing the proper quantity of insulin. The most typical side effects of semaglutide, similar to those of liraglutide, are diarrhea and nausea. Those who have had medullary thyroid cancer or have relatives who have, should not take semaglutide. Additionally, semaglutide should not be taken by those who have multiple endocrine neoplasia syndrome type 2 (MEN 2), an endocrine system disorder.

Tirzepatide is used to treat type 2 diabetes. It can help adults without diabetes lose a significant amount of weight over time. It also lowers the chance of endocrine and cardiac problems. Although tripeptide has not yet received approval for the treatment of obesity, this is anticipated to change soon. Low blood sugar, thyroid tumors, and pancreatitis are possible side effects. It should not be taken by people who have type 2 multiple endocrine neoplasia syndrome. Certain over-the-counter diet supplements, such as herbal remedies, assert to improve weight loss through boosting metabolism or elevating feelings of fullness. These supplements should be avoided as they have not been demonstrated to be beneficial and may include dangerous additives or stimulants (like ephedra, caffeine, guarana, and phenylpropanolamine).

10.2. Principles of Nutrition

Nutrition is an important aspect of healthcare that is essential for maintaining good health and preventing chronic diseases. Nurses play a crucial role in promoting and maintaining their patients' nutritional health.

1. **Balanced Diet**. A balanced diet includes a variety of foods from all the food groups in appropriate portions. This includes:

- **Carbohydrates:** These are the primary source of energy for the body and should make up the majority of a person's diet. Good sources of carbohydrates include fruits, vegetables, whole grains, and legumes.
- **Proteins:** Proteins are essential for the growth and repair of the body. Good sources of protein include meat, poultry, fish, beans, and dairy products.
- **Fats:** Fats are important for the absorption of fat-soluble vitamins, insulation of the body, and providing energy. However, it is important to consume healthy fats such as those found in nuts, seeds, fish, and vegetable oils.
- **Vitamins and Minerals:** These are important for maintaining good health and preventing diseases. They can be obtained from a variety of foods, including fruits, vegetables, whole grains, and dairy products.

2. **Caloric Intake**: Caloric intake refers to the amount of energy consumed through food and beverages. It is important to consume the right amount of calories to maintain a healthy weight and prevent chronic diseases such as diabetes, heart disease, and obesity.

The number of calories a person needs each day depends on various factors, including age, gender, activity level, and body weight. It is important to work with a healthcare professional to determine the appropriate caloric intake for each individual.

3. **Hydration**: Hydration is important for maintaining proper bodily function, especially during physical activity. It is recommended that individuals drink at least 8 glasses of water each day. Other beverages such as tea, coffee, and juice can also contribute to hydration, but water should be the primary source of hydration.
4. **Nutrient Density**: Nutrient density refers to the amount of nutrients in a food compared to the number of calories it contains. Choosing foods that are high in nutrient density, such as fruits, vegetables, whole grains, and lean proteins, can help maintain good health and prevent chronic diseases.
5. **Dietary Restrictions**: Some individuals may have dietary restrictions due to food allergies, intolerances, or medical conditions. Nurses need to understand these restrictions and provide appropriate dietary counselling and education.
6. **Malnutrition**: Malnutrition can occur when a person's diet lacks essential nutrients or when they consume too many calories. It can lead to a variety of health problems, including weakened immune function, delayed wound healing, and decreased muscle mass. Nurses should be able to identify signs and symptoms of malnutrition and provide appropriate intervention and education.
7. **Cultural and Religious Beliefs**: Cultural and religious beliefs can impact an individual's dietary habits and preferences. Nurses need to be aware of these beliefs and provide culturally sensitive dietary counselling and education.

Understanding the basic principles of nutrition is crucial for nurses to provide effective care to patients, promote good health, and prevent chronic diseases. A balanced diet, appropriate caloric intake, hydration, nutrient density, dietary restrictions, malnutrition, and cultural and religious beliefs are all important considerations when providing dietary counselling and education. Nurses should work with healthcare professionals to provide comprehensive nutritional care to their patients.

10.2.1. Importance of Nutrition in Healthcare

In the context of healthcare, nutrition is critical because it supports healing and recovery, prevents chronic diseases, and preserves overall health. Every bodily function, including the production of energy, the growth and repair of tissues, the operation of the immune system, and the maintenance of mental and emotional well-being, depends on adequate nutrition. Numerous health issues, such as malnutrition, obesity, heart disease, diabetes, cancer, and mental health issues, can be brought on by poor nutrition. In actuality, one of the main global risk factors for early death and disability is inadequate nutrition.

In healthcare, nutrition is important not only for preventing and treating illness but also for optimizing health outcomes and improving quality of life. For example, good nutrition is essential for:

- Promoting healing and recovery after surgery or illness.
- Managing chronic conditions such as diabetes, heart disease, and kidney disease.

- Supporting healthy growth and development in children and adolescents.
- Maintaining healthy weight and body composition.
- Boosting immune system function to prevent infection and disease.
- Supporting cognitive and emotional health.
- Preventing malnutrition and dehydration in older adults and hospitalized patients.

In the medical field, nurses are vital in promoting healthy eating. They are in a good position to evaluate patients' nutritional needs, offer nutrition education and counselling, and collaborate with other healthcare professionals to develop and carry out nutritional care plans because they are frequently the frontline healthcare professionals who have the most direct patient interaction. All things considered, the role that nutrition plays in healthcare cannot be emphasized. Sustaining optimal health outcomes, averting chronic illnesses, and promoting good health all depend on adequate nutrition. Promoting healthy eating and making sure patients receive the nutritional support they require to attain and maintain good health are important roles that nurses can play.

10.2.2. Role of Nurses in Promoting Good Nutrition

In the healthcare industry, nurses are essential in promoting healthy eating. As frontline healthcare providers, they frequently serve as patients' initial point of contact and are in a good position to determine their nutritional needs, offer guidance and education on nutrition, and collaborate with other healthcare providers to create and carry out nutritional care plans.

The role of nurses in promoting good nutrition includes:

- **Nutrition Screening and Assessment**: Nurses can screen and assess patients for nutritional risk factors and identify those who are at risk of malnutrition. This can include assessing patients' dietary intake, weight status, body composition, and medical history.
- **Providing Nutrition Education and Counselling**: Nurses can provide patients with nutrition education and counselling to help them make healthy food choices, manage dietary restrictions, and improve their overall nutritional status. This can include providing information on healthy eating patterns, portion sizes, and food preparation techniques.
- **Developing and Implementing Nutritional Care Plans**: Nurses can work collaboratively with other healthcare professionals to develop and implement nutritional care plans that are tailored to the individual patient's needs. This can include developing meal plans, recommending dietary supplements, and monitoring patients' nutritional status over time.
- **Addressing Cultural and Religious Beliefs**: Nurses can be sensitive to the cultural and religious beliefs of their patients when providing nutrition education and counselling. They can work with patients and their families to find culturally appropriate ways to meet their nutritional needs and preferences.
- **Providing Ongoing Support and Follow-Up Care**: Nurses can provide ongoing support and follow-up care to patients to ensure that they can maintain healthy eating

habits over time. This can include monitoring patients' weight and nutritional status, providing reinforcement of healthy habits, and making adjustments to nutritional care plans as needed.

The role of nurses in promoting good nutrition is critical to ensuring that patients receive the nutritional care they need to achieve and maintain good health. By assessing patients' nutritional needs, providing nutrition education and counselling, and working collaboratively with other healthcare professionals to develop and implement nutritional care plans, nurses can help improve health outcomes and prevent chronic diseases.

10.2.3. Strategies for Providing Effective Nutritional Care to Patients

Nurses must provide patients with effective nutritional care. Here are some strategies that nurses can use to provide effective nutritional care to their patients:

- **Assess the Patient's Nutritional Status**: Nurses should assess the patient's nutritional status using tools such as food diaries, dietary histories, and physical exams. This information can be used to determine the patient's nutritional needs and develop a nutritional care plan.
- **Provide Nutrition Education**: Nurses should provide patients with nutrition education that is tailored to their individual needs. This can include information on healthy eating habits, portion sizes, and food preparation techniques.
- **Use Motivational Interviewing**: Nurses can use motivational interviewing techniques to encourage patients to make healthy dietary choices. This involves asking open-ended questions and listening actively to the patient's responses to encourage them to identify their reasons for making dietary changes.
- **Involve the Patient's Family**: Nurses should involve the patient's family in the nutritional care process. Family members can provide support and help to reinforce healthy dietary habits.
- **Collaborate with Other Healthcare Professionals**: Nurses should work collaboratively with other healthcare professionals, such as dietitians, to develop and implement a comprehensive nutritional care plan.
- **Monitor and Evaluate Progress**: Nurses should monitor and evaluate the patient's progress in achieving their nutritional goals. This can involve regular follow-up visits, weighing the patient, and measuring other relevant indicators of nutritional status.
- **Address Barriers to Compliance**: Nurses should identify any barriers to compliance with the nutritional care plan, such as cultural or religious beliefs, and work with the patient and their family to find solutions that meet their nutritional needs.
- **Provide Emotional Support**: Nurses should provide emotional support to patients who may be struggling to make dietary changes. This can involve listening actively, empathizing with the patient's concerns, and providing encouragement and positive reinforcement.

Providing effective nutritional care to patients involves assessing the patient's nutritional status, providing nutrition education, using motivational interviewing techniques, involving the patient's family, collaborating with other healthcare professionals, monitoring progress, addressing barriers to compliance, and providing emotional support. By using these strategies, nurses can help patients achieve their nutritional goals and maintain good health.

10.2.4. Nutrition Screening and Assessment in Clinical Practice

Nutrition screening and assessment are essential components of clinical practice for nurses and other healthcare professionals. The purpose of nutrition screening and assessment is to identify patients who are at risk for malnutrition or who have nutritional deficiencies, and to develop and implement nutritional care plans that can help improve their nutritional status.

Here are some steps involved in nutrition screening and assessment in clinical practice:

- **Conduct a Screening**: A screening can help identify patients who are at risk for malnutrition. Common tools for screening include the Malnutrition Universal Screening Tool (MUST), Mini Nutritional Assessment (MNA), and Subjective Global Assessment (SGA). Screening tools usually assess factors such as weight loss, BMI, and recent changes in dietary intake.
- **Conduct a Comprehensive Assessment**: A comprehensive assessment is necessary to identify specific nutritional deficiencies and develop a nutritional care plan. The assessment can include a physical exam, dietary history, and laboratory tests.
- **Evaluate Dietary Intake**: Evaluating a patient's dietary intake can help identify nutrient deficiencies or excesses. This can include a 24-hour recall or food diary to evaluate the patient's usual dietary intake.
- **Evaluate Weight and Body Composition**: Weight and body composition can provide important information about the patient's nutritional status. This can include measuring BMI, waist circumference, or skinfold thickness.
- **Conduct Laboratory Tests:** Laboratory tests can help identify specific nutrient deficiencies or excesses. This can include tests for protein levels, serum albumin, and electrolytes.
- **Analyze the Data**: Once the data has been collected, it is important to analyze the results and develop a nutritional care plan that is tailored to the patient's specific needs.
- **Implement the Nutritional Care Plan**: The nutritional care plan should be implemented with the patient's cooperation and support. This can include dietary changes, supplements, and regular monitoring of the patient's progress.

Nutrition screening and assessment are critical components of clinical practice for nurses and other healthcare professionals. By using standardized screening tools, conducting a comprehensive assessment, evaluating dietary intake and weight, and analyzing laboratory results, healthcare professionals can identify patients at risk for malnutrition and develop effective nutritional care plans to improve their nutritional status.

10.2.5. Providing Nutrition Education and Counselling to Patients

Providing nutrition education and counselling to patients is an important responsibility for nurses and other healthcare professionals. The goal is to empower patients to make healthy dietary choices and achieve optimal health outcomes. Here are some steps that nurses can follow to provide effective nutrition education and counselling to their patients:

- **Assess the Patient's Knowledge**: Nurses should assess the patient's knowledge of nutrition and dietary habits to identify areas that require further education. This can include asking open-ended questions and using tools such as food diaries or dietary assessments.
- **Use Clear and Concise Language**: Nurses should use clear and concise language to explain complex nutritional concepts to patients. It is important to avoid using jargon or technical terms that the patient may not understand.
- **Provide Practical Advice**: Nurses should provide practical advice that the patient can incorporate into their daily routine. This can include tips on portion control, healthy food choices, and meal planning.
- **Use Visual Aids**: Visual aids such as food models, posters, or educational videos can help patients understand complex nutritional concepts and make healthier food choices.
- ***Individualize the advice***: Nutrition education and counselling should be individualized to meet the patient's specific needs and preferences. This can include taking into account the patient's cultural or religious beliefs, food preferences, and health goals.
- **Encourage Patient Participation**: Nurses should encourage patient participation in the nutritional care process. This can include setting realistic goals and involving the patient in the development of a dietary plan.
- **Monitor Progress**: Nurses should monitor the patient's progress and provide regular feedback on their dietary choices. This can include follow-up appointments and regular weigh-ins.
- **Address Barriers**: Nurses should address any barriers to compliance with the dietary plan, such as cultural or financial barriers. This can involve working with the patient and their family to find solutions that meet their nutritional needs.

Providing effective nutrition education and counselling to patients requires nurses to assess the patient's knowledge, use clear and concise language, provide practical advice, use visual aids, individualize the advice, encourage patient participation, monitor progress, and address barriers to compliance. By following these steps, nurses can help patients make healthy dietary choices and achieve optimal health outcomes.

10.2.6. Collaborative Approaches to Developing and Implementing Nutritional Care Plans

Collaborative approaches to developing and implementing nutritional care plans are essential for achieving optimal outcomes for patients. Nutritional care plans should be developed in collaboration with the patient, their family, and other members of the healthcare team. Here are some steps to follow for collaborative approaches to developing and implementing nutritional care plans:

- **Identify the Team**: The team involved in developing and implementing nutritional care plans may include the patient, their family, the nurse, the dietitian, the physician, and other healthcare professionals involved in the patient's care.
- **Assess the Patient**: The healthcare team should conduct a comprehensive assessment of the patient to identify their nutritional needs and risk factors for malnutrition. This can include a physical exam, dietary history, and laboratory tests.
- **Develop Goals and Objectives**: The healthcare team should develop goals and objectives for the nutritional care plan that are specific, measurable, achievable, relevant, and time-bound (SMART). Goals and objectives should be tailored to the patient's individual needs and preferences.
- **Determine the Interventions**: The healthcare team should determine the interventions that will be used to achieve the goals and objectives of the nutritional care plan. This may include dietary modifications, nutritional supplements, or other interventions.
- **Assign Responsibilities**: The healthcare team should assign responsibilities for implementing the nutritional care plan. This may include the nurse, who may be responsible for monitoring the patient's progress and adjusting the plan as necessary.
- **Communicate and Coordinate**: The healthcare team should communicate and coordinate regularly to ensure that the nutritional care plan is implemented effectively. This may include regular meetings, progress reports, and updates to the patient's medical record.
- **Evaluate Outcomes**: The healthcare team should evaluate the outcomes of the nutritional care plan to determine its effectiveness. This may include regular monitoring of the patient's nutritional status and adjustments to the plan as necessary.
- **Modify the Plan**: The healthcare team should modify the nutritional care plan as necessary based on the patient's response to treatment and changes in their nutritional status.

10.2.7. Addressing Cultural and Religious beliefs in Nutritional Care

Addressing cultural and religious beliefs in nutritional care is an important aspect of providing effective care to patients. Cultural and religious beliefs can affect food choices, food preparation, and the willingness to follow a prescribed diet. Nurses should be aware of these beliefs and understand their potential impact on the patient's nutritional status. Here are some steps that nurses can follow to address cultural and religious beliefs in nutritional care:

- **Identify the Patient's Cultural and Religious Beliefs**: Nurses should assess the patient's cultural and religious beliefs related to food and nutrition. This can include asking questions about their dietary habits, food preferences, and beliefs about the role of food in their culture and religion.

- **Respect the Patient's Beliefs**: Nurses should respect the patient's cultural and religious beliefs related to food and nutrition. This can include accommodating their dietary preferences and avoiding foods that are prohibited by their religion or cultural practices.
- **Educate the Patient**: Nurses should educate the patient about the importance of a healthy diet while respecting their cultural and religious beliefs. This can involve providing information about healthy food choices that are consistent with the patient's cultural and religious practices.
- **Collaborate with the Dietitian**: Nurses should collaborate with the dietitian to develop a nutrition plan that takes into account the patient's cultural and religious beliefs. The dietitian can provide guidance on alternative food choices that are consistent with the patient's dietary restrictions and preferences.
- **Provide Resources**: Nurses should provide resources that are culturally and linguistically appropriate to support the patient's nutritional care. This can include recipes, educational materials, and referrals to community resources.
- **Address Misconceptions**: Nurses should address any misconceptions that the patient may have about the role of food in their culture or religion. This can involve providing accurate information about the nutritional value of certain foods and dispelling myths about certain dietary practices.

Addressing cultural and religious beliefs in nutritional care is essential for providing effective care to patients. Nurses should identify the patient's cultural and religious beliefs, respect their beliefs, educate them about the importance of a healthy diet, collaborate with the dietitian, provide resources, and address any misconceptions. By following these steps, nurses can provide culturally sensitive nutritional care that supports the patient's health and well-being.

10.2.8. Motivational Interviewing Techniques for Promoting Behavior Change in Nutrition

Motivational interviewing is a counselling approach that can be used to promote behavior change in nutrition. It is a patient-centered approach that focuses on helping patients identify and overcome barriers to behavior change. Here are some motivational interviewing techniques that nurses can use to promote behavior change in nutrition:

- **Express Empathy**: Nurses should express empathy towards the patient by acknowledging their feelings and perspectives related to their dietary habits. This can help build a trusting and supportive relationship between the nurse and the patient.
- **Develop Discrepancy**: Nurses should help the patient identify discrepancies between their current dietary habits and their desired health outcomes. This can help

motivate the patient to make changes in their behavior.

- **Avoid Argumentation**: Nurses should avoid argumentation or confrontation when discussing the patient's dietary habits. Instead, they should focus on understanding the patient's perspective and helping them identify their own reasons for behavior change.
- **Roll with Resistance**: Nurses should "roll with resistance" by acknowledging the patient's ambivalence towards behavior change and helping them explore their reasons for maintaining their current dietary habits. This can help the patient identify potential barriers to behavior change and develop strategies to overcome them.
- **Support Self-Efficacy**: Nurses should support the patient's self-efficacy by helping them identify their strengths and successes related to behavior change. This can help build the patient's confidence and motivation to make further changes.
- **Use Reflective Listening**: Nurses should use reflective listening to demonstrate that they are actively listening and understanding the patient's perspective. This involves restating or summarizing what the patient has said to ensure that they feel heard and understood.
- **Elicit Change Talk**: Nurses should elicit "change talk" by asking open-ended questions that encourage the patient to discuss their reasons for behavior change. This can help the patient identify their reasons for change and develop a sense of ownership over their behavior change process.

Motivational interviewing techniques can be effective in promoting behavior change in nutrition. By expressing empathy, developing discrepancy, avoiding argumentation, rolling with resistance, supporting self-efficacy, using reflective listening, and eliciting change talk, nurses can help patients identify and overcome barriers to behavior change, and develop a sense of motivation and ownership over their dietary habits.

10.2.9. The Link Between Nutrition and Mental Health

The link between nutrition and mental health is increasingly recognized as an important aspect of overall health and well-being. Poor nutrition has been linked to an increased risk of mental health disorders, while a healthy diet has been shown to have positive effects on mental health. Here are some ways in which nutrition and mental health are linked:

- **Nutrient Deficiencies and Mental Health Disorders**: Deficiencies in certain nutrients such as vitamins, minerals, and omega-3 fatty acids have been linked to an increased risk of mental health disorders such as depression, anxiety, and ADHD. For example, low levels of vitamin D have been associated with an increased risk of depression.
- **Inflammation and Mental Health**: Inflammation is a key factor in the development of many mental health disorders. A diet that is high in processed foods, sugar, and unhealthy fats can lead to chronic

inflammation, which has been linked to an increased risk of depression, anxiety, and other mental health disorders.

- **Gut Microbiome and Mental Health**: The gut microbiome plays an important role in the production of neurotransmitters such as serotonin, which is a key regulator of mood. A healthy diet that is rich in fiber and plant-based foods can promote a healthy gut microbiome, which in turn can have positive effects on mental health.
- **Blood Sugar and Mental Health**: Fluctuations in blood sugar levels can affect mood and energy levels. A diet that is high in sugar and processed carbohydrates can lead to unstable blood sugar levels, which can contribute to mood swings, fatigue, and other symptoms of poor mental health.
- **Positive Effects of a Healthy Diet on Mental Health**: On the other hand, a healthy diet that is rich in whole foods such as fruits, vegetables, whole grains, and lean protein has been shown to have positive effects on mental health. For example, a Mediterranean-style diet has been associated with a reduced risk of depression and anxiety.

The link between nutrition and mental health is complex, and many factors contribute to this relationship. However, poor nutrition can increase the risk of mental health disorders, while a healthy diet can have positive effects on mental health. Nurses can play an important role in promoting good nutrition as a means of supporting mental health and well-being among their patients.

10.2.10. Nutritional Support for Patients with Chronic Conditions or in the Hospital Setting

Nutritional support is an important aspect of care for patients with chronic conditions or those in the hospital setting. Here are some strategies for providing nutritional support to these patients:

- **Individualized Care**: Each patient has unique nutritional needs, depending on their medical condition, age, and other factors. Nurses should work with the healthcare team to provide individualized nutritional care plans that meet the specific needs of each patient.
- **Oral Intake Optimization**: For patients who are able to eat and drink, nurses should ensure that they are receiving adequate nutrition through oral intake. This may involve offering a variety of foods that are nutrient-dense and easy to digest, and encouraging patients to eat and drink regularly.
- **Enteral Nutrition**: For patients who are unable to eat or drink, enteral nutrition may be necessary. This involves providing nutrition through a feeding tube that is inserted through the nose or directly into the stomach or small intestine. Nurses should monitor the patient's tolerance and response to enteral nutrition, and adjust the feeding regimen as needed.
- **Parenteral Nutrition**: For patients who cannot tolerate enteral nutrition or have a non-functioning gastrointestinal tract, parenteral nutrition may be necessary. This

involves providing nutrition through an IV, typically in the hospital setting. Nurses should monitor the patient's response to parenteral nutrition, and work with the healthcare team to adjust the regimen as needed.

- **Collaboration with Dietitians**: Dietitians can provide valuable expertise in developing and implementing nutritional care plans for patients with chronic conditions or in the hospital setting. Nurses should collaborate with dietitians to ensure that patients are receiving appropriate nutritional care.
- **Education and Counselling**: Nurses should provide education and counselling to patients and their families on the importance of nutrition in managing chronic conditions or recovering from illness. This may involve providing information on specific dietary recommendations, as well as strategies for improving oral intake and managing feeding tubes or IV nutrition.

Nutritional support is an important aspect of care for patients with chronic conditions or in the hospital setting. Nurses can play a key role in providing individualized care, optimizing oral intake, and managing enteral or parenteral nutrition, in collaboration with the healthcare team and dietitians. Providing education and counselling to patients and their families is also important for promoting good nutrition and supporting overall health and well-being.

10.2.11. Preventing Malnutrition in Older Adults and Hospitalized Patients

Preventing malnutrition is critical for older adults and hospitalized patients, as malnutrition can lead to a variety of health problems, including increased morbidity and mortality, longer hospital stays, and decreased quality of life. Here are some strategies for preventing malnutrition in these populations:

- **Screening for Malnutrition**: Healthcare providers should screen all older adults and hospitalized patients for malnutrition using a validated screening tool. This can help identify those at risk for malnutrition and allow for early intervention.
- **Early Intervention**: For patients identified as at risk for malnutrition, early intervention is crucial. This may involve providing additional nutritional support, such as oral nutritional supplements, enteral or parenteral nutrition, or working with a dietitian to develop an individualized nutrition care plan.
- **Collaboration Between Healthcare Providers and Dietitians**: Dietitians can provide valuable expertise in developing and implementing nutrition care plans for older adults and hospitalized patients. Collaboration between healthcare providers and dietitians is important for identifying those at risk for malnutrition, developing individualized care plans, and monitoring the response to nutritional interventions.
- **Education and Counselling**: Education and counselling can help older adults and hospitalized patients understand the importance of nutrition and make informed decisions about their dietary choices. This may involve providing information on specific dietary recommendations, such as increasing protein intake, and offering strategies for improving oral intake.

- **Patient-Centered Care**: Providing patient-centered care is important for preventing malnutrition in older adults and hospitalized patients. This may involve taking into account the patient's food preferences, cultural and religious beliefs, and other factors that may affect their nutritional intake.
- **Discharge Planning**: Discharge planning is critical for ensuring that older adults and hospitalized patients continue to receive adequate nutrition after leaving the hospital. This may involve providing information on how to prepare nutritious meals, recommending appropriate oral nutritional supplements, and scheduling follow-up appointments with a dietitian or healthcare provider.

Preventing malnutrition is critical for older adults and hospitalized patients. Strategies for preventing malnutrition include screening for malnutrition, early intervention, collaboration between healthcare providers and dietitians, education and counselling, providing patient-centered care, and discharge planning. By implementing these strategies, healthcare providers can help improve outcomes for older adults and hospitalized patients and support their overall health and well-being.

10.2.12. Integrating Nutrition into Patient-Centered Care

Integrating nutrition into patient-centered care is essential for improving patient outcomes and promoting overall health and wellness. Here are some strategies for integrating nutrition into patient-centered care:

- **Conduct a Nutritional Assessment**: To determine a patient's nutritional needs, healthcare providers should conduct a nutritional assessment. This assessment should include evaluating the patient's dietary intake, medical history, and physical exam. The information gathered from the assessment can be used to develop an individualized nutrition plan.
- **Develop an Individualized Nutrition Plan**: An individualized nutrition plan should be developed for each patient based on their specific needs and preferences. This may involve developing a meal plan, providing nutritional supplements, or recommending dietary changes to improve overall health.
- **Involve Patients in Decision-Making**: Patients should be involved in the decision-making process when it comes to their nutrition plan. This involves explaining the benefits and risks of different options and helping patients make informed decisions about their nutritional choices.
- **Educate Patients**: Educating patients about nutrition is essential for empowering them to make healthy choices. Healthcare providers should provide patients with information on healthy eating habits, portion control, and the importance of adequate nutrient intake.
- **Monitor Progress**: Monitoring progress is essential for ensuring that the nutrition plan is working and making adjustments as needed. This may involve regular check-ins with the patient or using biomarkers to assess progress.

- **Collaborate with a Registered Dietitian**: Registered dietitians can provide valuable expertise in developing and implementing nutrition plans. Collaborating with a registered dietitian can help ensure that patients receive the most appropriate nutritional care and support.
- **Sharma AM, Engeli S. Managing Big Issues on Lean Evidence**: Treating obesity hypertension Nephrol Dial Transplant. 2002; Integrating nutrition into patient-centered care can help improve patient outcomes, promote overall health and wellness, and support patient engagement and empowerment. By incorporating these strategies into clinical practice, healthcare providers can help ensure that patients receive the best possible nutritional care (Reinehr et al., 2005; Sharma et al., 2002).

A Closer Look

Metabolically Healthy Obesity

Metabolically healthy obesity (MHO) is a concept that describes individuals who, despite having a body mass index (BMI) classified as obese (30 or above), do not exhibit the metabolic complications typically associated with obesity. These individuals maintain normal levels of blood pressure, lipid profiles, glucose metabolism, and inflammation markers, effectively showing a reduced risk of developing conditions like type 2 diabetes, cardiovascular diseases, and metabolic syndrome compared to their metabolically unhealthy obese (MUO) counterparts. The prevalence of MHO varies widely depending on the criteria used for its definition and the population studied but is generally estimated to be around 10–30% of the obese population.

Thc factors contributing to MHO are multifaceted and not entirely understood. Genetic predisposition plays a significant role, in influencing how fat is distributed and stored in the body. Individuals with MHO tend to have a higher proportion of subcutaneous fat rather than visceral fat, which is more metabolically active and associated with greater health risks. Lifestyle factors also contribute; those classified as MHO often engage in higher levels of physical activity and maintain better dietary habits than those with MUO. This supports the idea that maintaining a healthy lifestyle can mitigate some of the adverse effects of excess weight.

Despite the seemingly better health profile, the concept of MHO is contentious. Longitudinal studies have shown that MHO individuals are at an increased risk of transitioning to MUO over time. Factors such as age, weight gain, and declining physical activity levels can contribute to this transition. The risk of developing metabolic diseases remains higher in MHO individuals compared to those of normal weight with a similar metabolic profile, indicating that MHO may be a temporary state rather than a permanent condition. This highlights the importance of continuous monitoring and lifestyle management even in those currently classified as metabolically healthy.

The clinical significance of MHO is critical in terms of public health messaging and medical management. While it might seem reassuring to classify a subset of obese individuals as metabolically healthy, it should not detract from the broader public health efforts aimed at addressing obesity as a major risk factor for numerous diseases. The focus should remain on promoting healthy lifestyles for all individuals, regardless of their metabolic status. Physicians should approach MHO with caution, recognizing the potential for future health risks and encouraging regular health screenings and proactive management strategies.

Research into MHO also emphasizes the need for more personalized approaches in obesity treatment. Understanding the mechanisms that allow certain individuals to remain metabolically healthy despite excess weight can inform more targeted interventions. For instance, enhancing physical activity and improving dietary quality is universally beneficial but might be particularly critical in maintaining metabolic health in obese individuals. Additionally, studying MHO can provide insights into the pathophysiology of metabolic diseases, potentially leading to novel therapeutic targets.

Metabolically healthy obesity represents a complex and nuanced phenotype within the obese population. While these individuals exhibit a favorable metabolic profile compared to their metabolically unhealthy counterparts, they are not immune to the long-term risks associated with obesity. Continuous lifestyle management, regular health monitoring, and a cautious approach to their metabolic health are essential. The concept underscores the need for personalized and sustained public health efforts to combat obesity and its associated risks effectively, ensuring that all individuals, regardless of their metabolic status, receive appropriate guidance and care.

Summary

- Obesity is a complex, chronic disease with several causes that lead to excessive body fat and sometimes, poor health. Body fat itself is not a disease, of course. But when your body has too much extra fat, it can change the way it functions.
- Obesity is a complex, multifactorial, and largely preventable chronic disease defined as abnormal or excessive fat accumulation. Body mass index (BMI), calculated as weight in kilograms divided by the square of height in meters (kg/m^2), is the current most widely used criterion for classifying obesity.
- Energy-dense foods, which are foods that have a large number of calories in a relatively small amount (volume), promote weight gain. Most of these foods contain more processed carbohydrates, more fat, and less fiber.
- Obesity is diagnosed by determining the body mass index (BMI). However, BMI has some limitations. The BMI does not take sex and age into consideration and makes only a few adjustments based on ethnic group. For people who are of Asian descent and some other ethnic groups, the BMI that is considered overweight is slightly lower.
- The BMI measures average body weight against average body height. As a generalization, healthcare providers associate a BMI of 30 or higher with obesity. Although BMI has its limitations, it's an easily measurable indicator and can help alert you to obesity-related health risks.
- Healthcare providers also use BMI to calculate obesity in children, but they calculate it relative to the child's age and assigned sex. A child older than 2 years may be diagnosed with obesity if their BMI is greater than 95% of their peers in the same category.
- Obesity specifically raises the risk of Type 2 diabetes seven-fold in people assigned male at birth and 12-fold in people assigned female at birth. The risk increases by 20% for every additional point you gain on the BMI scale. It also diminishes with weight loss.
- The dietary changes you personally need to make to lose weight will be individual to you. Some people may benefit from cutting portion sizes or snacks between meals. For others, it may be more about changing what they eat than how much. Almost everyone can benefit from eating more plants.

References

1. Akıs, N., Pala, K., Irgil, E., Aydin, N., & Aksu, H. (2003). Overweight and obesity among 6-14 year-aged schoolchildren at six elementary schools in Orhangazi-Bursa. *Journal of Uludağ University Medical Faculty, 29*(3), 17–20.
2. Bozbora, A. (2002). Surgical treatment of obesity. *Journal of ANKEM, 16*(3), 337.
3. de Onis, M., & Blösner, M. (2000). Prevalence and trends of overweight among preschool children in developing countries. *American Journal of Clinical Nutrition, 72*, 1032–1039.
4. Gurel, F. S., & Inan, G. (2001). Childhood obesity: Diagnostic methods, prevalence, and etiology. *ADÜ Journal of Medicine, 2*, 39–46.

5. Hedley, A. A., Ogden, C. L., Johnson, C. L., Carroll, M. D., Curtin, L. R., & Flegal, K. M. (2004). Prevalence of overweight and obesity among US children, adolescents, and adults, 1999–2002. *JAMA, 291*, 2847–2850.
6. Patel, S. R., & Hu, F. B. (2008). Short sleep duration and weight gain: A systematic review. *Obesity (Silver Spring), 16*(3), 643–653.
7. Reinehr, T. (2005). Clinical presentation of type 2 diabetes mellitus in children and adolescents. *International Journal of Obesity (Lond), 29*(suppl 2), S105–S110.
8. Sharma, A. M., & Engeli, S. (2002). Managing big issues on lean evidence: Treating obesity hypertension. *Nephrology Dialysis Transplantation, 17*, 353–355.
9. Sujoldzić, A., & De Lucia, A. (2007). A cross-cultural study of adolescents' BMI, body image, and psychological well-being. *Coll Antropol, 31*(1), 123–130.
10. Suzek, H., Ari, Z., & Uyanik, B. S. (2005). Prevalence of overweight and obesity among school children aged 6-15 living in Mugla. *Turkish Journal of Biochemistry, 30*(4), 290–295.
11. Wabitsch, M. (2000). Overweight and obesity in European children and adolescents: Causes and consequences, treatment and prevention: An introduction. *European Journal of Pediatrics, 159*, 5–7.
12. Whitaker, R. C., Wright, J. A., Pepe, M. S., Seidel, K. D., & Dietz, W. H. (1997). Predicting obesity in young adulthood from childhood and parental obesity. *New England Journal of Medicine, 337*, 869–873.
13. World Health Organization Technical Consultation. (2000). *Obesity: Preventing and Managing the Global Epidemic*. WHO Technical Report Series. Geneva: World Health Organization.

INDEX

D

E

F

G

H

I

MIX
Papier | Fördert gute Waldnutzung
FSC® C083411

Kolibri 360 GmbH
Ferdinand-Jühlke-Straße 7
99095 Erfurt, Deutschland
produktsicherheit@kolibri360.de